CONTEMPORARY PRACTICAL/VOCATIONAL NURSING

CONTEMPORARY PRACTICAL/VOCATIONAL NURSING

Third Edition

Corrine R. Kurzen, MEd, MSN, RN

Supervisor
Practical Nursing Program
School District of Philadelphia
Philadelphia, Pennsylvania

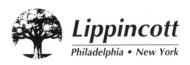 **Lippincott**

Philadelphia • New York

Acquisitions Editor: Lisa Marshall
Assistant Editor: Sandra Kasko
Project Editor: Gretchen Metzger
Production Manager: Helen Ewan
Production Coordinator: Nannette Winski
Design Coordinator: Doug Smock
Indexer: David Amundson

Edition 3

Library of Congress Cataloging in Publications Data

Kurzen, Corrine R.
    Contemporary practical/vocational nursing / Corrine R. Kurzen. – 3rd ed.
        p.   cm.
    Includes bibliographical references and index.
    ISBN 0-397-55363-3 (alk. paper)
    1. Practical nursing–Vocational guidance.   I. Title.
    [DNLM: 1. Nursing, Practical.   WY 195 K96c 1997]
    RT62.K871997
    610.73′069′3–dc20
    DNLM/DLC
    for Library of Congresss   96-9043
                                                                    CIP

Care has been taken to confirm the accuracy of the information presented and to describe generally accepted practices. However, the author, editors, and publisher are not responsible for errors or omissions or for any consequences from application of the information in this book and make no warranty, express or implied, with respect to the contents of the publication.

The author, editors and publisher have exerted every effort to ensure that drug selection and dosage set forth in this text are in accordance with current recommendations and practice at the time of publication. However, in view of ongoing research, changes in government regulations, and the constant flow of information relating to drug therapy and drug reactions, the reader is urged to check the package insert for each drug for any change in indications and dosage and for added warnings and precautions. This is particularly important when the recommended agent is a new or infrequently employed drug.

Some drugs and medical devices presented in this publication have Food and Drug Administration (FDA) clearance for limited use in restricted research settings. It is the responsibility of the health care provider to ascertain the FDA status of each drug or device planned for use in their clinical practice.

9 8 7 6 5 4 3 2

. . . to good friends, for their love and encouragement

Preface

Welcome to the third edition of *Contemporary Practical/Vocational Nursing.* This edition places an emphasis on healthcare facilities rather than on hospitals. This shift is in response to a greater emphasis on providing healthcare services outside the hospital. It is not intended to reduce the importance of hospital care but to expand the student's awareness of the vast array of places where healthcare is provided.

It is important for those entering the field of practical/vocational nursing to recognize that personal characteristics and qualities are as important as medical knowledge and nursing skills. The personal characteristics and qualities of nurses that contribute to quality nursing care are interspersed throughout the book.

The first two chapters focus on you as a student and offer suggestions on how to adjust to your role as a student nurse and how to continue meeting responsibilities to yourself and to your family while in school. Chapters 3, 4, and 5 provide a sense of where nursing is "coming from" and how nursing education and study of nursing theory will prepare you for your role as a nurse.

Chapters 6 and 7 provide an in-depth study of the current healthcare system and the healthcare team. Some calculated guesses are made as to the direction of healthcare in the future. These chapters are intended to enhance students' understanding of their place in our changing healthcare system.

Chapters 8, 9, and 10 concentrate on the patient. Cultural, social, and ethical concerns related to nurse interactions with patients are explored. In this third edition, the original Chapter 8 entitled "The Patient: Focus of Nursing Care" was divided into two chapters. The discussion of cultural diversity was greatly expanded and is now included in Chapter 8, while Chapter 9 discusses the nursing needs of special groups of patients. The content of these two chapters is particularly relevant when students are learning to individualize patient care.

Chapters 11, 12, and 13 discuss the practical/vocational nursing career, including legal controls affecting practice and leadership and management skills. These chapters help students develop an understanding of their professional role.

Chapters 14 and 15 are concerned with the student's future. Job-seeking skills, maintaining competence, and current issues and concerns affecting practical/vocational nurses are discussed.

Appendices provide resources that are valuable long after the basic practical/vocational nursing curriculum is completed.

Whether to call recipients of healthcare services *patients* or *clients* or *residents* continues to be discussed. In this book, I have generally referred to recipients of nursing care as patients. It would be more appropriate, but extremely cumbersome, to use the phrase *patient, client, or resident*. Regardless of the word used to describe someone who is seeking healthcare, each person should be viewed as an *individual*.

Your decision to become a nurse will undoubtedly change your life. Your experiences will expose you to the sorrows and joys of being human. You will acquire knowledge and learn nursing skills, but beyond that, you will learn how to care effectively.

Although our society does not place a lot of value on providing services or on caring for strangers, you have chosen a career that requires both. Your special ability to care and to provide care for others will be appreciated by the hundreds or even thousands of patients you will serve during your career in practical/vocational nursing.

Your faculty has designed an instructional program that will take you from where you are now to being a nurse — a process that is often challenging. You will spend many hours studying and preparing for clinical assignments. You will experience both success and frustration. You may occasionally wonder whether the effort is worth it. But you will persevere, and you will succeed because you have a special ability to care for others.

It is my hope that you will continue to care as much as you care today. Take pride in what you do and how you do it, and treat all people with dignity and respect. You will feel a tremendous self-satisfaction when you know you have done your best.

Corrine R. Kurzen, MEd, MSN, RN

Acknowledgments

My thanks to Robert Conosciani for reviewing history through the 18th century; to Mary Carriere, RN, Sharon Erickson, RN, BSN, MS Ed, Sylvia Mertens, RN, and Mary Thiel, RN, MS, for reviewing the manuscript; to students whose suggestions are always valuable; and to Lisa Marshall and Sandy Kasko of Lippincott-Raven for their assistance with the third edition.

Contents

Appendices

Adjusting to Student Life

1

OBJECTIVES

When you complete this chapter, you should be able to:

Design a schedule that includes time for study, personal needs, and family, social, and recreational activities.

Describe your role in learning through lectures, audiovisual presentations, computer-assisted instruction, and reading assignments.

Organize your notes and notebooks according to subjects and dates.

Use dictionaries, as well as tables of contents and indexes in textbooks, to find specific information.

Use library cataloging systems and library personnel to locate needed information.

Use test-taking skills when taking various types of tests.

Explain the relationship between classroom and clinical instruction.

Twenty-three women and men ranging in age from 19 to 53 years became suddenly silent as Mary Henderson entered the classroom. Mrs. Henderson, a registered nurse for "more than 20 and less than 30 years," as she liked to say, walked briskly to the front of the room. She was a handsome woman with a proud bearing that reflected her feelings about herself and her profession.

"I'm your instructor," Mrs. Henderson said with a serious look. "We'll be spending most of the next year together, much of it right here in this classroom. I won't apologize for the age of the building. I'll only say that both of us have seen our share of eager students enter—and more classes graduate than either of us would like to admit." She smiled brightly. The class responded with a laugh. Mrs. Henderson surveyed the students, face by face. "There are 23 of you in this class today," she continued. "How many of you expect to be here when we assemble on graduation day?"

The room became silent. The students looked around the room at one another. Slowly, 23 hands went into the air. Mrs. Henderson nodded approval. It was exactly the kind of confidence she liked in a new class. She had a good feeling about this group. The students' positive attitude was already beginning to show. She knew it would be invaluable later when they would be deep into their studies and might need a boost through the hard work that lay ahead.

"And how many think the others in this class will be here with you when you graduate?"

Every hand shot up without hesitation.

"Wonderful," Mrs. Henderson exclaimed. "That's exactly what I had hoped. And that's exactly the way it will be if we all work together to stay together. However, it's possible that some won't be here to graduate. I frankly doubt it, with such an enthusiastic group as this, but it could happen. The decision will be yours." She paused. "Every one of you has the potential to succeed in this program. You wouldn't be here if you didn't. And I would not be here if I didn't have faith in you, too. It won't always be easy. But I know the goal is worth it because I've been a nurse for..." She smiled. "I almost said how long, that time, didn't I?" The class laughed.

Once again Mrs. Henderson looked into the face of each student. "All right, class. We've made our decision. I, your program, and the administration will do everything we can to support that decision. We're all in this together to become nurses. Let's get to work to make it happen." The students broke into spontaneous applause. Now they were a class.

Your decision to become a licensed practical/vocational nurse can be one of the most fulfilling choices of your life. In approximately 1 year you will be ready to enter practice. The knowledge and experience you gain in school will prepare you for an important career that is valuable to society and is also personally rewarding.

The months ahead will be full. You will work on a busy daily schedule with new ideas, information, and people. You will be asked to make hard decisions. When asked to do something, you will be expected to do it. Much of what you do will be influenced by rules and regulations. In addition, you will have to balance the demands of your personal life with those of your student life. How well you adjust and learn will become the foundation of your career.

But you have been a student before. Whether that was last year or years ago, being a student again is not a totally new experience for you. A student nurse must work hard and be dedicated to achieving goals, but you have made the first step already. Your program will prepare you for the rest.

ORIENTATION

Student orientation sessions with faculty and staff are held to familiarize new students with their program's facilities and hospital affiliations. In these sessions, the rules and regulations for class, hospital, and residence conduct are explained. The program's courses and course content are described. If there is a student government, it is explained. Information about important student services, such as library, health, and counseling services, is given in detail.

The more you know about your program, its requirements, and what is expected of you, the better and quicker you will adjust as a student. Student orientation sessions are the perfect times to ask questions. If you have already had your student orientation, review the information you were given. If you have more questions, now is the time to ask an instructor for the answers.

ADJUSTING TO STUDENT LIFE

Adjusting to student life requires more than knowing rules and regulations. It is more than simply studying and learning. Self-awareness—being conscious of your own feelings and how well you fit in—is equally important. We'll discuss self-awareness in depth in Chapter 2.

Caring for others is a big responsibility. It is often demanding. Your program is preparing you to give nursing care to your patients. The better you understand yourself, the better that care will be.

Understanding oneself improves the quality of the care given because full attention is on what has to be done without interference from personal issues. If you cannot take care of yourself, your effectiveness as a nurse will diminish.

Taking care of yourself means to be aware of, to understand, and to provide for your own physical, emotional, and intellectual needs. These needs may be complex or simple.

Being aware of your needs and what to do about them is your responsibility. But you are not alone. Your instructors and program administrators know that personal, social, and scholastic problems can arise at any time.

Counseling services to help students make adjustments and solve problems may be available to you. Make use of them. If your program does not have special counseling services, discuss your needs with your program adviser, your instructors, or other members of the faculty or administration. Don't hesitate to ask for help or advice—the sooner, the better.

YOUR PROGRAM

Organization and Curriculum

Your program may vary somewhat from other practical/vocational nursing programs, but the foundation of most programs is similar. In general, basic nursing and healthcare theory and principles are presented in classroom lectures. Clinical instruction is provided in a variety of healthcare facilities, such as hospitals, long-term care organizations, rehabilitation centers, community health agencies, or mental health treatment centers.

Programs are approximately 1 year long. Some are sequential with classroom instruction followed by clinical instruction. Others offer a concurrent curriculum, which presents theory at the same time as the clinical rotation in that subject. Programs are usually sponsored by community colleges, vocational/technical schools, or by hospitals or other types of healthcare institutions.

Basic course curricula for programs include communications, anatomy and physiology, pharmacology, professional adjustments, contemporary health issues, fundamentals of nursing, sociology, psychology, mathematics, geriatrics, nutrition and diet therapy, maternal and child health, and medical-surgical nursing. Cardio-pulmonary resuscitation and first aid courses may also be required.

Program Structure

Your success as a student will be improved if you understand and use your program, its organization, and its personnel efficiently. Each part of your program has an objective.

Your school's objective is to provide the overall structure and services needed to be certain that graduates will be safe and competent nurses and that they will pass the licensing exam in practical/vocational nursing.

The administration's objective is to manage the program so that all school policies and procedures are adhered to and that the course of study meets the local, state, and national requirements.

Your instructor's objective is to guide you in applying the concepts of nursing that you learn in the different courses of study.

Learn why your program is structured the way it is. Find out why each course is included. Ask what you are expected to do. Much of your success will depend on how well you prepare. If you know what to prepare for, doing what is expected will go smoothly.

Get to know your institution and its administration. Learn who the people are who run it. Find out what they do. This information will be invaluable when you need help.

Know your instructors. Find out what they expect of you. Learn their views on class discussion. Knowing who welcomes discussion and who prefers to lecture without interruptions tells you when to ask questions and when to be a good listener. Find out how your instructors feel about their relationships with students. Some may like open, friendly associations. Others might prefer well-defined lines between teacher and student. When you know your instructors' preferences, you can avoid the mistake of trying to warm up to someone who views such friendliness as improper.

Familiarize yourself with the importance of grades, quizzes, and tests. Find out how tests are scored and which count more than others. Learn the value of class participation, homework, punctuality, and attendance. Ask whether typed papers are preferred over handwritten papers.

In other words, learn everything you can about your program and the people in it. The more familiar you are with your program, the easier it will be to adjust to it. Your immediate objective is to integrate your student life with your personal life so that you can concentrate on your long-term goal: to become a licensed practical/vocational nurse.

Scheduling Your Time

How you use your time can make the difference between being prepared and falling behind. Almost every day will be full. On occasion, you may wish there were more than 24 hours in a day. Finding the time to get everything done may take some ingenuity. And when you do find extra time, you'll treasure it. A written schedule is a good way to organize your time so that every hour can be put to its best use.

A good schedule should be realistic. To get the most out of your program and still have time for your personal life, make a schedule that fits the time you have, not how much you wish you had. Set your tasks and the amount of time to do them according to what you can reasonably expect to get done.

Use your class schedule as the basis for organizing the rest of your time. A well-organized schedule should let you see a full week, hour by hour, at a glance. For a sample schedule, see Table 1-1.

The easiest way to schedule your time is to buy a pocket- or purse-size calendar and use its organization as the basis for your own daily and weekly program.

LEARNING SKILLS

Learning and Intelligence

Simply defined, learning is acquiring knowledge, skills, or attitudes. How well one learns depends on the ability to study, the motivation to learn, and thinking, reasoning, and problem-solving skills. Evidence of learning can be observed in or through changed behavior.

Intelligence can be defined as the ability to adapt what one knows to new situations. Put another way, how easily one can solve problems is a measure of intelligence. Intelligence is a combination of memory, imagination, acquired knowledge, and judgment. It is partly dependent on what you already know and partly under your control to change.

Intelligence also reflects one's heredity and environment. Heredity is what you're born with and can't be changed. Environment is the surroundings in which you live and can be changed.

An ideal learning environment is one in which your whole attention can be directed to learning. Such an environment is unrealistic because life, for most people, is filled with a variety of interests and obligations that compete for time and attention. However, you can change the parts of your environment that interfere with your studies. Identifying them and changing them will improve your ability to learn.

Lectures

Much basic information is presented through the lecture method of instruction. During a lecture, your instructor will present information that will clarify those

TABLE 1-1 Typical Weekly Schedule of a Mother With Two Children

	Monday	Tuesday	Wednesday	Thursday	Friday	Saturday/Sunday
5:30	Get up, shower and dress, breakfast					Sleep
6:30	Drop children off at babysitter					Get up and dress
7:00	Travel to school—Memorize equivalents on flash cards					Study math
8:00	Anatomy class	Anatomy class	Anatomy class	Anatomy class	Anatomy class	Shopping and
8:50	Anatomy class	Anatomy class	Anatomy class	Anatomy class	Anatomy class	household
9:40	Psychology class	Psychology class	Psychology class	Psychology class	Psychology class	chores
10:30	Break	Break	Break	Break	Break	
10:40	Nursing class	Nursing class	Nursing class	Nursing class	Nursing class	
11:30	Lunch / Review lab procedures	Lunch / Review for math test	Lunch / Make flash cards	Lunch / Review lab procedures	Lunch / Meet with adviser	Recreation
12:30	Nursing class	Nursing class	Nursing class	Nursing class	Nursing class	
1:20	Math class	Nutrition class	Math class	Nutrition class	Nursing class	
2:10	Vocational Relations class	Sociology class	Vocational Relations class	Sociology class	Math class	
3:00	Travel from school—Memorize medical terminology on flash cards					
4:00	Pick up children from babysitter					
4:30	Household chores; dinner with children					Household chores / Dinner
6:00	Study Nutrition	Study Math	Study Nutrition	Study Math	Study Vocational Relationships	Recreation
7:00	Study Anatomy	Study Anatomy	Study Anatomy	Study Anatomy	Study Anatomy	Study Psychology
8:00	Study Nursing	Study Nursing	Study Nursing	Study Nursing	Study Nursing	Review all notes from past week
9:00	Study Sociology	Study Psychology	Study Sociology	Study Nursing	Study Psychology	Relax
10:00	Relax	Relax	Relax	Relax	Relax	Sleep
10:30	Sleep	Sleep	Sleep	Sleep	Sleep	Sleep

parts of the reading assignment that may need further explanation, identify important points that you should remember, and assist you in finding relationships in what you are learning.

Lectures will let you know what is expected of you. It is where you will have the best opportunity to ask questions. How much you get from lectures will depend on how good a listener you are and how well you have prepared yourself before the lecture.

Listening

Listening and hearing are not the same. Hearing is biophysical, the perception of sounds. Listening is intellectual, a conscious effort to interpret sounds. You may hear sounds being made by someone but you might not be interpreting those sounds. To understand sounds, you must use listening skills. In lectures and elsewhere, listening takes effort.

Being a good listener is one of a nurse's most useful skills. Throughout your nursing education and career, most of your interactions with instructors, other nurses, physicians, and patients will be verbal. Even the observations you make will depend heavily on what is said to you as well as what you see. Knowing what is said can affect how well you perform.

To listen effectively, fix your eyes on the lecturer's face. Pay close attention to the words, following them in your mind. Make your written notes while you listen but concentrate on what is being said rather than on what you're writing.

Taking Notes

Nobody is expected to remember everything but as a student, and later when you begin to practice, you will be expected to recall a surprising amount of information. The better your memory, the easier this will be. For most people, memory is imperfect. Everyone needs reminding from time to time. The best reminders are well-organized, written notes.

The goal of good note taking is to capture key words, ideas, and concepts in short phrases. Like good study habits, the best note-taking system is the one that works for you. If you already have a note-taking system, use it. If taking notes is not something you normally do, develop a system now. It will be indispensable to you as a student and will continue to work for you after you've graduated.

The advantages of good note-taking skills far outweigh the effort needed to learn to them. The main benefit is higher grades. Notes are short, written phrases that capture key points. Well-taken, clearly written notes record important facts and ideas that are buried in books, lectures, films, computer programs, and other instructional materials. Good notes will help you to review and remember what you've covered. They are especially helpful when you need them most—for study and review just before quizzes and tests.

Get into the habit of taking notes. Take them in lectures, when you read, when watching films, videos, and demonstrations, during clinical rounds, and in any other situation where you are being given information to learn and remember.

If note taking does not come naturally to you, or if you have problems keeping good notes, ask your instructor for help immediately. The sooner you begin a set of organized notes, the easier it will be to record, remember, and review the material being taught.

Following are some general rules for note taking:

1. Omit unnecessary words.
2. Use an outline format.
3. Don't repeat what is in a handout or your textbook.
4. If you highlight your textbook as you read, highlight information stressed in class in a different color.
5. Make a note of information that is confusing to you; clarify this with the instructor immediately after class.

An example of outline notes from a pharmacology lecture might be as follows:

I. 6 rights of drug adm.
   A. drug
   B. dose
   C. patient   (see pg. 75 Pharm. textbook)
   D. route
   E. time   MEMORIZE - PROBABLY ON TEST
   F. documentation

II. Dr. orders must contain
   A. pt. name
   B. date
   C. drug   (Ask instructor—What does the nurse
   D. dose   do if one of these parts is missing?)
   E. route
   F. frequency
   G. signature

III. Categ. of med orders
   A. stat (once - NOW)
   B. single order (once - specific time - ex 8 PM)
   C. standing order (for some period - ex 7 days)
   D. prn (as needed - ex. pain meds)

There are many kinds of notebooks. Individual preference will determine which type you use. Some students prefer keeping all their notes in one loose-leaf notebook with subject dividers. A single notebook keeps and organizes all notes for all classes in one place. Making additions or deletions, or moving pages or sections from one place to another, is simplified. Others prefer a notebook for each subject. An alternative to notebooks is index cards. They allow easy filing and cross-indexing but are less portable and convenient.

For legibility and neatness, use lined paper and write on one side only. The blank facing page can be used for additions or comments to the main notes. Date each set of notes. It's also a good idea to identify each page of notes by date, course, instructor, or subject, and to number them if they are in loose-leaf form so that they can be reorganized if they get out of sequence.

When taking notes in class, sit where you can be comfortable, as close to the lecturer as possible. Make sure you have a clear view of the chalkboard so that you can read what is written on the board. Sit comfortably. Good posture will help you keep alert.

Missed lectures mean missing notes. If you miss a lecture or class, make arrangements to get notes from a classmate to avoid blanks in your notebook and to keep up with the course. Tape recording a lecture can be helpful if you miss one, but regularly taping lectures wastes time, just as word-for-word notes do.

Note taking is easier when reading assignments are kept up-to-date because the information in one reinforces the other. A good general rule is to have your reading assignment done before a lecture. If possible, review assignments briefly so you will be prepared to take notes on new information that can not be found in your textbooks.

Guidelines for Taking Clear Notes
1. *Listen.* Pay attention to what is being said; avoid distractions; watch, as well as listen.
2. *List.* Write down the main ideas, facts, and supporting data; write down any chalkboard notes; write down your questions if something is not clear.
3. *Read.* Read your notes as soon as possible after taking them; fill in with any material you remember but didn't write down.
4. *Review.* Review your notes on the day they were made, just before the next class in that subject, and before exams.

When listening, keep your ears tuned for key words and phrases. Listen and watch for signals that indicate what is considered to be important. Phrases such as "will be on the exam," "studies have shown," "the main reason for," "the important thing to remember," and similar remarks are strong suggestions that what will be said next should be written down.

Other clues that the information is important are: pausing, repeating, slowing down, underlining, and emphasizing. If you pay attention, after a few lectures you'll learn the instructor's style and will know when to write and when to listen. During a lecture, be sure to record the notes, diagrams, charts, dates, and other data your instructor writes on the chalkboard.

Your note-taking style should be what is most comfortable for you. But information may come faster than you can keep up with while using normal writing. If you know shorthand or can improvise a personal shorthand, you will be able to devote your attention to the information. Use underlines or capital letters for emphasis. Number lists. Eliminate vowels in words to shorten them. Leave out unnecessary words. Shorten sentences.

The standard abbreviations and terms used in charting that you'll be learning can double as shorthand in your note taking. Be cautious when taking abbreviated notes. Although it is easy to abbreviate words, it is sometimes difficult to recall what your abbreviation means. This is especially true when you are building a medical and nursing vocabulary. Completely write or print words that are new to you. If you decide to abbreviate, write the abbreviation in parentheses next to the word. You can use the abbreviation for the new word from that point on because you have a record of what a particular abbreviation means to you.

Avoid doodling on your note pages and letting your attention wander. Concentrate on what is being said and condense what you hear into brief, legible notes.

An example of notes from a nursing lecture might read like this:

Warm Soaks

1. Normal saline solution (NSS)
2. Temp 105–110 degrees Fahrenheit (F)
3. 3 times a day (t.i.d.)
4. 20 min.

The next time the lecturer refers to normal saline solution, you need only write NSS in your notes; when reference is made to three times a day, you need only write t.i.d., and so forth.

Studying

Studying is the process of attentively applying the mind to learn or understand a topic or subject. How much time you have to study will be clear from your schedule. The choice of how to study is up to you.

Study habits are learning tools. Good study habits combined with a desire to learn are essential to success as a student. Both are under your control. If you have study habits that worked in the past with good results, use them. If your study skills are rusty or you don't have a study method, use these guidelines:

Study Suggestions

1. Set regular times for study and mark them in your schedule.
2. Establish an area with minimum distractions.
3. Set aside a minimum of study time for each hour spent in class.
4. Allow enough time to study each subject.
5. Schedule your study time by priorities.
6. Study the most important subjects first.
7. Study hard subjects before easy subjects.
8. Set the time you'll need for each subject by the difficulty of the material.
9. Revise your schedule and priorities according to need.
10. Take short rests every 45 to 60 minutes of study time.
11. Study just before and right after classes.
12. Study when your energy level is up.
13. Have all necessary books, papers, notes, and other study material on hand before starting.
14. Study dissimilar subjects in each session to help keep you and the material fresh.
15. Avoid distractions and interruptions; when they do occur, deal with them quickly.
16. Take advantage of instructor review sessions and student study groups.

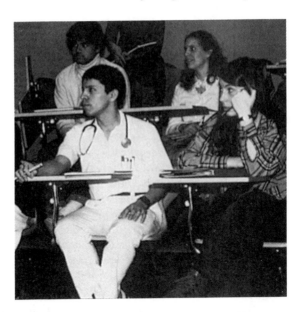

Good listening, notetaking, and study skills will help you succeed.

In general, shorter sessions are less tiring than long ones and allow better concentration. Limiting the length of each session makes sessions more productive.

Proper rest and nutrition are important to clear thinking. Be as comfortable as possible but avoid conditions that make you drowsy.

Where you study can be as important as how you study. Choose places where the lighting is good, the temperature is comfortable, and noise and distractions are at a minimum. Always resist temptations that interferes with scheduled study time.

Once you establish a study pattern, stick with it. There will be times when you will have to make adjustments. Handle them as they come along and return to your normal pattern when they're done.

Your study schedule should be a part of your life, not all of it. Allow yourself some free time to do the things you enjoy.

The better organized you are, the easier your life as a student nurse will be. This is especially true if school and study do not come easily for you. If getting organized is difficult, ask your adviser, an instructor, or another student who has these skills for help.

Computer-Assisted Instruction

The use of computer technology is an important component of your nursing education. The sooner you familiarize yourself with computers and what they do, the easier it will be to use them.

Completing computer learning assignments may be required as a part of your program of study. Instructional computer programs, which aid learning, display information on a screen. The user is given step-by-step instructions on how to move from one screen to the next. Ask your instructor, librarian, or computer lab assistant for help if you have problems using computer-assisted instruction.

A computer-assisted learning assignment is usually an independent learning activity, which means that you must do it on your own. Find out what hours you can use the computer and whether you need to schedule computer time. Be prepared for the session by having materials such as note paper, pencils, and textbooks with you.

In addition to required computer-assisted learning assignments, your library or computer lab may have many additional programs on file that will help with your studies. Ask what titles are available and make use of these programs often.

The computer can also provide access to the Internet, which contains a wealth of information. Dictionaries and encyclopedias, as well as a variety of medical topics, are included. You should be aware that some of the medical information may not be accurate so you might want to check other sources to verify the information you obtain from Internet data bases.

Electronic mail (E-mail) is an efficient way to send and receive information. Your E-mail address is similar to your postal address. Your faculty may use E-mail to send you messages regarding assignments, schedules, meeting locations, and so forth. If you are assigned an E-mail address, you should make it a habit to check your mail daily.

Distance learning, or learning some distance away from the primary classroom, is assisted by computer technology. Lectures, workshops, demonstrations and even entire courses of instruction offered in one location are broadcast to locations that may be some distance from the primary classroom. Participants can interact with the presenter through telephone and computer technology as though they were in the primary classroom.

If you are thinking about purchasing a computer, you should first make a list of what you want to be able to do with the computer. Do you want to be able to write reports and term papers? Do you want to be able to learn math and dosage

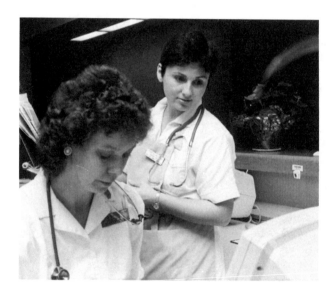

Computer use in healthcare facilities is increasing.

calculation skills? Do you want to be able to work through clinical simulations? Do you want to be able to access a computerized list of drugs and interactions? Do you want to take a simulated licensing examination? Do you want to access the Internet? Do you need a CD-ROM to run the programs you might purchase? After you decide what it is you want to be able to do, you need to find the software programs that meet your needs. Each software program lists the type of computer system needed to run that program. By taking this approach, you will purchase the hardware (computer and accessories) that can support the software you want to use. Your instructors may be able to recommend software titles that will contribute to your nursing education.

The National Council of State Boards of Nursing, the agency that administers nursing licensure examinations, conducts nurse licensing examinations by computer. Because computers are now, and will be in the future, used in so many areas of your nursing practice and in your personal life, it is important that you develop some skill in using this technology. Take advantage of every opportunity to learn to use computers.

Audiovisual Instruction

Audiovisual (A/V) instruction through cable television, videocassettes, films, filmstrips, and other visual media extends your classroom to places and people you might only hear or read about otherwise. Clinical demonstrations, nursing procedures, and your own performance in skills and techniques can be reviewed conveniently and as often as desired on videotapes.

Treat A/V presentations with the same approach as you do other sources of information by taking notes and periodically reviewing them.

ASSIGNMENTS

Most days you'll be given assignments to do before your next class session. These assignments are an important part of your preparation and are intended to introduce new material. When you complete assignments before class, you will be able to ask questions to clarify what you did not understand during class. A few simple guidelines will help you to effectively complete reading and writing assignments.

Reading Assignments

Good reading skills are the foundation of successful studying. Whether you are reading a textbook, a journal, or a computer screen, reading is more efficient if you are mentally and physically prepared. Review the guidelines for study on page 10 because studying and reading go hand-in-hand. In addition:

1. Read in a quiet place with a minimum of interruption or distraction.
2. Adjust temperature and lighting to a comfortable level.

3. Sit upright in a comfortable chair.

4. Avoid reading on a full or an empty stomach.

5. Place your book or computer screen at a comfortable angle.

To help you to concentrate on what you are reading in books and journals, to increase your reading speed, and to improve your ability to recall what you read, a popular shortcut called the SQ3R (survey-question-read-recite-review) method will be useful if you don't have a reading system of your own. Use it as follows:

Survey the title, objectives, key words, chapter heads, introduction, first and last paragraphs, italicized passages, graphs, illustrations, photos, and end-of-chapter questions before you begin normal reading.

Question what you will be reading. Think about it before you begin.

Read by skimming first to find and look up unknown words. Then read for content. Take notes as you read. Summarize your notes after you have finished reading.

Recite aloud or silently the substance of what you've read. Repeat it as often as needed to get the material firmly fixed in your mind.

Review the material before going on to the next task.

Written Assignments

Written assignments, usually in the form of term papers, case studies, and care plans, are a part of your education. You may be given a topic or be asked to choose one. Once you have a topic, the following five steps will help get you through most papers.

1. Collect the material—books, notes, papers, articles, and other reference matter—your paper is to be based on. The amount of reference material you need will be determined by the assigned length of the paper.

2. Organize and then outline the reference material. A sample outline for a short paper follows:

  I. Introduction (states purpose of paper). Say what you're going to say. Open with a topic sentence and follow with a short background or history.

  II. Body (states main ideas and details). Develop the paper's purpose, using research material to substantiate your case. State the main idea and then give details for each main idea you are presenting.

  III. Conclusion (states what was said). Briefly summarize what you've said in the paper.

3. Write your first draft from beginning to end. Avoid rewriting and editing the first time through.

4. Read your first draft, add notes, make changes and revisions, and then write the final draft.

5. Proofread your final draft and make corrections before handing in the paper.

Plan to complete written assignments before they are due. If you have a technical problem with your computer or typewriter or a personal problem requiring your attention, you will have a margin of time to cope with these unexpected events.

REFERENCE MATERIAL

Books

Beyond lectures, other sources of information you will need are found in books. Most of the books you will use will be recommended by your instructors and other authorities. Trust their judgment because they speak from experience. Choose wisely when buying books other than those your course requires. Nursing books are revised often to keep up with change.

Knowing how to use a book to find what you need is a basic tool for every student. Time spent familiarizing yourself with how to use a book now will save you hours of work throughout your program and career.

Textbooks, reference books, and most other nonfiction books are organized to simplify finding information. A table of contents at the front of a book lists each chapter by title, often with a brief description of the topic covered in that chapter. Page numbers indicate where to find the specific chapter.

An index will be found at the back of most books. The index lists specific items in alphabetical order. Names, subjects, and individual topic-related words are in a good index. If you want to find where in the book to look for psychologists, for example, look under P. The word psychologist will be listed, followed by the page or pages where it is used.

Use tables of contents and indexes to quickly obtain the information you need.

Appendixes (appendices) are separate sections of related material found at the back of books. A book may have an appendix in which the addresses of nursing organizations are listed, for example. Reference to an appendix is usually made in the body of the book. An item will be followed by a note in this form: See Appendix D, Drug Interactions.

Glossaries are separate sections listing vocabulary words special to the topic of the book, such as a glossary of nursing terms.

Other Materials

Other reference materials include journals, magazines, pamphlets, audiovisual programs, general reference books such as dictionaries and encyclopedias, and information accessed through computer programs or the Internet.

Official journals of nursing and journals from other healthcare organizations provide the latest news and information long before it can be published in books. Your program, library, or instructors may have copies of journals available. You may wish to buy your own subscriptions, but it is a good idea to become acquainted with various journals first to ensure buying those that fit your needs.

Health-oriented books and magazines and popular consumer magazine articles frequently present good, readable, general health information that can be used to supplement your other reading. Follow your instructor's advice regarding nontechnical sources.

When selecting reference material of any kind on your own, see that it's up-to-date, accurate, and reliable. Your instructor is the authority.

Using Libraries

A library is no longer a place just for books. Modern libraries include many different types of materials that provide learning resources. In fact, the term "Learning Resource Center" is often used to describe what used to be known as the library.

Your program may have its own library or may provide access to one at a nearby hospital or other healthcare facility. Public libraries, especially central libraries in larger cities, will also have nursing and medical reference material.

Using a library is not difficult. It requires familiarity with using a computerized catalog, which lists the titles of materials available in the library, It also requires some knowledge of how materials are cataloged. The process is systematized so that every library is organized in the same basic way.

If you have difficulty locating materials in a library, ask the librarian for help. He or she will be more than willing to assist you.

CRITICAL THINKING SKILLS

In your nursing education program, you will have to memorize the meaning of vocabulary words, normal lab values, usual drug dosages, and many other things.

But the ability to memorize facts is not enough. Every patient you care for will present new challenges and new problems. No two patient care situations will ever be exactly alike. You will need to take the facts you have learned and then apply critical thinking skills to each situation.

Using critical thinking skills will help you eliminate those things that don't fit the situation; associate things that go with the situation; put things in order; compare alternatives; contrast findings; evaluate alternatives; and think logically in assessing, planning, implementing, and evaluating nursing care.

You can learn to become a critical thinker by working at it. In a given clinical situation ask questions of yourself. Ask questions such as "What is the factual basis for my actions? What are the alternatives to my first thoughts? What should I do first and why? Why am I doing this procedure in this way? Did my actions achieve the desired result?"

Welcome questions from your clinical instructor about what you are doing and why. Developing your own questions and questions from your instructor will, with practice, help you take factual knowledge and adapt it appropriately to meet the needs of your individual patients.

Box 1-1 describes some of the characteristics of critical thinkers. Constantly working on your critical thinking skills will help you apply the factual knowledge you have attained in a variety of clinical settings and situations.

TAKING TESTS

Tests are a fact of life for students. Getting through them will be easier if you are prepared. The energy that tests stimulate can be used to your advantage. Direct the energy to preparing for the test, rather than wasting it in unproductive nervous activity.

Test Anxiety

Test anxiety is a term used to describe the psychological and physical feelings experienced before an examination. While for most students this actually increases performance, for some the anxiety is devastating. If the anxiety is overwhelming, following is a list of a few things you can try.

- Tell yourself that you studied the material.
- Tell yourself that you do not need to get all the answers right.
- Tell yourself that you will not panic when you don't know an answer.
- Avoid listening to other students talk about what they studied and what they think will be on the test.
- Avoid participating in a last minute review session with other students.
- Avoid taking sedatives or stimulants before the test.
- Get a good night's sleep before the test.
- Practice relaxation techniques (see Appendix A).
- Have confidence in your ability.
- Replace negative thoughts about yourself with positive ones.
- Don't panic when other students finish the test long before you.
- Don't change answers unless you are certain the first one was incorrect.
- Don't put pressure on yourself that doesn't exist. Not doing well on one test will probably not be the end of your enrollment in school.
- Use your reasoning ability and what you have learned in life to answer questions that you think you don't know the answer to.

If using these tips do not help you overcome excessive anxiety, consider professional help. A professional can offer many strategies that will be individualized to meet your specific needs.

Preparation for tests includes planned study and review sessions. Be sure of the exact location and time the test will be given. Know the kind of test it will be (eg, true/false, essay, multiple choice) and the subjects it will cover.

BOX 1-1. CHARACTERISTICS OF CRITICAL THINKERS AND HOW THEY THINK

Critical Thinkers Are:

- **Aware of their strengths and capabilities:** They're confident that they can use reason to find answers and make good decisions.
- **Sensitive to their own limitations and predispositions:** They know their weaknesses, values, and beliefs and recognize when these may hamper their ability to assess a situation or solve a problem.
- **Open minded:** They listen to new ideas and viewpoints and consider the situation from many perspectives.
- **Humble:** They overcome their own tendency to feel that they should have all the answers.
- **Creative:** They are constantly looking for better ways to get things done. They follow recommended procedures, however, they continually examine whether these are the best ways to meet goals and objectives.
- **Proactive:** They accept responsibility and accountability for their actions. They study situations, anticipate problems, and find ways to avoid them *before* they happen.
- **Flexible:** They recognize the importance of changing priorities and interventions when planned approaches don't seem to be getting results.
- **Aware that errors are stepping-stones to new ideas:** They turn mistakes into learning opportunities, reflecting on what went wrong and identifying ways to avoid the same mistake in the future.
- **Willing to persevere:** They know that sometimes there are no easy answers and that there may be time-consuming struggles to find the best answer.
- **Cognizant of the fact that we don't live in a perfect world:** They realize that sometimes the *best* answer may not be the *perfect* answer.

Critical Thinkers Also:

- **Maintain a questioning attitude:** They ask questions like, "What's going on here?"; "What does it mean?"; and "What else could it mean, and how else could it be interpreted?"
- **Ask for clarification when they don't understand:** For example, they say, "I'm not clear about this. Can you tell me more?" *or* ask questions like, "What do you mean by *better,* better in what way?"
- **Apply previous knowledge to new situations:** They see similarities and differences between one experience and another, between one concept and another.
- **See the situation from many perspectives:** They value all viewpoints and watch that their judgments are based on *facts,* not personal feelings, views, or self-interest.
- **Weigh risks and benefits (advantages and disadvantages) before making a decision:** They avoid risky decisions and find ways to reduce adverse reactions before putting a plan into action.
- **Seek help when needed.**
- **Put first things first:** They ask, "What's the most important thing to do here?"

Critical Thinkers Use Logic. They:

- **Test first impressions to make sure they are as they appear:** They doublecheck the logic of their thinking and the workability of their solutions.
- **Distinguish between fact and fallacy:** They take the time to verify important information to be sure that it's true.

(continued)

*BOX 1-1. CHARACTERISTICS OF CRITICAL THINKERS
AND HOW THEY THINK (Continued)*

■ **Distinguish fact from inference (what they *believe* the fact means):** For example, they recognize that because someone is sitting quietly in a corner may not mean that the individual *is withdrawn;* it means that he is sitting quietly in a corner and it would be helpful to find out why.

■ **Support views with evidence:** They wouldn't state that the person above is withdrawn without providing additional supporting evidence, such as the individual saying he wants nothing to do with anyone.

■ **Determine what's relevant and what's irrelevant:** They recognize what's important for understanding a situation and what's unimportant. For example, the fact that you're a nurse or studying to be a nurse is relevant to how I should write this book; the fact that you are female or male is irrelevant.

■ **Apply the concept of "cause and effect":** They look for what's causing a problem to more fully understand the problem itself. They anticipate responses to their actions before performing the action. For example, critical thinkers would attempt to find out the *cause* of pain before deciding how to *treat* it. They would determine how someone might *respond* to a medication before *administering* it.

■ **Withhold judgment until all the necessary facts are in:** They realize the dangers of jumping to conclusions.

From Alfaro-LeFevre R: Applying Nursing Process: A Step-By-Step Guide, Third Edition. Philadelphia, JB Lippincott, 1994.

Strategies for Taking Tests

A general strategy for test taking includes the following:

1. Before the exam begins, make sure you understand the directions and what you're supposed to do. If you're uncertain, ask questions before you begin.

2. Look over the whole exam before you begin to answer questions to estimate how much time each section will take. Make a note of your estimate so that you can gauge your progress once you are underway.

3. Be certain you understand the relative grading weights of different sections. Some parts of a test may count more than others. Use this information to determine where to spend more or less time.

4. Differentiate between hard and easy sections or questions.

5. Once you have done steps 2, 3, and 4, make a test-taking plan based on your evaluation and stick to it. For example, you can go straight through the test or do either the hard or easy material first.

6. When you have a plan, proceed with the test. Pay just enough attention to the time to keep to your plan.

Some test-taking hints are as follows:

On Mixed Easy-to-Hard Questions
- Do easy questions first to build confidence.
- Mark hard questions with an x and harder ones with xx, and answer them in order as time allows.
- Hard and easy are determined by what you know.

On Multiple-Choice Tests
- Find out before the test if you will be penalized for guessing.
- When guessing, trust your first response as correct.
- Eliminate two or more answers before guessing.
- Use what you learn from one question to help answer others.
- Answers with "all," "never," and "always" are generally incorrect.

On Essay Questions
- Think through each answer before writing.
- Make a brief outline.
- Allot an appropriate amount of time for each answer.
- Answer the easy questions first.
- If time is short, get important information down first.
- After completing an exam, use any remaining time to review your answers.

Standardized Examinations

Classroom exams are designed to test your knowledge of specific subjects learned over a limited time. Standardized tests show how much of a range of subjects you've learned through all or a portion of your education. They compare your knowledge with students around the country. The comparisons are usually given in percentile rankings. An evaluation of your progress can be based on the comparison.

No real method of preparation for taking standardized exams is possible because they draw on a broad range of material learned over a long time. However, before taking a standardized test, you may find it helpful to review a similar test to familiarize yourself with the format and types of questions asked. Also, a general review of material that is to be covered in a standardized test will help you recall what you have already learned.

When taking a standardized test, be sure you understand the directions and follow them. Don't make any extra marks on the answer sheet and be certain to mark the boxes or bubbles that go with the questions. If you get out of sequence, every answer will be wrong.

Standardized tests may penalize you for guessing. The test directions or the person administering the test will tell you. If you are uncertain, ask.

Read all the answers before making a mark on your answer sheet. If the test doesn't penalize for guessing, eliminate the answers you know are wrong and guess from those remaining. Avoid skipping questions even if you are not sure of the answer. If you finish the test before the time is up, go back and review the test.

CLINICAL INSTRUCTION

Clinical instruction is arranged by the faculty to give you practical experience in the care of people in various healthcare settings. Your first clinical assignment might be in a nursing home or in a hospital. Regardless of where you are assigned, you will be expected to integrate and apply what you learned in the classroom to the care of the patient.

Before you begin to care for your patient, you should review your textbooks and notes to be sure you correctly understand the patient's condition, the treatment being given, and the procedures you will be performing. In the beginning, your instructor will help you define what you are permitted to do. As you gain experience and clinical skills, you will be expected to identify those skills you can perform independently and those which require instructor observation.

Most often, your day will start with a short preconference. During this time, your instructor will review the instructional plan for the day. You and your classmates will be given an opportunity to ask questions about your assignments. Your instructor may give specific instructions about new treatments or procedures that you may be expected to complete during your clinical time. It is important that you write these notes on a pocket notepad. It is easy in the rush of the clinical environment to forget the directions your instructor gave you. It is also easy to forget what you are expected to do for your patients.

The majority of your clinical time will be spent learning to care for patients. Your instructor is usually responsible for your activities in the patient unit, and you

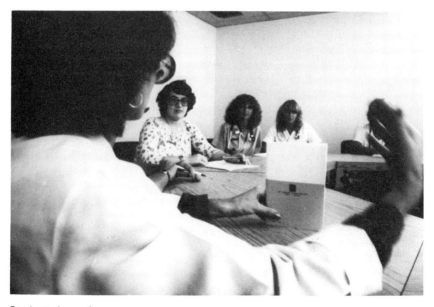

Students in conference.

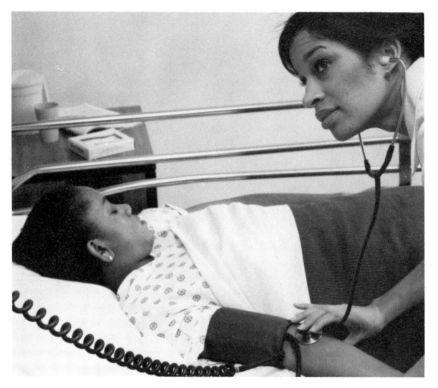

Learning to care for patients is the focus of your clinical experience.

must keep him or her informed of any changes in your patient's condition. Your instructor will frequently ask you questions about your patient's disease, treatments, procedures, family situation, and so forth. This is really an oral quiz. You should be prepared to answer these questions at any time.

Meal and break times are assigned by your instructor or the nurse in charge of the unit. Assignments are made to ensure that adequate nursing personnel are always present on the patient unit. It is easy to understand why it is important to plan your activities so that you can leave the unit on time and return on time.

Your clinical day may conclude with a postconference. A variety of activities usually occur during postconference. Students may present preassigned reports to the class; the instructor may discuss the care of a particular patient; a guest speaker may present a topic of special interest; or new equipment or procedures may be demonstrated. Note taking is important. You are responsible for learning the material presented during your clinical day, just as you are for learning the material presented during a classroom lecture.

Attendance during your clinical assignments is crucial to developing nursing skills. Your classmates and the nursing staff depend on you. Being late is disruptive to the care of the patient, to your own organization, to the nursing staff, to your classmates, and to your instructor. Your absence requires that your assignment be given to someone else, often at the last minute. Being on time is an essential personal trait of a nurse.

There are occasions when something unavoidable happens and you must be late or absent. Your instructor will tell you how to handle these situations. You will be expected to comply with your program regulations.

DISCUSSION QUESTIONS/LEARNING ACTIVITIES

1. What do you think will be the most difficult adjustment you will have to make to attend school? What do you think you will do to make the adjustment?

2. Construct a schedule for yourself similar to the schedule shown in Table 1-1 and follow it closely for 1 week. What changes do you think you should make in your schedule and why?

3. Compare your note-taking system with that of some of your classmates. Look for ideas that will help you with your notes.

4. Discuss study techniques with other students in your class. Which techniques might you be able to use that you had not thought of before?

5. What adjustments could you make in your study schedule to compensate for a short-term personal or family emergency?

6. What are the procedures for using library facilities and how can you get assistance in finding information in your library?

7. Share techniques that you and your classmates use to handle anxiety associated with taking exams.

READ MORE ABOUT IT

Alfaro-LeFevre R: Applying Nursing Process: A Step-By-Step Guide, Third Edition. Philadelphia: JB Lippincott, 1994.

Alfaro-LeFevre R: Critical Thinking in Nursing: A Practical Approach, First Edition. Philadelphia: WB Saunders, 1995.

Bandman EL, Bandman B: Critical Thinking in Nursing, Third Edition. East Norwalk: Appleton and Lange, 1995.

Chenevert M: Mosby's Tour Guide to Nursing School: A Student's Road Survival Kit, Third Edition. St. Louis: CV Mosby, 1995.

Fondiller SH, Nerone BJ: Health Professionals Stylebook: Putting Your Language to Work, First Edition. Publication No. 14-2551. New York: The National League for Nursing, 1993.

Goodall JH: A Survivor's Guide to Study Skills, First Edition. New York: Churchill-Livingstone, 1996.

Kesselman-Turkel J, Peterson F: Study Smarts: How to Learn More in Less Time. Chicago: Contemporary Books, 1981.

Kesselman-Turkel J, Peterson F: Test Taking Strategies. Chicago: Contemporary Books, 1981.

Kesselman-Turkel J, Peterson F: Note Taking Made Easy. Chicago: Contemporary Books, 1982.

Kesselman-Turkel J, Peterson F: Getting It Down: How to Put Your Ideas on Paper. Chicago: Contemporary Books, 1983.

Meltzer M, Palau SM: Reading and Study Strategies for Nursing Students, First Edition. Philadelphia: WB Saunders, 1993.

Miller MA, Babcock DE: Critical Thinking Applied to Nursing, First Edition. St. Louis: CV Mosby, 1995.

Palau S, Meltzer M: Learning Strategies for Allied Health Students, First Edition. Philadelphia: WB Saunders, 1993.

Regan JM: Springhouse Notes: A Guide to Surviving Nursing School, Second Edition. Springhouse, PA: Springhouse, 1996.

Vitale BA, Nugent PM: Test Success: Test-Taking Techniques for the Healthcare Student, First Edition. Philadelphia: FA Davis, 1995.

2

The Student Nurse as a Person

OBJECTIVES

When you complete this chapter, you should be able to:

Name the five levels of human needs described by Maslow.

Identify at least six factors that should enhance your personal health.

Describe several personal characteristics that contribute to maintaining good mental health.

Explain the role of socializing and of recreation in developing positive physical and mental health.

Describe your personal values and beliefs related to health.

Listen to the views and opinions of others with respect.

Recognize your own physical and mental limits and live within those boundaries.

Linda, an LVN working nights at a nursing home, was summoned to her patient's room by the blinking light over the room door. The corridors were silent. She stepped into the room, which was lighted by the glow of a small lamp. Her patient, Mrs. Mulrooney, was awake. "Can I help you?" Linda asked.

Mrs. Mulrooney nodded. "I'd like a glass of water," she said.

Linda poured a fresh glass and put it to Mrs. Mulrooney's lips. She noticed that the woman was trembling. "Is something wrong?" Linda asked.

Mrs. Mulrooney looked to the side of her bed. "The bedside rails are broken," she whispered.

Linda smiled. "No, Mrs. Mulrooney. They were repaired just today. Remember?"

The woman looked puzzled. "Was that today?"

Linda put the glass on the night stand. "Yes," she said. "You don't have to worry." She tucked the blanket under her patient's chin.

The woman smiled and said she felt safer with the bed rails up. She then touched the nurse's hand. "You make me feel so good," she said.

Linda returned the gesture with a gentle touch. "I'm glad," she said. "You're very important to me."

Mrs. Mulrooney beamed. "I am?" she asked. Linda stroked her patient's forehead. "Of course you are. You're important to all of us."

For a moment Mrs. Mulrooney said nothing. She was thinking. Then she smiled. "I guess I am," she said proudly. "I should be. I lived a good life. I have two wonderful children and five grandchildren..."

Linda stepped to the door as the woman's eyes began to close in sleep.

"I think I did with my life what I was supposed to," Mrs. Mulrooney said.

"I think so, too," Linda whispered into the room. Mrs. Mulrooney was asleep. Her face was calm. She was smiling.

HUMAN NEEDS

All people have needs. Because these needs are necessary for survival and health, they are called basic human needs. The story presented above illustrates five categories of human needs identified by Dr. Abraham Maslow, an authority in the field of psychology. They are as follows:

1. Physiological ("I'd like a glass of water.")
2. Safety and security ("I feel safer with the bed rails up.")
3. Love and belonging ("You make me feel so good.")
4. Self-esteem and recognition ("You're very important...")
5. Fulfillment ("I think I did with my life what I was supposed to.")

According to Maslow, these five categories of needs can be ordered from simple to complex. Figure 2-1 illustrates Maslow's different levels of human needs. Physical survival and safety come before love and belonging, followed by the need for self-esteem and for self-actualization or self-fulfillment.

Working with others requires understanding their needs. It also requires understanding your own needs. Unless your needs are recognized, it is difficult to give full attention to the needs of others. Ask yourself what your needs are in each

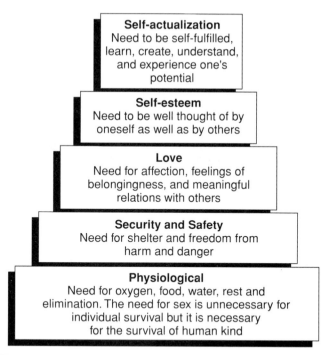

Figure 2-1. Maslow's five levels of human needs.

of Maslow's five levels. Are enough of your personal needs being met to allow you to be concerned about the needs of others?

The more you work with people, the more opportunity you will have to learn about yourself. The opportunity begins now. Your self-actualization will grow if you know what your needs are and what you must do to satisfy them.

YOUR PHYSICAL HEALTH AND WELL-BEING

Physical health is the absence of disease, pain, or abnormal conditions. It is in a constant state of change as the body adapts to conditions and events affecting it. Good physical health is important for anyone working in healthcare. Good health makes it easier for you to perform your duties. Being healthy is an example you should try to set for your patients. To be healthy, you have to pay attention to your body as though you were your own patient.

When you begin caring for patients, a question you often will ask them will be, "How are you feeling today?" The answers your patients supply will tell you what to do for them.

It isn't necessary to ask yourself this question. You already know the answer. But you do have to respond to what your body tells you. Waiting for a problem to develop is not the best way to ensure good health. Preventing problems, whenever possible, is. Health problems can be minimized through regular physical exams and dental checkups.

Your program may offer health-related services to its students that include exams and checkups. Make use of them. If medical services are provided, you will be expected to pay for them according to established policies. Whenever you have questions regarding charges for your own healthcare, don't be reluctant to ask about them ahead of time.

If charges for your medical care are reduced as a courtesy by a treating physician, it is a sign of good manners to express your appreciation. On the other hand, it is improper to ask for medical advice for yourself or your family from the physicians you work with while on duty.

Diet

"You are what you eat" is more than a clever saying; it is true. Your daily performance is directly affected by what you eat or don't eat. You'll learn the fundamentals of diet and nutrition. The consequences of poor eating habits versus balanced nutrition are a matter of scientific record. Your own experience tells you that heavy meals produce drowsiness, hunger disrupts concentration, too much caffeine causes jitters, alcohol impairs judgment, and too many calories lead to overweight.

Nurses and others whose work is demanding, often intense, and sometimes awkwardly scheduled, may be open to breaking the rules of good nutrition. Students may also adjust their eating habits to meet the daily requirements of classes, study time, and their personal life, even though both their mental and physical activity demand peak performance. As a student, you will benefit from good eating habits.

Start each day with a balanced breakfast. Eat small, balanced, nourishing meals to maintain energy and stamina through the rest of the day. Avoid snacks with high sugar content. They produce unstable blood sugar levels while adding calories. Whatever your weight, calories that don't help you to study, keep you alert, or ward off exhaustion have no place in your diet. Learn your ideal weight and maintain it. A nurse who is overweight will have difficulty advising patients to diet. If you have to diet, avoid crash diets and diets that exclude variety.

The U.S. Department of Agriculture and the Department of Health and Human Services issued guidelines on how to choose a healthy diet. These guidelines are presented in a food pyramid (Fig. 2-2). This pyramid indicates what foods should be included in a healthy diet and in what proportion each day. The food pyramid recommends 6 to 11 servings of bread, cereal, rice, and pasta; 3 to 5 servings of vegetables; 2 to 4 servings of fruit; 2 to 3 servings of milk, yogurt, and cheese; and 2 to 3 servings of meat, poultry, fish, dry beans, eggs, and nuts each day. At the top of the pyramid is fats, oils, and sweets. These foods should be sparingly consumed.

In 1990, the U.S. Department of Agriculture, along with the U.S. Department of Health and Human Services, published dietary guidelines for Americans. Figure 2-3 outlines these guidelines.

Following these guidelines and recommendations will help provide the energy you will need to study and concentrate, work and play, and maintain your nutritional health.

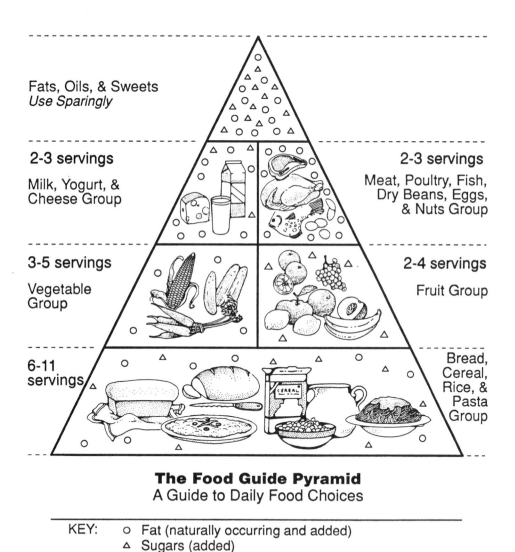

Fats, Oils, & Sweets
Use Sparingly

2-3 servings

Milk, Yogurt, &
Cheese Group

2-3 servings

Meat, Poultry, Fish,
Dry Beans, Eggs,
& Nuts Group

3-5 servings

Vegetable
Group

2-4 servings

Fruit Group

**6-11
servings**

Bread,
Cereal,
Rice, &
Pasta
Group

The Food Guide Pyramid
A Guide to Daily Food Choices

KEY: ○ Fat (naturally occurring and added)
      △ Sugars (added)
These symbols show fats, oils, and added sugars in food.

Figure 2-2. This guide is commonly used to evaluate the dietary status of individuals and to educate people about food choices.

Dietary Guidelines for Americans

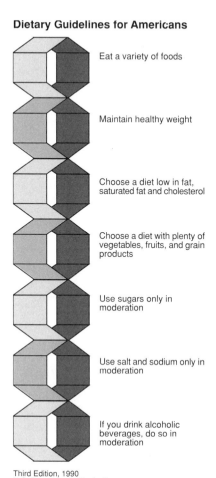

Eat a variety of foods

Maintain healthy weight

Choose a diet low in fat, saturated fat and cholesterol

Choose a diet with plenty of vegetables, fruits, and grain products

Use sugars only in moderation

Use salt and sodium only in moderation

If you drink alcoholic beverages, do so in moderation

Third Edition, 1990
U.S. Department of Agriculture
U.S. Department of Health and Human Services

Figure 2-3. Following these guidelines will help provide you with the energy you need to study and concentrate.

Rest and Exercise

Studying and clinical experience may create a double drain on your energy because of the demand for both physical activity and mental activity. Having to concentrate while keeping up with a busy schedule may make you more tired more than you're used to. You may require more rest. Watch for signs of fatigue, such as indifference, sluggishness, personality changes, or a drab physical appearance, to prevent the situation from growing worse.

Mental alertness and physical endurance are qualities you must have as a student and throughout your career. They depend in large measure on how well you rest. You can't "save up" on sleep. The amount of sleep needed varies with the individual, so only you will know if you're getting enough. Seven to eight hours a night is average, although some people manage on less and others need more. Experiment to learn your own limits and then stay within them to maintain a consistent level of energy.

Restful deep sleep is better than tense light sleep. How well you sleep is indicated by how rested you feel after you've been up a short time in the morning. How one prepares for sleep is a personal practice but, in general, to ensure quality sleep, relax before going to bed, avoid eating or drinking before retiring, sleep on a firm mattress, and provide comfortable temperature and ventilation.

To increase your endurance during the day, take scheduled rest breaks. It is not necessary to nap, but if you can, let your body and mind enjoy a few moments of peace by reducing or eliminating physical and mental activity.

A scheduled program of specific exercise also helps to keep the body working efficiently. Even though your work may be physically demanding, if parts of your body are neglected, the effect on them is the same as having no exercise at all. Walking, swimming, aerobic workouts, jogging, and bicycling are exercises that use a full range of body activity. To help keep your energy levels high, your body tone good, and your weight in control, engage in a sport or exercise that matches or slightly exceeds your ability. You may find it helpful to join a group of other students or friends in scheduled exercise sessions two or three times a week.

Oral Hygiene and Dental Health

You will be working closely with patients, staff members, and others who will appreciate the attention you give to keeping your teeth and breath attractive. A pleasant smile can be an asset.

Regular dental checkups will find problems such as cavities, decay, and gum disease, while daily brushing and periodic freshening will help to ensure a clean, healthy mouth. Consider seeing a dentist or orthodontist if cosmetic treatment is indicated for dentition problems (poor bite), particularly if they affect your self-confidence or the image you'd like to project.

Personal Hygiene

Cleanliness in health services begins with personal hygiene. It affects your image and may affect your susceptibility to cross infection and disease. Your personal care must reflect the higher overall standards expected from people in healthcare.

Basic personal care includes clean skin, clean, neatly combed or brushed hair, and the absence of body odor. Hands and nails must be clean. If your program (and later your employer) provide policies about the use of makeup and perfume, length of nails, use of nail polish, and types of hair styles, follow them. Perfumes, scented deodorants and hair sprays may create discomfort in patients and can aggravate allergies. If the decision on grooming aids is up to you, a moderate approach is best. If you are unsure, ask someone whose opinion you respect for advice.

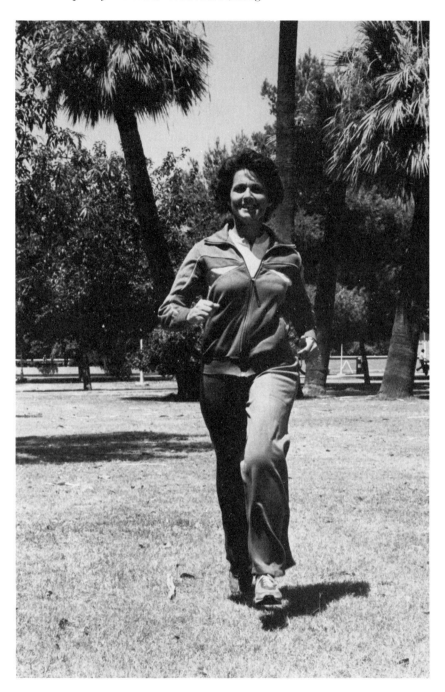

Regular exercise promotes physical and mental well-being.

Clothing and Uniforms

Your uniform is a symbol of your vocation. It is often the first thing people notice, especially patients, who identify it with their stay in a hospital or healthcare facility. It makes a statement about you, what you stand for, and your authority. It should be worn only at work.

Maintain a positive impression by wearing uniforms and other clothing that are clean, pressed, and fresh. Shoes are also a part of your uniform and should be clean and in good repair. They should be comfortable and of a style that is consistent with your work and image.

Pins, name tags, and other devices that identify you, your institution, or your affiliations should be worn in accordance with policies set forth by your employer, your state, or the associations they represent.

Posture

How you stand, sit, walk, and carry your body is a matter of habit by now. If your habits are good, there's no need to change them. On the other hand, if your posture is not good, your appearance, performance, and energy level usually improve if you change it.

Basic good posture is to hold your body straight. When standing, keep your back straight and your head up. Walk with your shoulders back and your head erect. When sitting, keep your back straight and both feet on the floor. Be relaxed in your posture, not rigid. Keeping muscles tense will tire you quickly.

Body language, which is how you hold and carry yourself, can reflect how you feel physically, some of what you feel about yourself, and some of what you feel about others.

For example, standing straight expresses self-confidence. Slouching reduces your authority. Talking to someone with your arms folded tightly across your chest puts people off. Facing them directly in a straightforward, relaxed manner encourages a positive response.

Smoking

People who smoke give many excuses for their habit, but nobody can claim it is good for health. The public is keenly aware of the negative effects of smoking. Studies clearly show that some heart disease, lung cancer, chronic obstructive pulmonary disease, and other ailments can be directly linked to smoking. You will learn more about the health dangers associated with smoking as your knowledge about health increases. You'll see patients whose only reason for being ill is related to smoking; some of them, tragically, are terminally ill. Others will have illnesses that smoking complicates by making manageable conditions worse and marginal sickness serious. In the air or on one's clothes, smoke is an irritant. For a patient whose well-being depends on optimum conditions, the smell of smoke, whether firsthand or secondhand, is contraindicated.

There is another side to the smoking question for you as a student nurse. As a highly visible member of the health professions, your example to others can affect how they view their own smoking. A health practitioner who smokes gives unspoken approval to the habit.

If you smoke, you have an obligation not to do so when or where it will affect others in any way. For your good health and the health and comfort of those you're around, look closely at your excuses for smoking and its consequences. You'll find plenty of reasons to quit. Groups are available for those who want to quit but have trouble doing so.

Chemical Dependence

The use and abuse of substances such as alcohol and narcotics, barbiturates, sedatives, tranquilizers, depressants, inhalants, hallucinogens, and cannabis can lead to serious problems, which affect people from every walk of life. For some, addiction (uncontrollable, compulsive dependence) and habituation (psychological and emotional dependence without addiction) occurs quickly and "just this once" may lead to untold misery and unhappiness.

Hardly a day goes by that we don't read or hear about the tragic effects of substance abuse. The drunk driver who kills an innocent person, the teenage who dies from an overdose, the apparently successful husband (wife, mother, father, sister, brother) who committed suicide because of an addiction, or the murder of a person for a few dollars to buy drugs are all indicative of the seriousness of the problems created by these substances.

The use and abuse of these substances can lead to the loss of family, job, and self-respect. Drug-related convictions can prevent a person from receiving federal student financial aid, from joining the armed services, from public office, and from a number of good jobs.

The illegal use or possession of controlled substances can also be cause for denying, suspending, or revoking a nursing license. Your school and the clinical facilities with which you affiliate have policies on drug use.

The firsthand knowledge of the effects of drug and alcohol abuse that you gain through your program should be a constant reminder to you to protect your health and career. Others who are not so fortunate may approach you because of your access to drugs in a hospital or institution. Make it very clear to them that you neither use, approve of, nor supply or administer any drugs for any reason unless prescribed by a physician for your patients.

There is a high rate of drug and alcohol abuse among nurses. Their dependence is doubly tragic because it affects not only their own lives, families, and careers, but the lives of their patients as well.

Whatever your personal beliefs and feelings about the use of alcohol and drugs, there is never justification for using these substances at work or for abusing them at any other time. Your education and the experiences you will have will demonstrate the disastrous effects of drug and alcohol abuse on people's lives and health. The likelihood of serious disciplinary action in your program or by an employer in the future (many use prehiring drug screenings) is ample reason for you to avoid their use and abuse.

As a nurse, your relationship with drug and alcohol use is twofold. You must be very cautious of it in your own life, and you must also empathize with your patients who have a problem with substance abuse.

Almost all State Boards of Nursing have a rehabilitative program for psychologically or chemically impaired nurses. These programs are designed to prevent the revocation of the nursing license by outlining and monitoring treatment programs. Those who do not comply with the voluntary program are subject to more severe disciplinary action including the loss of the nursing license.

Your local telephone directories can provide the names and telephone numbers of agencies that work with those who suffer from various addictions. Study the information presented in Appendix B to understand more about controlled substances.

Personal Illness and Your Patients

The same standards of care and protection you use when working with patients with transmissible illness apply to you when you are ill. The difference is that although you may be informed about your patient's health, they know nothing of yours.

It is your obligation to avoid contaminating the clinical environment when you have any illness that could harm or affect a patient's health or well-being. This applies to transmissible diseases, from common colds to serious infections, and to conditions that have a negative psychological effect, such as coughs, rashes, and other symptoms of disease.

Your program or clinical facility policies may be explicit on matters of personal illness. If not, your good judgment will tell you when to avoid exposing co-workers and patients if you are ill. Your awareness of the state of your health is your best guide to protecting yourself and others.

Sexually Transmitted Diseases

There are many sexually transmitted diseases (STDs). Once called venereal diseases, they include syphilis, gonorrhea, herpes, and others. Their complications can be serious and may lead to death. Those that are not directly life-threatening can lead to infections and illnesses that are. Many STDs can lead to sterility and other reproductive problems.

In 1995, there were an estimated 13 million new cases of STDs; the cost of treating these diseases was about $5 billion. The Centers for Disease Control estimate that more than 60 million people are affected with STDs other than the acquired immunodeficiency syndrome. These numbers are astounding; the seriousness of STDs should be of concern to everyone.

The emergence of acquired immunodeficiency syndrome in 1981, which now includes 32 organisms and 26 syndromes, greatly increased public awareness of STDs. However, there is still a lot of misinformation and fear about them. Providing health information to others is a service performed by nurses. As a student nurse, you may be asked questions about STDs. Your ability to answer them will increase as your education progresses.

Although some STDs can be transmitted by blood transfusion and other means, they are generally associated with human sexuality, a subject that many find difficult to discuss. Your willingness to be open, frank, and honest about STDs is important to patients and others who seek information because education is the best method to control these diseases. As a student nurse, what you have to say is valuable.

You should not make judgments that will keep information about STDs from those who need it. STDs can be acquired by anyone who is sexually active, and there are no social, economic, racial, or other barriers. Because STDs always involve two or more people, the sex partners of anyone with an STD should be informed so they can seek medical attention. Also, because reinfection of a partner is likely if only one is treated, all partners must get treatment to contain the chain of infection.

Learn accurate, scientific information about what causes STDs, what their incubation periods are, how they are transmitted, how to identify them, and what to do to prevent and treat them. Armed with this information, you can do much to promote good health for yourself and others. For further information on STDs, refer to Appendix C.

YOUR EMOTIONAL HEALTH

Mentally healthy people are able to effectively cope with the pressures and stresses that are a part of everyday life. It is essential that those who are aspiring to become nurses be mentally healthy so they can provide the compassionate nursing care that patients expect to receive.

As a nurse, you will be confronted almost daily not only with personal pressures and stresses but also those of your patients. The nurse who is focused entirely on his or her own problems and concerns will not be able to recognize the needs of the patient. Everyone experiences upsets in life. It is not the degree of upset but how it is handled that determines the state of one's mental health.

Many people have personality quirks that are managed appropriately and are not considered mental disorders. However, as many as 1 out of 10 Americans need professional help for mental disorders, whether they seek it or not. The degree of your own mental health will be evident in how you interact with others. It will influence your success in life and work.

Mentally healthy students are those who see a need to act and then act responsibly. They will act independently if the duty is clearly theirs or willingly under the direction of others when asked. If uncertain, they are willing to ask questions and request help when needed. They deal with problems as they are, not as they wish they were. When confronted by an unfamiliar task, they know not to attempt it without consulting their instructor or a supervisor.

Mentally healthy students also have the ability to accept constructive criticism. Students who use correction and comment to improve themselves and their work do not personalize the criticism but recognize it as a part of the education they have paid for and expect.

Mentally healthy nurses keep an open, analytical mind. They see the positive side in situations and people that others may not see and work to promote it. They are open, caring, and friendly, and they respect their peers, supervisors, and other members of their health and administrative team.

Because nurses have the responsibility to care for people whose attention is fully on themselves and the effects of their illness, they must continually work to maintain their own mental health. Some techniques for maintaining good mental health are to understand yourself; to assess your personality; to examine your personal values, beliefs, and prejudices; and to learn to cope effectively with stress. See Appendix A for tips on managing stress.

Understanding Yourself

One gains or develops maturity and good mental health through self-understanding. A willingness to look at yourself and your life objectively (self-evaluation) and squarely face what you find will influence how well you succeed.

All of life's experiences, whether good or bad, affect how one sees oneself and provide the opportunity for self-understanding and self-improvement. For example, adapting to divorce can lead to better self-understanding, just as adjusting to being married can. Raising a child alone can provide valuable lessons for living, just as sharing the responsibility with a spouse can. When you evaluate yourself, look at every side and use what you see to build yourself up, rather than tear yourself down.

Without self-understanding, you cannot reasonably expect to understand others and therefore to help them. You are not expected to be fault free—nobody is. But your obligation as a nurse is to care for others. To do that you have to make the effort to limit your self-concerns during your workday so that they don't prevent you from attending to the needs of your patients.

Developing self-awareness is a lifelong process that produces rewards from the beginning. How deeply you probe is a matter for you to decide. To start, ask yourself how well you really know yourself. Does what you know agree with how others see you? Are you willing to make changes?

Personality

Personality is the collection of behaviors and attitudes that sets one person apart from everyone else. You were not born with the personality you have today. You developed it gradually—consciously and unconsciously—as a way of adapting to the circumstances of your life and environment. Personality is not character. Character relates to the conscious, consistent way one reacts to ethical and moral customs and the standards of society.

It is easier to change personality traits than character traits, but neither is altogether easy. It is your personality that interacts with others. Your personality is where to look for traits that need to be refined, changed, or eliminated.

As a nurse, how well you interact with others is important. The personal nature of your work requires you to do more than just get along. You also must inspire positive relationships. Supervisors will expect you to work with minimum supervision. Peers and associates will expect you to do your share of what needs to be done. Your patients will expect you to see to their physical and emotional needs without being asked. To relate positively takes conscious effort, especially in a healthcare setting, where there is a broad mix of age, culture, and background. Your personality will not work on "automatic pilot" with such diverse populations. You have to be willing to adapt as new situations occur.

Changing personality traits, especially those that are deep-seated, takes time, but they can be changed if you know what they are. Study yourself as though you were someone else. Make notes of traits you think are positive and those you think detract from a healthy personality. Look among the people you respect for traits that make them stand out, and use them as models. You don't have to adopt them entirely, just use the parts that suit you.

Get input about how others see you from people whose opinions you respect. Make it clear how important their insight is and that you are not looking for flattery. Be willing to accept what they tell you whether you agree with it or not. Use what you learn to change the parts of your personality that would hinder you from becoming a better person and a better nurse.

Personal Values and Beliefs

As individuals we behave independently, but much of our behavior is a result of learned social customs. These learned social customs taken as a whole provide a simple definition of culture. Culture is the sum of values, ideas, customs, attitudes, roles, behaviors, and arts of given groups of people during specified periods. It is the pattern of overall behavior that is passed from generation to generation.

Within a culture, there are social groups that share a religion, a race, a common ancestry, or other specific similarities. These groups are subcultures and are termed *ethnic groups.* An example of a cultural custom is the institution of marriage. The way a given group of people within that culture celebrates weddings is an ethnic difference. Many people spend much of their lives in the comfort of their own ethnic or cultural heritage, with people who share their deep-seated similarities. However, as a nurse, you will come into contact with people from widely differing backgrounds.

Because of the nature of nursing, nurses are confronted with a full range of people from cultures and ethnic groups different from their own. How you handle patient differences will be a measure of your compassion, understanding, and maturity. It will also depend on your willingness to accept individual differences regardless of your personal opinion.

The foundation of your service to your patients is the acknowledgment that their basic needs are the same as everyone else's, including your own. Your patients experience hunger but their choice in food may differ from yours. They need clothing but the style they wear may not be found in your wardrobe. They need shelter although they may not be your neighbors. They need human kindness but they may be strangers to you. Everything about your patients may be a "world" away from your own, but when all their cultural and ethnic differences are removed, you are their nurse, they are your patients, and you live in the same world.

To be an effective nurse, it may be necessary for you to examine yourself to see if you have any prejudices that might compromise how much and what kind of care you provide to those in need.

Prejudice

The term *prejudice* describes the attitude of people who reject another person or ethnic group's differences in favor of his or her own group's values. A prejudiced person believes his beliefs and values are right and those who don't hold the same values or beliefs are inferior.

Prejudice is not something one is born with but a behavior learned from others usually early in life. It comes easily because it takes no work or effort. It only needs one's willingness to go along with someone else's negative beliefs about individuals or groups of people. The result is widely accepted misinformation and misunderstanding about an ethnic group's values, customs, and behaviors.

To effectively provide nursing care, a nurse must work to consciously value the differences inherent in different cultures and ethnic groups. Learning about other groups and incorporating cultural sensitivity in your nursing practice will enhance communication with your patients. When your patient trusts you to respect their beliefs and values, the resulting plan of treatment will be culturally acceptable to the patient, as well as medically sound. Learning to work with and care for people from many different backgrounds and beliefs requires special skills and is the topic of Chapter 8.

Coping With Stress

Stress is a condition of tension between two opposite forces. The forces can be physical, psychological, economic, or social, alone or in combination. A simple yet descriptive example of physical stress is a hot air balloon tied to the ground by a rope. The balloon wants to rise. The rope wants to hold it down. Tension created by the opposition between the force to rise and the force holding the balloon down makes the rope stretch. If a rope is stretched too far, it will break.

So many situations in life are so similar to this analogy that stress has become a word in everyone's vocabulary. A child who wants to go outside but is stopped by a parent because the weather is wet and cold experiences stress. A student facing an important exam experiences stress. A stomach that is overfilled with a holiday meal produces stress. A couple having an argument undergo stress.

Not all stress is harmful. Limited stress before an exam can raise energy levels, for example. But too much stress may result in anxiety, physical illness, psychological distress, fatigue, and other emotional and physical responses. Stress requires a response. The nature of the response—how one copes—determines whether the stress is relieved or worsened.

The connection between the mind and body is underscored by stress. A stressful situation always produces a reaction in the body. If the reaction is too great, the odds increase that something will hurt or break. Tension headaches are stress-related, as are some ulcers. Nervousness and anxiety result from stress. It is to anyone's advantage to learn to control stress.

The most effective way to control stress is to release the tension before it gets out of hand. Periods of rest will reduce fatigue. A light snack will reduce hunger. Telling someone what is bothering you relieves psychological tension. Confronting a personal fear reduces anxiety.

Managing stress, whether your own or your patient's, can be accomplished by a number of techniques combining physical and mental relaxation. In principle, they cause the mind and body to slow down for a brief period or quietly force a change of attention. A progressive relaxation technique, for example, uses a 15- to 30-minute process in which one's attention is put on every part of the body, one part at a time, while one is consciously thinking and feeling relaxation. Another technique, called guided imagery, is one in which the person who wishes to relax uses the imagination to think himself into a pleasant situation, such as lying in the warm sun on a sandy beach. Deep breathing exercises are a part of most stress management techniques.

You can practice stress management techniques on your own or in groups. Group sessions are helpful because they let you share an experience with others, which itself reduces tension. As an individual, you can use simple breathing exercises, such as taking a few deep breaths before an exam or when facing a stressful situation, without elaborate preparation or the need for a quiet, private place.

Stress that gets out of hand can be harmful. When anxiety or other stress-related conditions begin to dominate your life and your efforts to manage stress by yourself are not working, look to others for help. Talking to a friend may be enough. A chat with your instructor may help. Professional counseling is always a good idea when the stress in one's life exceeds the ability to cope. Some stress management techniques are provided in Appendix A. You may find these suggestions useful for yourself and your patients.

COMMUNICATION

Good communication skills are absolutely necessary in nursing because how you communicate affects what you communicate. Both will influence your relationships with peers, supervisors, and patients.

Communication can be defined as the exchange of information. Dr. Albert Mehrabian identified the components of the communication process to be verbal, vocal, and nonverbal. The verbal part of the communication process is the words; the vocal part of the process is the tone of voice; the nonverbal part is the gestures and expressions accompanying the verbal and vocal part of the communication process. Dr. Mehrabian estimates that 7% of communication is verbal, 38% is vocal, and 55% of communication is nonverbal.

Verbal Communication

The following diagram describes the verbal communication process:

SENDER → MESSAGE → RECEIVER

The exchange can be one-way, as in the above diagram, two-way, or multidirectional. An example of one-way communication is a news broadcast. The sender is the news announcer, the message is the news, and the receiver is receiving the message. Two-way communication occurs when the sender of the message and the receiver can both send and receive messages. An example of two-way communication is a telephone conversation. Both parties can send and receive messages as the following diagram illustrates:

SENDER	→	MESSAGE	→	RECEIVER
↑				↓
RECEIVER	←	MESSAGE	←	SENDER

Multidirectional communication involves more than two people. Several different people send messages to and receive messages from several different people who also send messages and receive messages.

In face-to-face communication, the sender uses verbal, vocal, and nonverbal communication skills to send a message to the receiver. Verbal communication is language expressed in speaking and in writing. Whether the language is English or another language, spoken and written words constitute verbal communication.

Vocal Communication

How you speak can be as important as what you say because the sound of your voice and the style of your delivery can communicate hints of hidden meaning, just as nonverbal communication does. Important messages lose their impact when delivered in a wishy-washy way, and annoying characteristics of speech, such as whining, shouting, or slurring words, detract from what is being said.

Self-consciousness is a big obstacle to clear speaking. If you are uncomfortable when talking, now is the time to analyze your speech habits. Learn which habits are reducing your effectiveness as a speaker and replace them with new ones. Practice your new behaviors alone at first and then with a friend or classmate. When you begin to feel secure, try them out on strangers. Clear speaking is a skill that can be learned, just as poor speech habits can be unlearned. In a vocation where you will be "on stage" when you work, the sooner you perfect your technique, the more effective you will be.

To improve your vocal communication skills, study the way that you speak. For example, you can use a tape recorder to hear how you sound to others, and speaking in front of a mirror will show you how you look when talking.

When speaking, face the person you're addressing. Keep eye contact and state your words clearly without skipping syllables or slurring their pronunciation. Use words you're comfortable with to avoid using terms that sound out of place, even though you understand their meaning. Your words, tone, rhythm, inflection, and posture should work together when you communicate. The failure of any one aspect of communication will detract from what you are saying and may create a wrong impression.

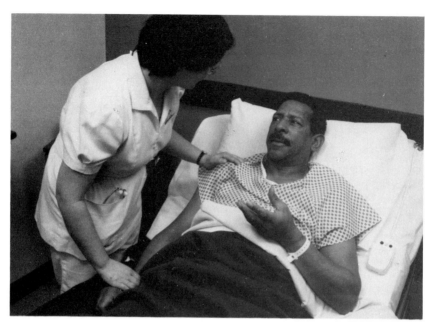

The nurse uses touch to communicate caring.

Nonverbal Communication

Nonverbal communication is body language that includes facial expressions, postures, body positions, and other actions that do not use words. Examples of nonverbal communication include averting your eyes when speaking or being spoken to; tapping a foot; frowning; yawning; putting your hand on your hip; gently touching a crying patient; smiling when entering a room; looking in the eyes of your patient; and presenting a clean, neat personal appearance. As you can see, nonverbal communication can be both positive and negative.

The Message

The message is information you want to communicate. It is important that you use correct vocabulary, grammar, medical terminology, and abbreviations when speaking and writing. Speaking clearly in a pleasant voice, using good judgment in what you say, giving simple, straightforward answers to questions, expressing confidence in what you say, listening without interrupting, and using accurate descriptions all contribute to presenting an effective message. It is important that you use words in your message that the receiver can understand. Nursing team members will understand medical terminology while your patient may not.

In general, to improve the quality of what you say so that you can be understood easily:

Organize your thoughts before speaking.
Avoid set speeches that sound memorized.
Keep your listener in mind when you're speaking.

Keep your opinions and values out of communications where they
    don't belong.

Use proper technical terms when speaking with colleagues.

Give complete explanations in words your patients understand when
    giving technical information to patients and families.

Restate or repeat in your own words questions or statements by others
    to make sure you understand what they've said.

Ask your listener for an opinion or other response.

Address people appropriately, as Mr., Mrs., Miss or Ms., according to
    their wishes.

Avoid trite terms of endearment, such as honey, dear, or Grandpa,
    when addressing patients and families.

Avoid teasing, even if your intention is to raise spirits.

Never be sarcastic.

Avoid giving false reassurances to anyone about your patient's condition.

Keep personal opinions out of communications where they don't
    belong.

Do your best to sound cheerful even when you don't feel it.

The Receiver

The receiver's role is to listen to the message being sent. Hearing and listening are two distinct activities. Hearing is biophysical and occurs when sound waves strike the structures in the inner ear. Listening is an active process requiring concentration and attention to the components of verbal, vocal, and nonverbal messages.

Effective listening skills can make a major difference in your expertise as a nurse. How good a listener you are affects communication between yourself and others. It can also influence how well you do your work. By listening closely and attentively, you will focus your attention on the information being communicated to you. When you are given directions to do something, for example, knowing exactly what your instructor or supervisor is telling you will help you work with confidence.

A good listener also gains the confidence of the speaker. Where instructors and supervisors are concerned, this translates into approval of you and your performance. Establishing confidence with patients makes working with them easier and, equally important, is therapeutic for them as well.

Good listening skills do not come naturally for everyone but they can be learned. In conversation or at other times when listening is important, most people focus their attention on what they themselves are saying or thinking, not on the speaker. This normal egocentricity (focus on the self) conflicts with the need for nurses to be exceptional listeners. There are two steps to good listening: (1) focus your attention on the speaker and what is being said, and (2) interpret what is said to understand what to do. As an important person in your patients' lives, you will be someone they will turn to to express their hopes, fears, opinions, and personal concerns. By listening closely to what they say, you will provide an outlet for feelings that they might otherwise keep bottled up. This can help to relieve their stress, which is often a component of illness. And by listening between the lines, you will know what they really need or want to say.

Being a good listener does not mean to insert yourself or your opinions into your patient's life the way one does in daily social conversation. It also does not mean you have the right to pry. Accept what they tell you without judging what they say. Treat information with total confidentiality. Remember that you are not the patient's only audience but only one of many people in his or her life at the moment. You should be receptive and open, but it is not your role to be an adviser.

Sharing experiences is a normal part of ordinary conversation, but a patient who relates a significant life event is not looking for a similar story from you, and you should not offer any. Nod, smile, and acknowledge that you are listening. Be there for your patients without interrupting. Ask questions as a way to show your interest, but don't ask questions that don't relate to what has been said or questions that can be construed as prying. Don't let boredom or lack of interest show. Be courteous, interested, and nonjudgmental in your conversations with patients.

Effective communication skills improves the quality of care while ineffective communication skills are the root of many errors in patient care. Thinking about and practicing to improve verbal, vocal, nonverbal, and listening skills is as important to you as a nurse as it is to you as a person.

Writing

Writing can be considered a part of verbal communication. Writing something down may be less threatening to you than telling someone directly, but writing requires the same attention as speaking.

You are already learning the importance of good writing from your note taking. Clear, legible notes release their information whenever it is needed without having to dig it out. Muddled, scribbled, and erratic notes take more time and work to translate than rereading the original material from which they were taken.

The need to write clearly does not end when you leave your program. Your ability to write well will be more important to you than ever when you enter practice. Once you begin to record on patients' charts, fill out forms and applications, write requisitions, and do the other writing your daily work will require, how well it is done will have a bearing on your patients' well-being, health, and life. Neatness, legibility, and precise meaning in as few words as possible are the basics of good writing.

Charting is a special kind of writing skill that has a direct bearing on patient care. Long, vague, or meaningless written observations do not communicate the hard information required to manage patient care. Use specific, concise terms and phrases that tell the facts, not opinions. Think about what you've observed, what you want to say, and then how you're going to say it before writing anything. This will become habit with time, but developing the habit requires thought and effort at the start.

It is permissible to use approved abbreviations when charting, but the abbreviations must be those in general use in your program. Learn them and use them. Don't use a shorthand that nobody else can understand.

Reading

Although reading is not considered to be a direct communications skill, it is a talent that puts you in direct touch with the information and ideas you need to perform your job well. Your education from now on will depend heavily on how well and what you read. Reading is and will be required in your education and work. Developing good reading habits now will help you throughout your program and career.

How fast you read and how well you understand what you read are the essentials of effective reading. Both can be improved with practice.

How fast you read depends on what kind of material you're reading and how efficiently your eyes travel over the page. A textbook or nursing manual goes slower than a mystery story or a general-interest magazine article because their purposes are different. Technical reading requires more concentration than recreational reading, but it does not have to be hard.

Your reading speed is also affected by how many words you read in a single glance, by whether you read each word, and by distractions, such as mouthing each word or reading aloud.

Observe how you read. Do you mouth or speak the words? Do you keep your place by running your finger along sentences as you read? Do you read each word separately? Do you go back over what you've read again and again? Your reading speed and comprehension will suffer if you do. If you have reading problems, ask for help. Changing poor reading habits will make learning easier.

How well you understand what you have read depends a great deal on the extent of your vocabulary. If you know the words, you will generally understand what is said; not knowing a key word may make the rest of a sentence meaningless. An excellent way to improve comprehension is to build a good vocabulary. Nurses require two vocabularies, each having their own dictionaries: one for common language and the other for medical terms.

When you find an unfamiliar word, look it up immediately, read the definition and the correct pronunciation, repeat the word, and then say it in your own words. Then go back and read the sentence where it was found. To increase word retention and make new words a part of your active vocabulary, use them soon and frequently.

You will use medical terms extensively in much of your reading and in communications with colleagues and patients. Medical terminology has its own special rules, particularly regarding root words, suffixes, and prefixes. Learn them well now so that you can figure out meanings of new words on your own. Then look them up to verify your definition.

Communicating Empathy and Sympathy

As a nurse, you will be in a position to give your patients emotional support, encouragement, and understanding. The source of this support comes from inside yourself, where your feelings reside.

Feelings require energy, and energy is a resource you cannot afford to waste. At times, just meeting the daily physical demands of your work will take more energy than you think you have. Add to that the emotional drain of working with patients who depend on you for many of their needs, and you will quickly see how the con-

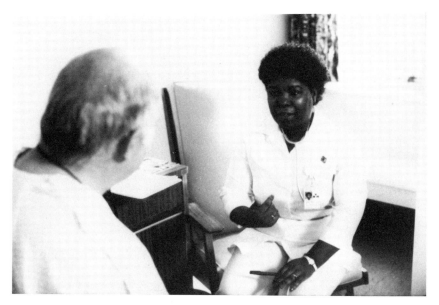

Empathy is communicated through verbal and nonverbal communication.

servation of physical and emotional energy is the only way to avoid exhaustion and loss of interest.

The way to provide emotional support to your patients and not deplete your own emotional reserves is to avoid becoming personally involved while still sharing with them their thoughts, feelings, and fears. This behavior is called empathy.

To empathize with someone is to project yourself into their situation to understand what they are experiencing, without experiencing it yourself. It lets you say to yourself, "How would I feel if I were my patient with this illness?" and not "How do I feel as my patient with this illness?" The latter is sympathy, which is to have another person's feelings or emotions.

Empathizing with patients lets them have their experience without interference but with the benefit of having someone who understands how important or serious it is. Sympathizing with a patient takes away from their experience and forces them to share it with you. It is unfair to them because they, not you, must actually deal with the experience and its consequences.

Being empathetic is not callous or hard-hearted. It lets you keep the distance you need from the patient's problem so that you can think and act in the patient's best interest.

PROBLEM SOLVING

A problem is not knowing exactly what to do in a specific situation. Problems can be complex, with many parts and many consequences, or simple, with just one answer. As a nurse you will have your share of each kind of problem. Knowing how to solve them will make your job easier.

It is not a good idea to respond to a problem without thinking about it first. Although it may sometimes be faster to act without thinking, you will do better if you use a system to solve all problems to avoid making errors. The first step to problem solving is making sure you understand the problem. State the problem in your own words as accurately as you can. Once you know what the problem is, determine its cause. There may be more than one reason for the problem. Find as many reasons as you can before attempting a solution. Make sure your information is accurate to avoid acting on hearsay, rumor, or someone else's misinterpretation of facts.

After pinpointing the causes, see whether there is more than one solution to the problem. If so, study each to find which one will solve the problem with the least negative effect on those involved, with particular attention to your patient. Avoid letting your own motives or emotions influence the solution unless the problem is a personal one.

Once you have a solution that best fits the problem, check your institution's practices and rules to avoid conflict. Then decide who is best suited to put the solution into action. Be careful not to use automatic solutions that are based on presumption. You may not have all the facts, or you may be seeing the problem or its solution from an inaccurate point of view. You can use your own past experiences to evaluate new problems, but avoid the trap of assuming that the solution that worked in the past will work every time. It may, but if you don't look closely at the problem, you could miss a key difference.

When you must question someone's authority to solve a problem, do so carefully. Give a clear, intelligent statement of the problem and its solution in a way that will keep the issue neutral. Problems can be worsened if the people involved are forced to defend their position or attack yours.

The following is a general guide to problem solving. Use it, but treat every problem as unique and solve each on its own merits.

Problem-Solving Hints
1. Define the problem in your own terms.
2. State your own objectives realistically.
3. Get as many facts as possible.
4. Get advice from your instructor and others if necessary.
5. Examine alternative solutions carefully.
6. Give yourself room to change solutions if necessary.
7. Choose the best solution in your judgment.
8. Take responsible action.
9. Evaluate the consequences of your action.
10. Choose another solution if your action did not solve the problem.

DISCUSSION QUESTIONS/LEARNING ACTIVITIES

1. List between 10 and 15 human needs and then place them in one of the five categories of human needs described by Maslow.

2. What are first impressions and how are they formed?

3. Describe hidden messages that people give by posture, appearance, and body language.

4. Think about how you might handle a situation when you know for certain that a classmate is using illegal drugs or is addicted to drugs or alcohol.

5. Describe the personal traits or characteristics that contribute to becoming an effective nurse.

6. What can you do to identify and adjust your personal prejudices?

7. What are some effective methods you might be able to use to reduce stress and anxiety?

8. Using forms other than verbal communication, try getting a message across to a friend or classmate.

9. Select a problem related to either school or your personal life and use the problem-solving techniques presented in this chapter to find one or more solutions. Did this process clarify your thinking?

READ MORE ABOUT IT

Barry PD: Mental Health and Mental Illness, Fifth Edition. Philadelphia: JB Lippincott, 1994.

Bennett D: Substance Abuse, Second Edition. Albany, NY: Delmar, 1991.

Blonna R: Coping with Stress in a Changing World, First Edition. St. Louis: CV Mosby, 1996.

Haas K, Haas A: Understanding Sexuality, Third Edition. St. Louis: Mosby, 1993.

Kahn S, Saulo M: Healing Yourself: A Nurse's Guide to Self Care and Renewal, First Edition. Albany: Delmar, 1994.

Long MA: Understanding/Responding: A Communication Manual for Nurses, Second Edition. Boston: Jones & Bartlett, 1992.

Milliken ME: Understanding Human Behavior, Fifth Edition. Albany, NY: Delmar, 1993.

Northouse PG, Northouse LL: Health Communications: Strategies for Health Professionals, First Edition. East Norwalk: Appleton and Lange, 1992.

Payne WA, Hahn DB: Understanding Your Health, Fourth Edition. St. Louis: Mosby, 1995.

Sampson EE, Sampson-Marthas M: Group Process for the Health Professions, Third Edition. New York: Wiley, 1990.

Sherman KM: Communication and Image in Nursing, First Edition. Albany: Delmar, 1994.

Shives LR: Basic Concepts of Psychiatric-Mental Health Nursing, Second Edition. Philadelphia: JB Lippincott, 1994.

Sullivan EJ, et al: Chemical Dependency in Nursing: The Deadly Diversion, First Edition. Reading, MA: Addison-Wesley, 1988.

Zawid C: Sexual Health: A Nurse's Guide, First Edition. Albany: Delmar, 1994.

3

Nursing From Past to Present

OBJECTIVES

When you complete this chapter, you should be able to:

Give the dates of the major historical periods and identify a significant event in each period.

Describe the contributions of Florence Nightingale to the development of modern nursing.

Trace the development of practical nursing from the late 1800s to the present time.

Name the two organizations primarily concerned with practical/vocational nursing education and practical/vocational nursing practice.

OCTOBER 1854

The British Light Brigade was under attack at Balaclava, Turkey, by Russian troops. It was a bloody war, this war in the Crimea. Cannons blazed under the heavy gray skies of late autumn. Muskets cracked, spitting fire and sudden death. Many soldiers would die in the Crimean War. Some would die needlessly.

The British field hospital in Scutari smelled of dirt, blood, and death. Thousands of sick and wounded soldiers, many still in their blood-caked uniforms, lay helpless and cold on filthy straw beds. The hospital was understaffed and short of supplies. Hunger and disease added to the soldiers' suffering. The death rate soared. In London, 2000 miles and many days' travel away from the battle, the London Times told the awful story of misery at the war front. The public was outraged but felt helpless. No organized care for British victims of war yet existed.

A brave young woman offered her services. She was a nurse. Although she had been raised in comfortable surroundings, the woman gave no thought to her own well-being or safety in volunteering to go to Turkey to care for the sick and dying. Her offer was accepted immediately.

In November, a group of 38 women accompanied the nurse to Scutari. They were appalled by what they found. Suffering was everywhere. Wounds festered for lack of soap and clean dressings. Rats, mice, bedbugs, and lice crawled amid the moaning men, adding to their torment. To many, death was a relief—and death came to many. More than half the men were dying.

Every night, the nurse walked the cold corridors to comfort the sick men. They could hear her footsteps, softly at first and then growing louder. But only when the flickering glow of her lamp brightened the darkness did they know that the kind lady with the lamp was not a dream.

The next months were a miracle. Using her own money, the nurse bought supplies and food. The small group of dedicated women scoured the dingy hospital. The kitchen prepared hot, nutritious meals for the patients. There were organized activities for the men. The death rate decreased with astonishing speed. Six months after the women's arrival, only two percent of the patients were dying.

The courageous young nurse who volunteered her services in the Crimean War was Florence Nightingale. Her lamp, still burning brightly after more than 140 years, is the beacon of modern nursing.

Nursing is deeply rooted in history, even though it is relatively new as a career. Today nursing is a contemporary, rapidly growing, highly skilled service that is as technically sophisticated as the latest discoveries in science and medicine. But people have practiced nursing for ages, and the tradition of serving persons in need can be traced far into the past.

The historical record of nursing in very early times is vague, but the conditions for nursing have always existed. New babies, illness, injury, aging, and the need for personal care are facts of life. One can assume that people have always needed what today is called nursing.

There is also no clear record of who in a group, tribe, or society performed the functions of nursing. Modern medicine can trace its primitive origins to the skills and wisdom of witch doctors, shamans, and medicine men. They performed healing rituals and administered herbs and roots that were known for their medicinal value. Their knowledge of the natural world came from tens of thousands of years of observation and experience passed down from generation to generation. That knowledge evolved into the traditions and tools of health care as it is practiced today. Your role in nursing has been defined by long experience.

NURSING IN ANCIENT CIVILIZATIONS

As cultures developed and the civilizations based on them flourished, guidelines for behavior were made into rules. The rules were intended to protect people and guarantee group survival. They governed sanitation, hygiene, diet, sexual relations, fitness and disease, and other areas of life.

Like many early civilizations, ancient Egypt developed on the banks of a river. Waterways such as the Nile were a source of life. But when large numbers of people lived together and used the river for drinking, washing, and sanitation, the need for personal hygiene and public sanitation became evident. Rules—early versions of community health laws—were made.

Egyptian physicians were skilled in treating fractures, filling teeth, and classifying drugs. Midwives practiced obstetrics, and friends or attendants served as nurses at births.

In ancient Babylonia, illness was seen as punishment for displeasing the gods. It was believed that atonement was possible through purifying the body with herbs and chants. Purification was performed in special temples that, in a sense, were care centers.

The Old Testament refers to many dietary, hygienic, and health laws. For example, it was forbidden to eat meat after the third day because in a hot climate without refrigeration, the meat would spoil. People with communicable diseases were isolated in sick houses. Provisions were made for the aged. Variations of those laws are still practiced today. Health, healing, and a tradition of caring for the sick and homeless are parts of an ancient heritage that continues.

Other early cultures practiced health and healing principles that were also forerunners of today's medicine and nursing. Over 3000 years ago, the *Vedas* (sacred Hindu books of India's earliest cultures) told of major and minor surgery, nervous afflictions, and urinary system diseases. Later, in India, advances were made in medicine, surgery, prenatal care, hygiene, and sanitation. They included public hospitals that were staffed by male nurses who would be qualified by today's standards to be practical nurses.

In ancient China, acupuncture, medical diagnosis by a complex pulse theory, and a vast knowledge of medicine and drugs were well known. This knowledge has survived and, in various forms, is still practiced today.

Hippocrates

A physician of the late fifth century B.C. named Hippocrates (460–370 B.C.) is referred to by early Greek writers as the Father of Medicine. He is still called that today. He taught at a medical school on Cos, a small Greek island. Little is known of his ideas and discoveries, and much of his life is unknown. The Hippocratic

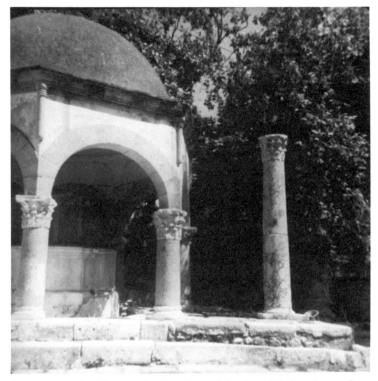

Legend says that Hippocrates taught medicine from this location on Cos.

oath, which is taken by medical school graduates today, is attributed to Hippocrates.

As the teachings of the school at Cos and another at Cnidus gained acceptance, the dominance that magic held in early medicine declined. The study of medicine shifted to a more scientific course.

Hippocrates' followers believed diseases always had specific causes that could be discovered by examination and analysis. The causes they sought were often wrong: they blamed disease on "humors" in the body, such as blood, phlegm, and yellow and black bile.

The idea that it is not magic or wrongdoing that causes illness was a big step forward. *Diagnosis* (the process of identifying a disease or medical condition scientifically) and *prognosis* (predicting the probable outcome of a patient's disease), rather than *cure* (restoration to health), were the foundations of Hippocratic medicine. It would be more than 2000 years later that scientists would discover the germ theory of disease.

The healing method taught by Hippocrates' followers was to help nature do its work. This was similar to what Florence Nightingale would write about nursing in her *Notes on Nursing: What It Is and What It Is Not* in 1859, more than 2000 years later. She said that nursing would "put the patient in the best condition for nature to act upon."

Practitioners of Hippocratic medicine were men who did not train nurses to do the nursing that their method ("help nature do its work") suggested. They did it themselves. Women in Greek society were subordinate to men. It was believed that women were not worthy of medical or nursing education. Greek nurses were little more than household servants, usually slaves, who took care of the children and family.

The rise of the vast Roman Empire (476–1096) was based on military might. Military hospitals to care for wounded soldiers were established, but Roman medicine was still based on superstition. This was a setback from advances made earlier by the Greeks. The Romans held their women in greater esteem than the Greeks did theirs. Roman women enjoyed a liberated position for the times but organized nursing care was not yet established.

NURSING IN THE EARLY CHRISTIAN ERA
(FIRST TO FIFTH CENTURIES A.D.)

Nursing by women who were dedicated to its practice began with the acceptance of Christianity, which taught caring for others. Deacons and deaconesses—men and women with equal rank in the church—served the sick, the poor, the aged, orphans, widows, slaves, and prisoners. They fed and clothed the needy, cared for the sick, visited prisoners, sheltered the homeless, and buried the dead. All were works of mercy.

Deaconesses were frequently well-bred, cultured widows or daughters of Roman officials. They performed services similar to today's community health or visiting nurses, carrying baskets of food and medicine to needy homes. Phoebe, a friend of St. Paul, who lived about A.D. 55, is considered to be the first deaconess and visiting nurse. She is mentioned in the New Testament.

Two other women's groups, the Order of Widows and the Order of Virgins, were also dedicated to the principle of merciful care for those in need. Like the deaconesses, they lived in humble, selfless service to others. They are sometimes called the first organized public health service nurses.

The deaconess movement reached its peak at about A.D. 400 in Constantinople (today's Istanbul, Turkey), which was an important center of the early Christian church. The movement diminished when the church took away the role of the deaconesses, but not before spreading as far west as present-day France and Ireland.

In A.D. 380 in Rome, a beautiful and wealthy woman named Fabiola founded the first public hospital. She had divorced her first husband and was remarried when she converted to Christianity. Her second husband died. Because remarriage after divorce was considered a sin, Fabiola atoned by dedicating her life to charity. To the dismay of others, she personally cared for the sick and injured, often cleaning and dressing sores and wounds with her own hands.

THE EARLY MIDDLE AGES
AND THE MONASTIC ORDERS (A.D. 476–1000)

The influence of the Roman Empire peaked at the time of the birth of Jesus. It ended in A.D. 476 after hundreds of years of attacks by barbarians. Europe was split into many separate kingdoms. The next 500 years are called the Dark Ages because learning almost stopped. Christians retreated to walled monasteries while the world was plunged into war, rivalry, and ignorance. The teachings of the early Greek Classical period were saved by the dedication of monks who lived in relative safety in monasteries. They kept learning alive and preserved the record of the past in handwritten books.

The idea of caring for those in need was also preserved. The emphasis in medicine shifted from a scientific interest in anatomy, physiology, and the healing effects of nature's drugs to personal care and comfort, which is the foundation of nursing. Monks and nuns performed nursing tasks in the monasteries under the direction of the church.

The first hospitals were founded at monasteries in Lyon in A.D. 542 and Paris in A.D. 650. Santo Spirito Hospital was founded in Rome in A.D. 717. The first nursing order of nuns, the Augustinian Sisters, staffed the hospital in Paris.

THE HIGH MIDDLE AGES (1000–1475)

The small states that emerged from the High Middle Ages were dominated by the church, which had slowly filled the vacuum left by the collapse of the Roman Empire. Almost everything in life, from philosophy, politics, art, and architecture to everyday activity, was deeply influenced by the church.

During this time, huge cathedrals were built and universities were founded. Some of the universities are still in existence today. A lengthy series of religious wars, the Crusades, began. The High Middle Ages had closed off much of Western civilization for almost 500 years; the Crusades reopened it.

The military orders of the Knights Hospitalers and the Knights Templars were priests, brothers, and knights who sought to reclaim the Holy Land from the Moslems. At the same time, they established a hospital to care for pilgrims of Jerusalem.

The Moslems used organized facilities for the care of their sick and wounded. The Crusaders saw this and adopted this method of treatment to care for their own casualties. They built hospitals near the battlefields. While some knights fought on the battlefield, others cared for the injured in the hospitals. The insignia of the Knights Hospitalers of St. John of Jerusalem, also known as Knights Hospitalers, was a bright red cross. It is now the symbol of the International Red Cross.

The Knights Hospitalers' strict principles of discipline, obedience, and devotion became an important part of organized nursing for hundreds of years. Knights who returned home from the wars in the Holy Land created a new version of society based on a middle class. The deaconess movement vanished and was replaced by monastic nursing orders, such as the Franciscans, the Alexians, the Brothers of Mercy, and the Knights of St. John, a military order that was formed to fight the Crusades.

Hospices

Monasteries continued to play an important role in nursing during the Middle Ages. Hospices were established within their walls. As places of safety from the outside world, hospices welcomed travelers, the poor, and the sick. The idea of separate hospitals for the sick was begun later. They were based on the hospitals of the Persians and Arabs, whose ideas were brought back to Europe by the Crusaders. The hospitals were staffed by both secular and religious orders.

Two early orders are still active. The First Order of St. Francis and the Second Order of St. Francis were regular monastic orders. Order members lived secluded lives under strict vows of poverty and chastity. The First Order of St. Francis was founded by Saint Francis of Assisi. The Second Order, now called the Poor Clares, was founded by his disciple, St. Clare. St. Francis also founded the Third Order of St. Francis for laypersons who wanted to follow his teachings but did not want to give up normal life for the strict discipline of the monastery. The Poor Clares continue to serve the poor and the aged today, but they do not perform nursing functions.

Nursing Orders and Church Influence

Nursing during the Middle Ages was an important way of life to its practitioners and a valuable service to those in need. Its practice reinforced its place in the slowly growing science of medicine. Its strict organization was also important. When new members joined nursing orders, they first had to spend a probationary period before they could wear the white robe that symbolized their work. After an additional novitiate period, they were allowed to wear the hood of the order. A nursing director, called a *maîtresse,* supervised their activities. Order members were expected to be obedient, unselfish, and totally devoted to the performance of their duties. These and other regulations are the roots of traditional nursing.

During this time, the power of the Catholic Church grew. Because the church sponsored the nursing orders, their strength and status also grew. The numbers of women entering nursing increased. Nursing was a popular and acceptable occupation for women.

At the same time, medicine as an occupation declined. The church did not favor medicine in the way it did nursing. The church, not medicine, held authority over nursing. What a nurse could and could not do was dictated by the church. For example, because it was believed that the human body was basically unclean, procedures such as perineal care, enemas, and douches were not performed. A nurse's priority was to serve her patients' spiritual needs. However, her duties included feeding, bathing, and washing patients, administering medications, changing dressing and linens, and all-around cleaning.

The nurse, not the physician, provided most health care in hospitals, even though the care was more custodial and centered on reducing discomfort than it was centered on treatment.

The church's authority and dominance began to decline. The kingdoms that were formed after the end of the Roman empire grew in power. The merchants had returned to Europe with ideas from the Moslem world and ancient Greece. They also brought the deadly black death (bubonic plague), a highly contagious, epidemic disease that swept Europe from 1347 to 1350. One fourth of the entire population died, while famine and war killed many more people and economies faltered. With such chaos affecting their lives, people's religious fervor turned to cynicism and hope was lost. The times were ripe for change.

THE DECLINE OF NURSING: THE RENAISSANCE (1400–1600) TO THE NINETEENTH CENTURY

An Augustinian monk named Martin Luther opposed many of the teachings of the Catholic Church. His protests led to the Reformation and the foundation of a new view of religion, Protestantism, which ended the absolute domination of the Catholic Church. It also opened the way for new ideas in areas other than religion. Some had a dramatic effect on nursing.

Monasteries were closed and the religious orders that ran them were disbanded. Nursing work once performed by women in hospitals virtually stopped. Women's role in society changed dramatically. Under the influence of the church, women had been revered. They were encouraged to do charitable work outside the home. Women from Europe's finest families had became nuns who taught and nursed.

Under Protestantism, women were considered to be subordinate to men. They were expected to stay at home to bear and raise children and to care for the home. Respectable women did not work in hospitals. Instead, nursing was done by "wayward" women of low status, such as prostitutes and alcoholic women who were given the work in place of going to jail.

Nursing fell to a low state, and its practitioners were reduced to poorly paid servants. The disruption of society by plague and famine meant that there were more sick and poor persons than ever. The early Greeks and Romans had developed wonderful ideas, but the ideas had been lost for centuries. Now the ideas were replanted.

In a burst of collective creative genius known as the Renaissance (meaning rebirth) that lasted until the sixteenth century, classical thought was raised to near perfection. The idea that the world could be studied became the foundation of a new science of discovery and exploration. That idea is still alive today.

Medicine took a lead among the sciences. Anatomy, physiology, and the scientific basis of healing were studied. Nursing went into a further decline. Nursing had been neglected during the Greek era, when Hippocratic medicine prevailed. It rose to dominate medicine during the monastic period. Now, during the Renaissance, it fell once again. Except for the hope represented by dedicated people such as St. Vincent de Paul, a French priest who, with follower Louise de Marilac, founded the Sisters of Charity, nursing remained dormant until the early 1820s.

THE EMERGENCE OF MODERN NURSING (NINETEENTH CENTURY)

Social conditions had deteriorated sharply by the end of the 1700s. Industrialization was replacing familiar agricultural society. Cities with large populations were breeding grounds for poverty, poor hygiene, and disease. Societies treated their members badly. The sick, insane, poor, and homeless were put into hospitals, jails, asylums, and poorhouses that were little more than warehouses for the needy. Living, health, and sanitary conditions were deplorable. Change was desperately needed, setting the stage for social reform. All that was needed were people with social vision.

A Londoner, John Howard (1726–1790), fought for reforms in public health. He had visited many foreign countries and had seen firsthand how prisoners were treated. He pushed for prison reforms that resulted in dramatic improvements in prison conditions and increased public awareness.

Howard's work was carried on by a London philanthropist, Elizabeth Fry (1780–1845). She organized a group called the Protestant Sisters of Charity, later called the Institute of Nursing Sisters, to provide nursing care for London's poor.

In Germany, a minister in Kaiserswerth was concerned with the problems of poverty faced by his parishioners. Pastor Theodor Fliedner (1800–1864) visited England, where he was impressed by Elizabeth Fry's work in British prisons. With his wife, Friederike, Fliedner opened a school in Germany to train deaconesses, the Kaiserswerth Deaconess Institution. It marked a revival of the deaconess movement that had ended 400 years earlier. It was the first real nursing school.

Pastor Fliedner opened his hospital in Kaiserswerth in 1836. Its first deaconess was Gertrude Reichardt. Many women were trained as deaconesses at the school. They became the core of the movement that would lead to modern nursing. Graduates of the Kaiserswerth Deaconess Institution founded similar programs to train women around the world. One of them, Florence Nightingale, opened the way to the new age of nursing.

Florence Nightingale (1820–1910)

Florence Nightingale was the younger of two sisters. She was born May 12, 1820, in Florence, Italy, and was named after that city. Her parents were visiting there from their native England. She returned to England with her family when she was one year old. As a daughter of wealthy parents, she was given an excellent classical education in languages, history, mathematics, and philosophy. She was taught the social manners and customs of the privileged class and grew up to be a cultured, attractive young lady. Her family expected her to become the wife of an equally eminent gentleman and live a life of comfort and plenty. Her own goals were decidedly different.

From childhood on, Miss Nightingale was a sympathetic and sensitive girl with a great affection for animals and people. As a youngster she visited the sick and poor. Her visits were a hint of her growing ambition to serve humanity. She began to think of a career as a nurse. She declared her intentions in 1844, when she was 24 years old.

The idea astounded her parents. Not only did such work not fit her social rank, but at that time women in nursing were often disreputable. The more her family objected to her calling, as she believed it to be, the more determined she became.

Miss Nightingale traveled to foreign countries. She visited hospitals and orphanages where she observed how nursing was performed by untrained individuals. She became an authority on public health and hospitals.

Dr. Elizabeth Blackwell, a close friend who was also America's first woman physician, encouraged Miss Nightingale to pursue her ambition to be a nurse. In 1851, at 31 years of age, Florence Nightingale went to the Kaiserswerth Deaconess

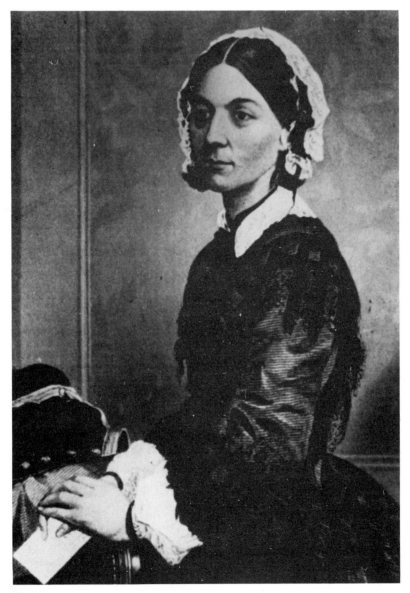

Modern nursing began with Florence Nightingale. (Courtesy of The Center for the Study of the History of Nursing.)

Institution, which she had heard about from friends. She studied there for 3 months. After her training, she worked in Paris with the Sisters of Charity. She also observed skilled French surgeons operate. Although she was pleased with her training, she knew it was not enough for the kind of nurse she wanted to be.

Florence returned to London, where she became superintendent of a small institution, the Establishment for Gentlewomen During Illness. Her family had still not accepted her independent attitude. Then, in 1854, the Crimean War broke out. This dark moment of history would certify her behavior. It would also help her leave her mark on the world.

British newspapers told of appalling conditions in the Crimea, where England, France, and Turkey were fighting against Russia. Ill and injured British soldiers lay neglected, while both allied and enemy soldiers were treated and cared for by organized groups of nurses. French casualties were taken care of by the Sisters of Charity. The Russians were cared for by the Sisters of Mercy. The English public was outraged. Miss Nightingale volunteered to take a group of nurses to the Crimea to care for English and Turkish soldiers. Her friend Sidney Herbert, Britain's secretary of war, had already written to her requesting her services.

On October 21, 1854, Florence Nightingale left for the front with 38 women. Some were trained as nurses and others were not. They took with them a stock of badly needed supplies. Conditions at the front were disgusting. Wounded soldiers, still in bloody uniforms, lay crowded into filthy wards on dirty straw. Sanitation was poor to nonexistent. There was no soap, clean linen, or even tables and chairs. The food was often inedible.

Adding to the horror, the reception the women received from army medical officers was characterized by resentment. Miss Nightingale took matters into her own hands. With her nurses, she tended to ill and injured soldiers. She fought red tape to obtain supplies and hired people to clean the hospitals. She set up laundries, organized kitchens to turn out nutritious meals, and personally made endless rounds to comfort wounded and sick soldiers. She even used her own money to purchase supplies.

Within 6 months, Florence Nightingale's labors paid off. Deaths dropped dramatically, from 420 per 1000 to 22 per 1000. Discipline and organization took over from neglect and disorder. She had become the "Lady with the Lamp" to her patients. It was an endearing reference to the nightly rounds she made with a lamp in hand to see to their comfort and care.

Florence Nightingale returned to England in July 1856. She was the unchallenged heroine of the war. But her own strength was sapped by sickness and exhaustion. She remained a semi-invalid for the remaining 54 years of her life. Florence Nightingale did not stop her work, however. Her powerful influence was felt in civilian and military hospitals and in nurse training. She also wrote books. Her best-known work is *Notes on Nursing: What It Is and What It Is Not*. She was awarded medals and jewels by grateful admirers who included England's Queen Victoria and the sultan of Turkey. A fund contributed by soldiers and citizens alike was used to establish a training school for nurses, the Nightingale School, which opened in 1860. The school became the model for modern nursing schools. Florence Nightingale died in 1910 at 90 years of age.

NURSING DURING THE LATE NINETEENTH AND EARLY TWENTIETH CENTURIES (1870–1960)

Nursing was changed forever by Florence Nightingale and the methods she introduced. The old practices fell away as major advances in nursing were made around the world.

J.H. Dunant was instrumental in founding the International Red Cross in Switzerland in 1864. Like Nightingale, Dunant had been horrified by the almost complete lack of care for the sick and wounded in wartime. Until that time there was no neutral international health organization that nations could turn to in time of war or after natural disasters. One of the Red Cross's early accomplishments was to make rules for the treatment of the wounded and for the protection of medical personnel and hospitals. Today, most countries have their own Red Cross organization that also belongs to the International Red Cross.

There were no formal programs to train nurses, and there were scarcely any trained nurses at all in the United States. War and other social conditions were major influences in the reform of the haphazard nursing practices that did exist. Government agencies became aware of the problem, and important changes were made. The Civil War (1861–1865) dramatized the need for skilled nurses. People realized that society was responsible for its own health.

The status of women was improving; Florence Nightingale's example led to advances in nursing education and practice. Women were beginning to assume new roles in public affairs, including nursing. In New York City, Bellevue Hospital opened the New York Training School in 1873, which was organized along the lines of the Nightingale School model.

Fifteen years later, the Mills School of Nursing, a school for training male nurses, was opened at Bellevue Hospital. Other schools were opened as the new nursing movement grew. Textbooks, uniforms for secular nurses, and a growing appreciation of nurses by a grateful public for their devotion to duty encouraged the growth.

Science and medicine made gigantic strides. The germ theory of disease was developed in 1876 by Robert Koch, a German bacteriologist. He said that bacteria, not "bad air" carry anthrax and other disease. Louis Pasteur's discoveries in chemistry and microbiology (pasteurization is named for him), Joseph Lister's aseptic surgical techniques, Ignaz Philipp Semmelweis's conquest of puerperal sepsis (childbed fever), and other scientific developments were changing humankind's ability to do something about its health.

Emergence of Nursing Leaders

Nursing also flourished during this time and a number of eminent women emerged as leaders of the growing reform.

Dorothea Lynde Dix (1802–1887) was concerned by the inhumane treatment of mentally ill persons. She traveled over the United States to encourage legislators to pass protective laws. As an untrained volunteer nurse in the Civil War, she was appointed to be superintendent of women nurses for all military hospitals. She was the first U.S. Army nurse.

Clara Barton (1821–1912) was a dedicated teacher at a time when few women held such jobs. She obtained permission from the U.S. government to take volunteer nursing to field hospitals during the Civil War. She cared for the ill and wounded of both sides, North and South, black and white, with equality. She was given the name *Angel of the Battlefield.* Miss Barton formed the American

Association of the Red Cross in 1881 after seeing the awful conditions of soldiers on the battlefield.

The first nurse to be trained in the United States was Linda Richards (1841–1930), who graduated from the New England Hospital for Women and Children in Boston after a 1-year training program. She developed a system for writing accurate patient reports that later became the basis for nursing and hospital recordkeeping. She was a lifelong student of nursing and taught its methods. She traveled extensively, studying, lecturing, consulting, and opening schools. The Linda Richards Award is given every 2 years by the National League for Nursing to an active nurse who has significantly contributed to nursing.

Mary Eliza Mahoney (1845–1926) was the first African-American graduate professional nurse in the United States. Her work for integration in nursing and improved working and health care conditions was a lifelong endeavor. The Mary Mahoney Award, first instituted in 1936, is given by the American Nurses' Association to recognize her accomplishments.

Lavinia Dock (1858–1956) was instrumental in the beginning of what is now called the National League for Nursing. Her book, *History of Nursing*, coauthored with Mary Adelaide Nutting, is the classic text on nursing history.

Mary Adelaide Nutting (1858–1947) graduated from the first class of the Johns Hopkins School of Nursing. She founded the first college-level department of nursing at Columbia University Teacher's College and was instrumental in raising the standards of nursing education. She wrote the four-volume *History of Nursing* with Lavinia Dock.

Isabel Hampton Robb (1860–1910) advocated nurses' rights, a 3-year training program, 8-hour instead of 12-hour workdays, and licensure to protect patients.

Lillian Wald (1867–1940) opened public health nursing in the United States when she founded the Henry Street Settlement in 1893 to provide free nursing care for the poor on the Lower East Side of New York City.

Annie W. Goodrich (1876–1955) was a strong-willed advocate of nursing training and the need to raise nursing to professional status. When World War I created the need for more nurses, she wrote plans for the Army School of Nursing.

Clara Maass (1876–1901) was a former volunteer contract nurse with the U.S. Army. She gave her life in an experiment to discover the cause of yellow fever. As a test subject, she was infected twice by mosquito bites and died at 25 years of age.

As the need for nurses, appropriate training, and better standards grew through the years, the American nursing community produced dedicated members to meet each demand. The number of nurses has risen during times of national emergency and war. In less critical times, the number has fallen. But there is always a need for well-trained, qualified nurses in good times and bad.

Before the 1870s and the foundation of professional nursing schools, nursing in America was done by women who learned by experience rather than by formal education. The nursing schools that opened in the last quarter of the nineteenth century changed that. Professional nurses have been educated in formal programs ever since.

THE DEVELOPMENT OF
PRACTICAL/VOCATIONAL NURSING

Practical nursing education has had a similar history, although formal education programs came somewhat later. The Industrial Revolution of the mid-1800s began a population shift from rural to urban areas of the United States. Many of the people who left the farm for the city were untrained and very often were also uneducated. The young women who arrived in the cities were particularly disadvantaged because there were few job opportunities for them. Men could find work in factories, but women were limited to domestic service.

Emergence of Practical Nursing Schools

To train women so that they could increase their opportunity to compete for jobs, the Young Women's Christian Association (YWCA), a church-affiliated organization that originated in Europe, gave classes in cooking and domestic chores. It is likely that simple home nursing skills and child care instruction were included.

In 1892, a formal 3-month YWCA course in practical nursing was offered for the first time in the United States in Brooklyn, New York. Its objective was to teach practical nurses how to care for children, invalids, and the elderly. Practical nurses were often in demand to fill nursing shortages. The Ballard School, named for its sponsor, Lucinda Ballard, opened in 1897 in response to the need for another school to train practical nurses.

Fifteen years later, in 1907, the Thompson School in Brattleboro, Vermont, was opened. In 1918, the Household Nursing Association School of Attendant Nursing was founded in Boston. The objective of these schools' programs was to train practical nurses in home nursing skills. The training emphasized cooking, cleaning, and other household duties. Some early practical nursing programs also provided hospital experience. If the program was affiliated with a hospital, it paid its students for their services.

By 1930, there were 11 schools of practical nursing in the country. Between 1930 and 1947, 25 more schools were opened. Probably as a result of World War II and the serious shortage of registered nurses, 260 more schools were opened between 1948 and 1954.

Rise of National Organizations

There were few controls, little educational planning, and minimum supervision of practical nursing schools before 1940. Standards were nonexistent and the programs varied widely. It was only after state agencies that were subject to legislation took over that controls were established. Although Mississippi offered licensing for practical nurses in 1914, it was not until 1938 that New York passed the first mandatory practical nurse licensing law. The Minneapolis Girls' Vocational High School offered the first high school vocational practical nurse program in 1919. It was not until 1941 that a national association for practical nursing was formed.

The Association of Practical Nurse Schools was organized in Chicago in 1941 to address the needs of practical nursing education. Hilda M. Torrop, director of

BOX 3-1. HISTORY OF PRACTICAL NURSING

1892	YWCA opened a 3-month training program for practical nurses in Brooklyn, New York.
1897	Ballard School for practical nursing education was opened in New York. Funding was provided by Lucinda Ballard.
1907	Thompson School for practical nurses was opened in Brattleboro, Vermont.
1914	Mississippi passed the first law that provided practical nurses the option to be licensed.
1918	Household Association School of Attendant Nursing was opened in Boston.
1918	National League for Nursing Education was founded.
1938	New York was the only state to mandate the licensure of practical nurses.
1940	Six states had passed laws that provided practical nurses the option to be licensed.
1941	Association of Practical Nursing Schools (later known as the National Association for Practical Nurse Education and Service [NAPNES]) was founded.
1944	U.S. Department of Education, Division of Vocational Education studied and made a number of recommendations that resulted in a significant increase in the number of practical nursing programs.
1949	National Federation for Licensed Practical Nurses (NFLPN) was organized by Lillian Kuster.
1950	The National League for Nursing was created by combining the National League for Nursing Education, the National Organization of Public Health Nurses, and the Association of Collegiate School of Nursing.
1951	The *Journal of Practical Nursing* was first published by NAPNES.
1955	All states had licensure laws for practical nurses.
1957	The National League for Nursing established a Council of Practical Nursing Programs.
1961	The National League for Nursing began offering accrediting services for practical nursing schools.
1965	The American Nurse's Association issued a position paper on nursing education. The ANA position was that professional nurses should be educated in colleges and universities and that technical nurses should be prepared in junior colleges. The ANA position proposed that practical nurse be replaced by the technical nurse. The ANA's position remains unchanged.
1965	Controversy surrounding the education of professional nurses and the role of the practical nurse began in earnest in 1965 and continues to be discussed by nursing organizations, non-nursing healthcare organizations, judical bodies, state boards of nursing, healthcare providers, and individual nurses.
1979	NLN published the first edition of a document listing the competencies of graduates of practical/vocational nursing programs.

(continued)

BOX 3-1. HISTORY OF PRACTICAL NURSING (Continued)

1984	NAPNES discontinued providing accrediting services for practical/vocational nursing schools.
1989	The American Medical Association (AMA) proposed a 9-month training program for a Registered Care Technologist (RCT). This "new" worker would perform many professional and practical nurse functions. Opposition from the nursing community prevented the implementation of this training program.
Early 1990s	The nursing shortage decreased and the job market for all nurses declined.
1994	April—The first computerized adaptive test (NCLEX-PN) for license nurses was administered.
1995	Economic pressures on hospitals changed the locus of care from hospitals to the community and the home. Hospitals implemented staffing patterns that reduced the number of full time employees and the nurse/patient ratio.
1996	The National Council of State Boards of Nursing, along with the National Association for Practical Nurse Education and Service, began offering a certification examination for licensed practical/vocational nurses in long-term care.

the Ballard School; Etta Creech, director of the Family Health Association in Cleveland; and Katherine Shephard, executive director of the Household Nursing Association in Boston, were the association's officers. Its name was changed to the National Association of Practical Nurse Education (NAPNE) in 1942 when membership was opened to practical nurses.

A service for accrediting practical nursing schools was begun by the Association in 1945 and was ended in 1984. In 1959, NAPNE organized a summer school and workshops for directors and instructors of practical nursing programs. Its journal, the first one for practical nursing and now called *The Journal of Practical Nursing,* was first published in 1951.

The Association changed its name in 1959 to the National Association for Practical Nurse Education and Service (NAPNES). By then it was sponsoring summer courses at colleges and universities, was emphasizing continuing education for practical nurses, and had established a Department of Education and a Department of Service for State Practical Nursing Associations. Membership in NAPNES is open to anyone who is interested in promoting the interests, concerns, and occupation of practical nursing.

In 1949, Lillian Kuster organized and became executive director of the National Federation of Licensed Practical Nurses (NFLPN), the official membership organization for practical and vocational nurses. Membership in NFLPN is limited to licensed or student practical/vocational nurses.

These two organizations, NAPNES and NFLPN, set standards for practical/vocational nursing practice; generally promote and protect the interests of practical/vocational nurses; and educate and inform the general public about practical/vocational nursing.

DISCUSSION QUESTIONS/LEARNING ACTIVITIES

1. Discuss how the changing role and status of women may have influenced the development of nursing.

2. Identify some of the personal characteristics of the nurses who made important contributions to nursing between 1820 and 1920.

3. Use library resources to explore in detail the contributions of a particular nurse.

4. Write to NAPNES and NFLPN to obtain information on membership in these organizations.

5. Compare early practical nursing journal articles with articles in current journals. Try to identify changes in the articles in these journals that reflect changes in practical nursing.

READ MORE ABOUT IT

Dietz LD, Lehozky AR: History and Modern Nursing, Second Edition. Philadelphia: FA Davis, 1993.

Dock LA, Nutting MA: History of Nursing, Four Volumes. New York: GP Putnam's Sons, 1907 and 1912.

Dock LL, Stewart IM: A Short History of Nursing, Third Edition. New York: GP Putnam's Sons, 1938.

Dolan JA, et al: Nursing in Society: A Historical Perspective, Fifteenth Edition. Philadelphia: WB Saunders, 1983.

Donahue MP: Nursing: The Finest Art: An Illustrated History, Second Edition. St. Louis: Mosby, 1995.

Ellis JR, Hartley CL: Nursing in Today's World: Challenges, Issues, and Trends, Fifth Edition. Philadelphia: JB Lippincott, 1995.

Fitzpatrick ML: Prologue to Professionalism, First Edition. East Norwalk: Appleton & Lange, 1983.

James J, Reverby S (eds.): A Lavinia Dock Reader. New York: Garland, 1985.

Kalisch BJ, Kalisch PA: The Advance of American Nursing, Third Edition. Philadelphia: JB Lippincott, 1995.

Lynaugh J: Nursing History Review: Official Journal of the American Association for the History of Nursing, Volume 4. Philadelphia: University of Pennsylvania Press, 1996.

Nightingale F: Notes on Nursing: What It Is and What It Is Not, Replica Edition. Philadelphia: JB Lippincott, 1946. (Originally published in 1859.)

Education for Nursing

4

OBJECTIVES

When you complete this chapter, you should be able to:

Explain the difference between professional and nonprofessional in terms of education.

Describe the educational preparation for registered nurses.

Describe the educational preparation for practical/vocational nurses.

Describe the educational preparation for certified nursing assistants.

List at least three types of institutions that can sponsor practical/vocational nursing programs.

Explain the difference between the terms "program approval" and "program accreditation."

Explain the purpose of student organizations.

(continued)

Paraphrase the major points of either the NFLPN or the NAPNES Standards for Practical/Vocational Nurses.

Describe the procedure for obtaining a license as a practical/vocational nurse.

List some of the reasons why a nursing license can be suspended or revoked.

> It was Rose's first visit to her high school since her graduation a few years earlier. She breathed deeply as she opened the door of the red brick building. The familiar smells of oiled wood floors and pine cleaner assaulted her nostrils. The long rows of lockers still lined the hallway. Even the paint on the walls was the same color. Nothing had changed.
>
> Suddenly the hall was filled with girls and boys rushing to their classes. She watched them hurry by. Then the metallic clang of a bell sounded and, as if by magic, the long hall became deserted. Rose walked slowly down the hall. She knew exactly where she was going. "Locker 213," she said aloud. There was her old locker, nestled against the wall in a line of others that had seemed a mile long when she used to run to it between bells.
>
> "Rose?"
>
> A woman in a nurse's uniform threw her arms around Rose. "Terri!" laughed Rose. She hugged the woman tightly. They had been classmates in this very school.
>
> "Come to my office," Terri said, "so we can talk."
>
> Rose looked around the tidy office. A student lay on a cot with a thermometer in her mouth. A boy was weighing himself on a scale in the corner. A nurse was talking to the boy. Rose turned to Terri. "Remember how I wanted to be a nurse when we were in school?" she said. "Now it's too late. I've got two kids..." Terri smiled. "So do I," she said. "and I've been a nurse for only 2 years. I went back to school 3 years ago and..." Rose rubbed her eyes. "It only takes 1 year to be a nurse?" she asked.
>
> "One year of hard work," Terri said. "I'm a licensed practical nurse," she added proudly. "And you can be, too, if you really want to be."
>
> "I do!" Rose said excitedly. "But how? Tell me all about it."

It would take more than a short meeting in a busy nurse's schedule to describe practical/vocational nursing today. The vocation has come a long way since the first school of practical nursing in the United States opened in 1892. The YWCA program at the Ballard School in New York was a mere 3-month course.

Other programs to educate nonprofessional nurses and nurse's assistants, such as those developed to train Red Cross nurse's aides in World Wars I and II, were also short. For example, the World War II program consisted of only 35 hours of lecture and 45 hours of supervised clinical experience.

It was already clear that there was a permanent place for practical nurses in American healthcare. A number of schools were in operation, but before 1940 they operated with minimal educational planning and supervision. With the establishment of a practical nurse association, the National Association of Practical Nurse Education (NAPNE), now known as the National Association for Practical Nurse Education and Service, Inc. (NAPNES), in the 1940s to regulate education and practice, programs for training nonprofessional nurses became more nearly uniform. Laws for certification and licensure were also established, so that today, virtually every program in every state is governed by regulating agencies.

DEFINING "PROFESSIONAL" AND "NONPROFESSIONAL"

The term *professional* generally implies someone who is competent and qualified to perform a specific occupation. Examples are a professional electrician, a professional secretary, and a professional painter. In this context, professional refers to someone who is an expert in his or her occupation. When someone refers to a person as "a real professional," it means that the person approaches the occupation with seriousness, has a high level of integrity, and can be trusted to maintain high personal standards when performing that occupation.

When the term professional is used in education, it has a somewhat different meaning. A professional education requires a minimum of 4 years of college; more often, a total of 6 or 8 years of formal study beyond high school is required. A person who studies theory and the application of theory in a specific occupation; subscribes to an occupational code of ethics; participates in the development of the occupation through organizational activities and research; and works independently of others is a professional.

The term *nonprofessional,* therefore, refers only to a nurse's educational preparation. All nurses should approach their responsibilities with a professional attitude. That is, any nurse, regardless of educational preparation, should be serious about the occupation, have a high level of integrity, be trustworthy, and maintain high standards.

TYPES OF NURSING PROGRAMS

Four-Year Professional Nursing Programs

A professional nurse is one who has completed at least 4 years of college and has passed the registered nurse licensure examination. He or she has studied nursing theory and its application to practice; performs responsibilities according to a strict code of ethics; and participates in the development of nursing through membership in nursing organizations. In addition, the professional nurse engages in nursing research and often works independently, without direct supervision. Many registered nurses who have completed a professional nursing education program have advanced to positions of leadership in nursing education and nursing service.

Two-Year Associate Degree Programs

The nurse who prepares for the occupation of nursing in 2 years and passes the registered nurse licensure examination is sometimes called an associate-degree or a technical nurse. These 2-year programs are sponsored by community, technical, and junior colleges. The development of 2-year nursing programs has grown rapidly since the first programs were established by Mildred Montag in 1952.

Diploma Nursing Programs

Nursing education programs sponsored by hospitals are called diploma nursing programs. These programs vary in length from 2 to 3 years. Graduates of these programs who pass the registered nurse licensure examination are sometimes called diploma nurses. The programs of study vary greatly; however, the emphasis is on developing skills in clinical nursing practice. Many diploma programs are affiliated with colleges and universities so that students in these programs also have 40 to 80 college credits upon graduation.

Practical/Vocational Nursing Programs

A practical/vocational nurse is prepared for this occupation in approximately 1 year. The emphasis in practical/vocational nursing education is on learning basic nursing skills that can be applied to patients in a variety of healthcare settings. The practical/vocational nurse, in most healthcare situations, functions under the supervision and direction of a registered nurse.

Most adult programs are between 10 and 18 months in length. Practical/vocational nursing programs are classified as adult practical/vocational nursing programs if the program is for adults and is not part of a high school curriculum. Secondary school practical/vocational nursing programs are those offered to high school students. Extended high school programs require additional classes after high school graduation. In 1994, there were 1094 adult, 35 secondary school, and 66 high school extended practical/vocational nursing programs in the United States.

A number of sponsoring institutions administer practical/vocational nursing programs. In 1994, the percent of programs by sponsoring institutions were as follows:

Technical/vocational schools: 49.7%
Junior/community colleges: 38.5%
Secondary schools: 6.2%
Hospitals: 3.7%
Government agencies: 0.5%
Senior colleges and universities: 0.9%
Independent agencies: 0.5%

Certified Nursing Assistants

On December 22, 1987, the federal government passed the Omnibus Budget Reconciliation Act (OBRA). This act required states to establish specific educational programs for nurse aides working in Medicare funded long-term care facilities and for Homemaker-Home Health Aides.

In addition to the OBRA mandated minimum 75-hour training program, each state was required to develop a mechanism for measuring competency. To do this, most states require that those nurse aides who have completed an approved course of study also pass a written and practical examination. The names of those who successfully pass the written and practical examination are placed on the state Nurse Aide Registry. To remain on the registry, each nurse aide must document completion of a minimum of 12 hours of continuing education each year.

Educational programs for nurse aides are offered by long-term care facilities, hospitals, vocational schools, community colleges, and private and governmental agencies.

A nurse aide whose name appears on a state registry can request to be placed on the registry in another state. Provided the original educational program, competency evaluation procedures, and work history meets the state requirements, the nurse aide requesting permission to work in a different state may be exempt from additional educational and testing requirements.

Depending on individual state laws, professional and practical/vocational nursing students who have completed specific course work may be eligible to apply for placement on the nurse aide registry. Professional and practical/vocational nursing students often find that working part time as a nurse aide is an excellent way to earn valuable experience in nursing as well as supplemental income while in school.

Nursing Education Statistics

The latest figures from the U.S. Department of Labor (Bulletin 2450, 1992) reported that LP/VNs held about 659,000 jobs, of which 25% were part-time positions.

The following figures compiled by the National League for Nursing indicate that more men graduated from basic registered nursing programs in 1995 than in the previous 15 years. While the number of admissions to practical/vocational

Basic RN Programs	1979–80	1989–90	1993–94	1994–95
Number of programs	1,385	1,470	1,493	1,501
Admissions	105,952	108,580	126,837	129,897
Graduations	75,523	66,088	88,149	94,870
	1981	**1991**	**1993**	**1994**
Men Admitted	7.3%	10.7%	11.1%	11.1%
Men Graduated	5.8%	8.4%	8.9%	9.6%
Basic P/VN Programs	**1979–80**	**1989–90**	**1993–94**	**1994–95**
Number of programs	1,299	1,154	1,159	1,084
Admissions	56,316	52,969	60,749	60,632
Graduations	41,892	35,417	44,822	45,083
	1981	**1991**	**1993**	**1994**
Men Admitted	4.4%	9.7%	8.2%	11.0%
Men Graduated	4.6%	9.4%	6.8%	8.5%

Source: National League for Nursing, Division of Research. Published and unpublished data, 1995.

nursing programs has remained fairly steady over the past 2 years, admission to basic RN programs has increased slightly.

PRACTICAL/VOCATIONAL NURSING EDUCATION

The philosophy, objectives, and curriculum of a practical/vocational nursing program are developed by the faculty. This basic framework of your educational program is periodically reviewed, evaluated, and revised by the faculty to ensure a program of instruction that will prepare you for your first position as a practical/vocational nurse.

Since most changes in philosophy, objectives, and curriculum proposed by the faculty of a practical/vocational nursing program must first be approved by the state board of nursing, it is important to understand the approval and accreditation process.

Approval and Accreditation

Each state has a board of nursing composed of nurses, consumers, and others interested in healthcare. It is this organization that is responsible for nursing services to citizens within its jurisdiction. As part of their responsibility for safeguarding the well-being of their constituents, the various state boards of nursing evaluate and approve nursing education programs within their state. Schools or organizations offering nursing programs must have the approval of the state board of nursing to operate nursing education programs. Part of the approval process includes specific regulations governing the length (in hours) of nursing education programs. Graduation from a state-approved school of practical/vocational nursing is one of the prerequisites for taking the practical/vocational nursing licensing examination.

In addition to mandatory approval by the state board of nursing, many schools voluntarily seek accreditation from the National League for Nursing (NLN). The key words *approval* and *accreditation* are essential to understanding the difference between the purpose of the state board of nursing and the purpose of the NLN. Approval by the state board of nursing is mandatory; accreditation by the NLN is voluntary.

Accreditation of a program by the NLN is often an indication that a particular nursing education program exceeds minimum requirements for conducting a program. This does not imply, however, that programs not accredited by the NLN do not exceed minimum standards established by a state board of nursing. Since the accreditation process is voluntary, some schools, for their own unique reasons, do not seek NLN accreditation. The nonaccredited program may exceed minimum standards by far, and it may offer an outstanding education program. One must be careful when using the term "approval," which is required, and the term "accreditation," which is voluntary, when discussing the quality of a nursing education program.

Your school may be scheduled for a program review by the state board of nursing or the NLN during the time you are enrolled. Having an approval or accreditation visit is an important process and one in which your participation will be expected.

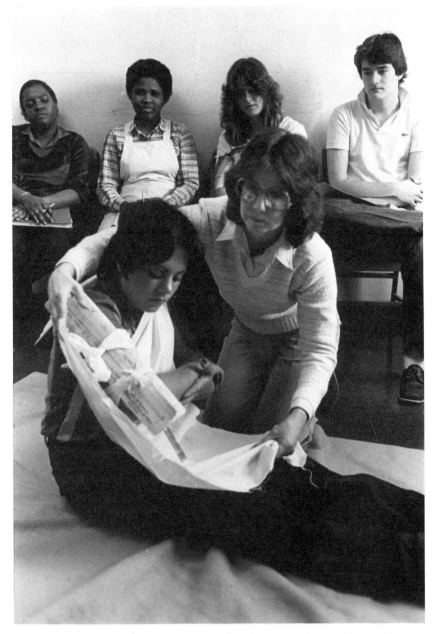

Classroom demonstrations prepare you for clinical practice. (© Richard Wood, Taurus Photos.)

Program Curriculum and Objectives

Generally, the early practical/vocational nursing programs were combined courses of theoretical (classroom) and clinical (institution) instruction that took approximately 2000 hours or 1 year to complete. The classroom phase took about one third of that time and consisted of lecture and laboratory classes. The remainder of the course was given to the clinical phase, with supervised experience in approved hospitals and institutions, in combination with some home care nursing experience.

It is no longer believed that classroom instruction, followed by clinical instruction, is educationally sound. The trend today is to relate classroom theory, laboratory practice, and clinical experience by offering integrated sections over the length of the entire program. However, there is considerable variety in the actual organization of individual programs around the country in this regard, just as there is in the specific courses that are offered.

A typical program starts in the fall (or first semester) with an introduction to basic nursing. Subjects covered through the year include fundamentals of nursing, communication skills, anatomy and physiology, nutrition, mental health, microbiology, maternity nursing, medical and surgical nursing of adults and children, diet therapy, pharmacology, and geriatrics. Elective courses in the humanities and the behavioral sciences may also be offered.

On successful completion of a practical/vocational nursing course, a graduate should have the following:

1. The education and experience needed to qualify for and pass the licensing exam in practical/vocational nursing.
2. The knowledge and skills to perform entry level tasks under appropriate supervision.
3. The knowledge and skills to help to meet a patient's physical, emotional, social, and spiritual needs.
4. Up-to-date information about health and disease prevention to teach to the community.
5. Familiarity with social, medical, health, and technological change.
6. Awareness of local and national nursing associations and what they do.
7. A desire to continue the process of learning and growing in the field.

ORGANIZATIONS

Organizations are groups organized for a specific purpose. You can probably think of many examples of organizations that were formed for a specific purpose.

Organizations require bylaws and procedural rules (rules of order) if their stated purpose is to be met. Meetings also follow established procedures or run the risk of accomplishing nothing. Meetings generally follow recognized rules of order, the most familiar being Robert's Rules of Order. These rules define the duties and responsibilities of the officers and organize discussion, vote taking, and other procedures. Minutes, which are detailed notes of the business conducted in a meeting, become a permanent record of an organization's meetings.

Two types of organizations are important to you as a nursing student: student organizations and nursing organizations. Nursing organizations will be discussed in Chapter 14.

Student Organizations

Your nursing program may be an integral part of a larger institution, or it may be small and independent. The type, complexity, and size of its student government will reflect the nature of its affiliation. A program that is a part of a college, for example, must take into account the regulations that apply to living on campus, whereas a vocational school program with only day students does not. The bylaws of the student governments of each will be either complex or simple, according to the needs and purposes of the group.

A student council is the most common form of student organization. It is a group made up of student and faculty members who serve as representatives of the student body to the sponsoring organization. Student members are elected by the student body. A faculty member elected by the student body serves as adviser to the student council.

The student council's function is to make recommendations to the sponsoring organization on matters affecting students. Such matters include the rules that govern students; their social, recreational, and extracurricular activities; and student discipline. The council also serves as a disciplinary board for infractions of school regulations. The precise manner in which each council operates is set by its bylaws. Secure a copy of your student council's bylaws and read them because they relate directly to your student life.

Involvement with your student council or government is an opportunity for you to have a voice in the daily affairs of your education and a chance to learn and exercise leadership skills. Involvement does not mean that you must be on the council. It means participating as an active, interested member of a student body with a common goal. It can also mean volunteering to be on special committees.

Practical/vocational nursing students in programs sponsored by larger organizations may have an opportunity to join other student organizations. These other organizations may emphasize politics, photography, journalism, or drama, to name a few possibilities.

One student organization of interest to practical/vocational nursing students is Health Occupations Students of America (HOSA). HOSA is a national organization with state affiliations and local chapters in secondary and postsecondary schools that offer courses in the field of healthcare and related services.

The purpose of this organization, which held its constitutional convention in 1976, is to assist students in developing vocational understanding, an awareness of social intelligence, civic consciousness, and leadership skills. HOSA chapter members participate in local, state, and national competitions in health-related areas.

If your school does not have a HOSA chapter, you might want to ask your faculty to consider sponsoring this worthwhile activity. Details on how to begin your own chapter are available from the national HOSA office (see Appendix D for the address).

Alumni Associations

If your program or school has an alumni (graduates) association, you and your classmates will have the opportunity to join other graduates of your program or school after graduation. By becoming active, you can keep in touch with one another and with the activities, programs, and progress of the school. Your experience will become valuable to those who follow you, just as the suggestions and help of those who have gone before you have been of benefit to your education.

Keeping in touch with your school and classmates can also provide you with networking opportunities and access to continuing education programs, job opportunities, information on advances and changes in practical/vocational nursing, and other developments of special interest to you.

STANDARDS FOR THE LICENSED PRACTICAL/VOCATIONAL NURSE

Three national organizations are primarily concerned with the practice of practical nursing. Membership in the National Federation of Licensed Practical Nurses (NFLPN) is only open to licensed and student practical/vocational nurses. NAP-NES accepts for membership anyone interested in promoting the practice of practical/vocational nursing. The American Licensed Practical Nurses Association (ALPNA) represents the interests of licensed practical/vocational nurses through lobbying and legislative activities. Membership in this organization is open to anyone interested in promoting the practice of practical/vocational nurses. Both NFLPN and NAPNES have issued statements defining the standard of nursing that the public can expect from a LP/VN.

In 1970, the NFLPN approved the "Statement of Functions and Qualifications of the Licensed Practical Nurse," which was written to help clarify the responsibilities of an LP/VN. It was revised in 1972 and again in 1979. In 1987, that statement was replaced by a new statement titled "Nursing Practice Standards for the Licensed Practical/Vocational Nurse."

The most recently revised NFLPN statement defining LP/VN nursing practice standards was published in 1991. This document basically outlines the standards of performance expected of LP/VNs in the areas of education, legal and ethical status, practice, continuing education, and specialized nursing practice. The full text of this statement is in Appendix E.

NAPNES has set the standards for nursing practice of LP/VNs since 1941. The most recently revised "Standards of Practice for Licensed Practical/Vocational Nurses" was issued in 1992. The full text of the NAPNES Standards is in Appendix F. The NAPNES Standards outline the competencies expected of the LP/VN in individual and family-centered nursing care. These Standards also discuss the moral, ethical, and legal components of practical/vocational nursing.

JOB RESPONSIBILITIES

The broad objective of an LP/VN education is to prepare the student to become legally qualified to work under the supervision of a medical or osteopathic doctor, registered nurse, or dentist as a responsible member of a healthcare team, performing basic therapeutic, rehabilitative, and preventive care for anyone who needs it.

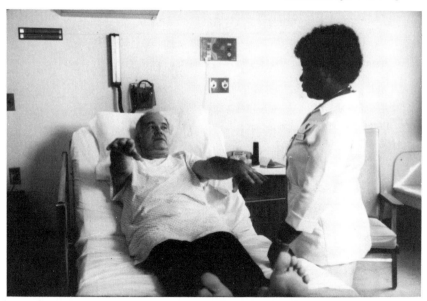

Range of motion exercises are some of the skills routinely performed by LP/VNs.

On successful completion of an LP/VN program, the new graduate is expected to be competent in a number of general areas. These competencies define the minimum expectations for graduates and were first outlined in competency statements developed by the NLN in 1979. The most recent NLN *Entry Level Competencies of Graduates of Educational Programs in Practical Nursing* are reprinted in Appendix G. Each state has additional nurse practice acts or administrative rules that further define an LP/VN's role and function in that state. In addition, some state associations of education are also defining entry-level competencies.

The range of specific nursing services provided by practical nurses is extensive and continues to grow as the increasing sophistication and specialization of healthcare keeps up with discoveries in science and technology and the needs of an ever-changing population.

An LP/VN's job responsibilities are also set by the employer and the charge nurse or physician for whom the LP/VN works. The responsibilities may change according to institution policies regarding the LP/VN's role at different patient illness levels. What an LP/VN can do for a patient may be restricted if the patient's condition worsens. The skills an LP/VN may be expected to perform are listed in Table 4-1.

LICENSURE QUALIFICATIONS

One of the major goals of your practical/vocational nursing program is to prepare you to pass the licensing examination. This examination measures your knowledge of nursing practice in a number of areas and requires that you retain information

TABLE 4-1 **Beginning LP/VN Skill Inventory**

Admit patients

Assist in transferring and discharging patients

Help patients with bathing

Help patients ambulate

Assist adults, children, and infants with meals

Perform range-of-motion exercises

Maintain traction

Assist in positioning patients in bed

Care for dying patients and their families

Provide skin care

Care for ostomy sites

Give enemas

Perform urinary catheterizations

Monitor oxygen therapy

Supervise coughing and deep breathing exercises

Teach and supervise postural drainage

Perform nasopharyngeal and endotracheal suctioning

Obtain specimens

Perform cardiopulmonary resuscitation

Administer compresses, sitz baths, and therapeutic baths

Measure temperature, pulse, respiration, blood pressure

Administer oral and intramuscular injections

Provide preoperative and postoperative care

Administer medications

Care for patients with infectious diseases

Assist patients in elimination needs

Assess neurological status

Document nursing care on patients' records

Contribute to patient care conferences and nursing care plans

Check emergency equipment and supplies

Initiate, administer, and monitor intravenous therapy

Administer skin tests

Collect venous blood samples

Use the nursing process to administer care

you were taught during your entire educational program. Many graduates spend some time reviewing their textbooks and notes before taking the licensing examination. Even though the examination can be taken more than once, you and your faculty expect that you will pass the licensure examination on your first attempt.

The *Test Plan for the National Council Licensure Examination for Practical Nurses* is a publication developed by the National Council of State Boards of Nursing (NCSBN) to assist student practical/vocational nurses in preparing for the examination. This publication is probably available in your school library, or you can obtain a copy for a fee by writing to the NCSBN. The address can be found in Appendix D under "Other Nursing Organizations."

The laws governing who qualifies to be licensed as a practical/vocational nurse are set by each state, but the trend is toward uniformity in all states. Most states require that an applicant be a graduate of a state-approved practical/vocational nursing program. The director of the school of practical/vocational nursing is required to sign an application for licensure for each graduate who has met all of the objectives of the school's program. The director's signature on the application indicates to the state board of nursing that the candidate for licensure has met the theoretical and clinical requirements of that school and is considered to be ready to enter the practice of practical/vocational nursing. State boards of nursing charge a licensure application fee that in most cases must be paid by the applicant.

Originally, each state had its own licensing exam. Today, however, there is one licensing examination for practical/vocational nurses in all states. This examination is developed by the NCSBN and is called the National Council Licensure Examination for Practical Nurses (NCLEX-PN). An overview of the NCLEX-PN Test Plan is in Appendix H.

Before April 1994, the NCLEX-PN written examination was given in April and October. Since April 1, 1994, the NCLEX examination for licensure as a registered nurse or a practical/vocational nurse is administered by computer at a local test center. There is a scheduling fee for the NCLEX examination and this fee is usually paid by the applicant. First-time applicants must be scheduled for the NCLEX-PN test within 30 days from when they call to schedule it. Repeat applicants must be scheduled for the NCLEX-PN exam within 45 days from when they call to schedule it.

The NCLEX-PN examination, using computerized adaptive testing technology, provides a fair, efficient way to test candidates. Computerized adaptive testing examinations are individualized so that each examinee takes a "customized" test. The maximum number of questions on the NCLEX-PN examination is 205 questions. Examinees may need to answer fewer than 205 questions to either pass or fail. The reason for this is that when an examinee answers a question correctly, the next question is slightly more difficult. If the more difficult question is answered correctly, the examinee gets a slightly more difficult question. If this question is answered incorrectly, the examinee gets a less difficult question. This process continues until, using statistical analysis, each examinee reaches a point in the examination where the competency level on answered questions indicates that the candidate has either passed or failed the NCLEX-PN examination. Candidates who are not successful on their first attempt to pass the NCLEX-PN examination must wait 91 days before being permitted to take the examination again.

The testing agency provides the state board of nursing with a list of people who have passed or failed the NCLEX-PN examination. The state board of nursing then determines who will be issued a license as a practical/vocational nurse. In general, state boards of nursing will not issue a nursing license to a person who has been convicted of certain crimes, a person who is mentally ill, or a person who is addicted to drugs or alcohol. Nurses who are issued licenses in California and Texas are known as licensed vocational nurses; all others are known as licensed practical nurses.

Licenses are issued for a period determined by the issuing authority. A license must be kept current. It is a violation of the nurse practice act or administrative rules to continue to practice after a license has expired or been revoked. Some states require licensees to provide proof of acceptable continuing education before a license can be renewed.

State boards of nursing have the authority to issue licenses and the right to revoke or suspend them for a variety of reasons. This authority protects patients and nurses alike by eliminating those who are incompetent or unfit for practice. The standing of practical/vocational nurses is upheld when all members of the group have the same high standards.

LICENSING

A license to practice as a licensed practical/vocational nurse is issued by the state in which the nurse practices nursing. The license gives legal authorization to perform (permission to practice) the skills learned in a practical/vocational nursing program. A license is valid for the life of the person it is issued to unless it is revoked or suspended. A nursing license must be renewed periodically (usually every 2 or 3 years) as required by that state's regulations.

Like all licensed persons who serve the public, practical/vocational nursing is governed by laws that protect those providing service, as well as the safety and welfare of the people being served. Laws that govern nursing are called *nurse practice acts* or *administrative rules*. The nurse practice acts or administrative rules of each state are administered by boards called by various names, such as board of nursing, board of nurse examiners, or nurse registration board. There are 62 boards of nursing in the 50 states, the District of Columbia, and the five U.S. territories. The six states that have separate RN and PN/VN boards are California, Georgia, Louisiana, Texas, Washington, and West Virginia. The five U.S. territories are the Virgin Islands, Puerto Rico, American Samoa, Guam, and the Northern Mariana Islands.

Board members include experienced nurses as well as consumers. The primary way to become a board member is to be appointed by an elected official, an elected body, or both. For example, the governor appoints members of 32 boards. The governor, with the confirmation of the Senate, appoints the members of 19 boards. The board members of the District of Columbia Board are appointed by the mayor, while those in North Carolina are elected by the public in general elections. The number of members on each board varies from 5 in the Northern Mariana Islands to 25 in New York. The average number of board members is ten.

These boards of nursing operate under their own state laws but cooperate with one another and belong to the NCSBN. This organization develops the licensure examinations. State boards of nursing are authorized to perform certain duties. Some of these duties include nursing program curricula and standards development; approval of nursing schools; issuing, renewing, and endorsing licenses; and disciplinary actions, such as license suspension or revocation. Anyone found in violation of the state's nurse practice act is subject to investigation and prosecution by the state board.

Legal Title

The legal title granted when a person successfully passes the licensing examination is either licensed practical nurse (LPN) or, in California and Texas, licensed vocational nurse (LVN). A license entitles the holder to enter the practice of practical/vocational nursing as described by the state. Persons holding a license have demonstrated to the issuing authority (state board) that they have the knowledge and ability to provide the minimal safe practices required to fulfill the duties of a practical or vocational nurse in that state.

A license belongs only to the person it is issued to. It cannot be transferred to anyone else for any reason. The unqualified use of a license is subject to legal prosecution. Reporting anyone known to be practicing without a license preserves the integrity of the license and the licensing procedure; protects the investment of the license holder; and guards unknowing consumers from potentially dangerous care. Forty-nine boards of nursing mandate reporting of nurse practice act/administrative rules violations.

All states require practical/vocational nurses to be licensed before they can practice. Called *mandatory licensing*, it helps to keep unqualified persons out of the healthcare system. Mandatory licensing protects the public from untrained people and upholds nursing standards set by law and nursing organizations.

Licensure by Endorsement

LP/VNs must be licensed by the state in which they practice. Nurses who move to or want to work in a state in which they are not licensed must apply for licensure in that state. In most cases, this process must be completed before the nurse can work in that state. You can obtain the information you need on how to apply for licensure in another state by writing to the state board of nursing in the state in which you want to work. See Appendix D for a list of addresses of state boards of nursing.

Disciplinary Sanctions

State boards of nursing, through nursing practice acts, have the authority to suspend or revoke nursing licenses for just cause. A nursing license can be revoked or suspended when the board of nursing finds a licensee guilty of an offense. Examples of offenses include:

1. Mental incompetence.
2. Conviction of a felony.
3. Guilty of fraud or deceit in obtaining a license.
4. Conviction of a crime involving moral turpitude or gross immorality.
5. Guilty of willful neglect of a patient.
6. Unfit by reason of negligence.
7. Habitual use and/or chemical dependence on drugs or alcohol.
8. Violations of the nurse practice laws of the state.
9. Suspended or revoked license in another state.

A nurse whose right to practice is being questioned must first be notified of the charges by the state board and must be given a hearing in which to enter a defense, either in person or through an attorney, before a license can be revoked or suspended.

In addition to revoking and suspending practical/vocational nursing licenses, the state board of nursing can also, for just cause, issue letters of reprimand, refuse to issue a license, refuse to renew a license, or place a licensee on probation.

Your license to practice practical/vocational nursing is a valuable document. Always conduct yourself in a manner consistent with the standards and ethics of your profession; this will assure you of a long and rewarding career as a licensed practical/vocational nurse.

DISCUSSION QUESTIONS/LEARNING ACTIVITIES

1. What is the name of the agency that approves your practical/vocational nursing program?

2. Write to your state board of nursing and request a copy of the laws governing the practice of practical/vocational nursing. When you receive your copy, read it carefully.

3. Review the bylaws of your student organization if you have one. Do they clearly state the purpose of the organization and its rules of operation? Should the bylaws be revised?

4. Discuss with your classmates how the Standards published by the NFLPN or NAPNES may affect your nursing practice.

5. How do you think you might handle a situation in which you are asked to perform nursing skills you are not legally permitted to do?

6. How might you handle a situation in which you observe a nurse (either a registered nurse or a licensed practical/vocational nurse) working while obviously chemically impaired? Does your state board of nursing offer anonymous reporting of impaired nurses?

7. You have read in the local newspaper that a nurse has been convicted of child abuse. Do you inform the state board of nursing? Give the reasons for your answer.

READ MORE ABOUT IT

American Nurses Association: Facts About Nursing, 43rd Edition Revised. Washington, DC: American Nurses Publishing, 1996.

Ellis JR, Hartley CL: Nursing in Today's World: Challenges, Issues, and Trends, Fifth Edition. Philadelphia: JB Lippincott, 1995.

Harrington N, et al: LPN to RN Transitions, First Edition. Philadelphia: JB Lippincott, 1995.

Kalisch PA, Kalisch BJ: The Advance of American Nursing, Third Edition. Philadelphia: JB Lippincott, 1995.

National Council of State Boards of Nursing: Issues. Volume 16, Number 1. Chicago: NCSBN, 1995.

National League for Nursing: Nursing Data Review 1995. Publication No. 19-2686. New York: The League, 1995.

National League for Nursing: State-Approved Schools of Nursing: LPN/LVN-1995. Publication No. 19-2692. New York: The League, 1995.

Robert HM: Robert's Rules of Order, Ninth Edition. New York: HarperCollins, 1991.

Nursing Theory and Nursing Process

5

■ ───

Nightingale
Henderson
Orem
Roy

Neuman
Nursing Theory and Its Relationship
   to Nursing Practice
Nursing Process

■ ───

OBJECTIVES

When you complete this chapter, you should be able to:

Name the four concepts included in any theory of nursing.

Briefly describe one nursing theory.

Describe the five steps of the nursing process.

Describe the benefits of the nursing process.

Explain the function of NANDA.

Discuss three ways in which a nursing care plan may be developed and/or revised.

"What are you doing to my father?"

   Vera looked up from her chart into the face of a very angry young man. She recognized him at once. He was the son of her patient in Room 410, Walter Simpkins. The son's name was Ray. Vera had met Ray a number of times when he was visiting his father.

   Vera closed the cover on the chart she was writing and stepped outside the nurse's station. "What's the trouble, Mr. Simpkins?"

   "I want an explanation, and I want it now," the man said loudly. The RN who was Vera's team leader had left the unit for a moment. Vera, an LPN, was the only healthcare staff member there. She was much younger than the man, but she spoke with authority.

   "I really don't know what you mean," Vera said. "Can you tell me more?"

The man calmed down. "I went to my father's room, like I do every day, to take him to the lobby, where we can talk," he said. "He told me you people are making him drink gallons of water all day long."

"I think I understand," she said. "And it isn't really gallons, Mr. Simpkins. It's more like a half a glass every 2 to 3 hours."

Ray appeared sheepish. "I-well, Dad was upset . . ."

"We know he's upset," Vera said. "But he was becoming dehydrated." Ray nodded approval. "I'm glad to know the nursing staff is on top of things." He turned and calmly walked down the hall to his father's room.

Vera returned to her charting. "If they only knew how carefully we assess our patients," she said to herself. She opened the chart. It was filled with notations and observations. "How else could we plan what to do for our patients to help them back to health?"

What Ray and most others unfamiliar with the practice of nursing do not know is that virtually everything Vera and all nurses do is based on a broad body of knowledge and thought developed from the thinking of many professional nurses over many years of careful research and study. What may appear to a patient or a patient's relative to be random care is in reality the precise application of practices that have been thought out thoroughly, applied, and constantly revised. These practices, derived from nursing theories, are the foundation of contemporary nursing.

As you learned in Chapter 3, in earlier times, nurses depended on the clergy to guide their activities. Until as recently as 30 years ago, nurses relied on other disciplines, such as medicine, to define their practice. Nurses were not encouraged to make independent decisions based on their own objectives. Today, however, nurses view nursing as a profession distinct from other professional occupations.

For any profession to advance, its educational programs and its practices must be based on a unique body of knowledge. As part of the process of becoming a separate, distinct profession, nursing has developed a body of knowledge and thought referred to as *nursing theory.*

A theory is an explanation of the nature of something. A nursing theory attempts to describe or explain the nature of nursing. Nursing theory guides the practice of nursing by providing a focus from which the nurse cares for other human beings.

You may hear the term *nursing model* used interchangeably with the term *nursing theory.* Although there are some differences between theories and models, both attempt to describe or explain the nature of nursing. Therefore, in this book, nursing theory and nursing model are used to mean the same thing.

Beginning with Florence Nightingale, a number of nurses have developed nursing theories. Although each theory is unique, all are similar in that they explain how nursing approaches four basic concepts: the person, the environment, health, and nursing.

During the late 1950s and early 1960s, several theories were developed. Since then, many more theories have been advanced by nursing scholars. Several of these theories are summarized in Table 5-1.

An understanding of nursing theory will help you as a student and as a practitioner. A specific nursing theory or a combination of nursing theories have been

TABLE 5-1 Selected Nursing Theories and Models

Theorist	Theme	Person	Environment	Health	Nursing
Nightingale, Florence 1859	Environment affects health	Has physical, intellectual, and spiritual attributes	Those aspects outside the person that affect health	Being free of disease	Putting the person in the best condition for nature to act upon him or her
Henderson, Virginia 1955	Fourteen principles or components of nursing care	Mind and body are inseparable	Can be either a negative or positive influence on the person	Ability to function independently in the physiological, environmental, and social aspects of life	Deliberate plan to meet the 14 components of nursing care
Orem, Dorothea 1958	Basic human needs are met through self-care activities	An integrated whole, with physiological, psychological, and sociological components	Created by society; includes values and expectations	Ability to meet self-care needs	Nursing education gives nurses the legitimate right to assist patients to meet self-care needs
Roy, Sister Callista 1964	Stressors affect how a person adapts	Biopsychosocial being in a changing environment	All internal and external influences that affect the human being	Health and illness are relative terms and exist at different times in differing degrees	Nurses' role to help the person adjust to changes in stimuli
Neuman, Betty 1972	Systems approach to meeting human needs	An integrated whole in a constant state of change because of dynamic inter-relationship of many variables	An external and an internal environment, both of which constantly affect the development of the person	Health seen as relative, depending on physiological, psychological, sociocultural, and developmental state of the person	Concerned with total person and attempts to either reduce or minimize effects of external or internal stress on the person

used as a basis for the design of your educational program. Theory also provides the perspective from which nursing service is designed in healthcare facilities. By understanding how nursing theory guides your activities in nursing, you are better able to be an active participant in your educational program and, in practice, a stronger contributor to the nursing team.

By studying the thinking of nursing theorists, you will begin to be able to refine your own beliefs about person, environment, health, and nursing. You will be challenged to grow in your understanding of yourself and your role as a member of the nursing team.

Nursing theories have become the guidelines of the nursing profession. The first theory was that of Florence Nightingale in 1859. Her views on nursing prevailed for almost 100 years. It was not until the early 1950s that new theories were developed. Since then, many theories have been advanced by nursing scholars.

Nursing education programs, including yours, are based on one or more nursing theories. Nursing theory is also used to design nursing service in healthcare facilities. Because these two applications of nursing theory—education and service—are the foundation of your nursing career, it is important for you to have a working understanding of nursing theory.

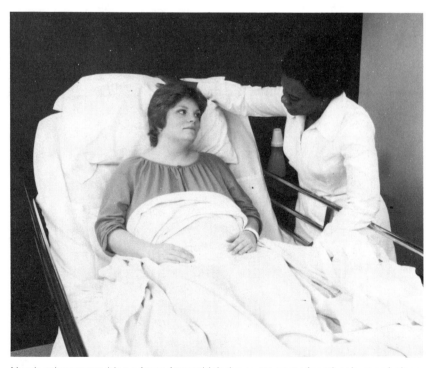

Nursing theory provides a focus from which the nurse cares for other human beings.

NIGHTINGALE

Nursing care in the United States and in England was based for many years on Florence Nightingale's nursing theory. It was a framework of her ideas about what she believed nursing should be, based on her observations and experiences. Her best-known work was originally published in 1859.

Florence Nightingale believed that nursing care delivery should be based on the laws of health, which said that in the right environment, a patient would get better through natural healing processes. A nurse's duty was to provide the right environment. This was done by providing physical care and attention to the environment.

Environment was emphasized in Nightingale's time because people lived in crowded, unsanitary conditions, epidemics of disease were common, social conditions were strained, and medicine as a science was still in its infancy. There was little that could be done except to make a patient comfortable in a clean environment.

HENDERSON

Virginia Henderson described her theory of nursing in her book titled *The Nature of Nursing: A Definition and Its Implications, Practice, Research, and Education,* which was first published in 1955. In the second edition, published in 1966, she defined nursing as follows:

> The unique function of the nurse is to assist the individual, sick or well, in performance of those activities contributing to health or its recovery (or to a peaceful death) that he/she would perform unaided if he/she had the necessary strength, will or knowledge. And to do this in such a way as to help him/her gain independence as rapidly as possible.

Henderson believes that health is basic to human functioning, and an individual's ability to function independently depends on health. She listed 14 components of basic nursing care that are intended to contribute to a patient's independence; they are as follows:

1. Breathe normally.
2. Eat and drink adequately.
3. Eliminate body waste.
4. Move and maintain a desirable position.
5. Sleep and rest.
6. Dress, undress, and select suitable clothing.
7. Maintain body temperature by adjusting clothing and environment.
8. Keep the body clean and well-groomed and protect the skin.
9. Avoid changes in the environment and personal safety.
10. Communicate to express emotions, needs, fears, or opinions.
11. Worship.
12. Work to acquire a sense of accomplishment.
13. Play or participate in various forms of recreation.
14. Learn, discover, satisfy curiosity for normal development and health, and use healthcare facilities.

Each of these components, according to Henderson, should be individualized to accommodate the uniqueness of each patient. The goal of nursing care is to assist the patient until he is able to perform these components independently.

OREM

Self-care—the things people do "on their own behalf in maintaining life, health, and well-being"—is the main theme of Dorothea Orem's nursing theory, first published in 1958. Orem sees humans as functioning biologically, symbolically, and socially, with specific needs in each of these areas. To her, health means being able to meet these needs for oneself. Orem's universal self-care requisites or needs are somewhat similar to the 14 components identified by Henderson. When a person's ability to perform self-care is impaired, in whole or in part, nursing care is indicated to compensate for this deficiency and to increase the person's potential to live in his or her environment. How much nursing is required is determined by the person's specific needs. Orem divides nursing intervention into three categories:

1. In wholly compensatory nursing, the nurse provides virtually all of the patient's self-care needs, as in intensive care and total care situations.
2. In partly compensatory nursing, the patient and the nurse work together to make up for the patient's limitations. As an example, the patient may be able to bathe unassisted but needs someone to change a dressing.
3. In supportive-educative nursing, the patient can provide self-care or could learn how to do so but needs help to learn or to adjust. Teaching a patient how to live normally within the limits of a diabetic diet is an example of this type of nursing.

In Orem's theory, nurses, by virtue of their education and training, have a legitimate role in helping the patient meet his self-care needs.

ROY

Sister Callista Roy proposes that a person's ability to adapt to his or her environment is the basis of an effective nursing model. Her adaptation model, which she began in 1964, says that people face a constantly changing environment and must adapt to it. Conflict between the changing environment and the need to adapt to it produces stress. A person's response to stress is observable behavior combining physiological, intellectual, and behavioral reactions. How well or how poorly the person copes with stress determines how much stress is reduced or eliminated, which, in turn, affects health.

Health, for Roy, can be represented by a continuous line from very ill to very healthy. Successful coping with stress produces better health; unsuccessful coping produces worse health. The nurse's goal is to help the client cope so that better health can be gained. The nurse does this by first assessing the patient's needs and then intervening to see that those needs are fulfilled. This is done with the client's active participation.

NEUMAN

In Betty Neuman's healthcare systems model (first published in 1972), the client is viewed as a whole being of many parts in an environment consisting of internal, external, and interpersonal elements. The combination is a system in which all its parts are constantly interacting. This healthcare model implies that to understand one thing about a person, you must take into account everything about that person, not only what the person is experiencing but how he is responding to the experience.

Forces or *stressors*, as Neuman calls them, act on people from both inside and outside. They may benefit or harm the individual they act on, and they can be either strong or weak. They tend to upset the individual's stability, which is the ideal condition to be in.

To remain stable, the person reacts to stress by using energy. A person's health is defined by the amount of energy available to respond to stress. It is determined by comparing normal conditions with present conditions. High energy is good health; low energy is illness; no energy is death. A person maintains good health, called *stability* or *harmony*, by using energy to balance the effects of stress.

In this model, nursing's aim is to identify a client's stressors being produced by any part of the system and then to intervene to reduce or eliminate them. Interventions should: (1) prevent stressors from reaching the client; (2) treat stressors after they reach the client; or (3) return the client to good health after treatment.

NURSING THEORY AND ITS RELATIONSHIP TO NURSING PRACTICE

Some trends in nursing theory development can be identified, and are evident in today's nursing practice. Early theorists (eg, Florence Nightingale) were more concerned with environment than with person, health, or nursing. Henderson's and Orem's models emphasize the concept of nursing as a patient/nurse relationship. Neuman's healthcare system model emphasizes the patient/healthcare system relationship. Physiological, psychological, sociological, and developmental factors are identified as some of the stressors that may have a positive or negative effect on the individual.

As nursing theory has developed from mostly environment-centered toward more person-centered, nurses have placed more emphasis on concern for the patient as a person. Total patient care and primary care (see Chapter 7) are intended to meet the unique needs of individual patients rather than groups of patients.

One of the most significant outcomes of nursing's increased interest in the uniqueness of each human is an attempt to meet the nursing and healthcare needs of that person. Who is the person? What are his or her health goals? How can nurses help the patient or client achieve those goals? These are some of the questions asked by contemporary nurses.

Madeleine Leininger, a nurse and an anthropologist, is the founder and leader in the field of transcultural nursing. Through her initial efforts in the mid-1960s, nurses began to consider their patients' and clients' cultural differences. Transcultural nursing encourages appreciation of all cultures and discourages imposing your own cultural practices on others. This means respecting other cultures and adapting nursing care to meet the needs of people from cultures other than the nurse's. Transcultural nursing is indeed the application of those nursing theories that stress understanding the whole person in the context of total environment. Nurses who consider their patients' political, spiritual, economic, and cultural values before planning nursing care are practicing transcultural nursing.

The United States is made up of people from diverse cultural backgrounds. In the 1700s, people emigrated primarily from Great Britain and Germany; in the early 1800s, most immigrants were from Ireland and Germany; and in the late 1800s, most immigrants came from southern and eastern Europe. In the early 1900s, a large number of people came to the United States from Italy, Russia, and central European countries. From 1970 to today, the largest number of immigrants have come to the United States from Asia and North America.

The Asian immigrants are predominately from China, India, Korea, Laos, the Philippine Islands, and Vietnam. The North American immigrants are predominately from Mexico, Cuba, the Dominican Republic, Haiti, Jamaica, and El Salvador.

Adapting to the culture and customs of the United States is often difficult, and immigrants have special needs when they require healthcare. Your sensitivity when caring for patients, regardless of their country of birth, can help you learn about different cultures and how to adapt your nursing knowledge and skills to the uniqueness of each patient.

NURSING PROCESS

Translating nursing theories and models into practice is accomplished through the nursing process. The nursing process is a systematic, organized method of practicing nursing. The nursing process consists of five steps:

1. Assess the patient
2. Formulate the nursing diagnosis
3. Plan nursing care
4. Implement the plan
5. Evaluate the effectiveness of nursing care

The first step, assessment, is done by observing the patient and asking questions of the patient or client or of his or her family or significant other. Things you can see are called *objective observations;* things that a patient says are called *subjective reports.* Objective observations include vital signs, skin condition, body language, and physical characteristics, such as height and weight. Subjective reports include a patient's description of pain, symptoms, or discomfort.

The second step in the nursing process is formulating a nursing diagnosis, a statement describing an existing or potential health problem that nurses can treat separately from a physician's order. A nursing diagnosis is made on the basis of information collected during the assessment phase.

To improve communication among nurses and to assist in nursing research, an organization called the North American Nursing Diagnosis Association (NANDA) was formed in 1973 to develop a standardized list of nursing diagnoses. Members of this organization discuss, review, and study research reports on proposed nursing diagnoses before including them in the NANDA-approved list of accepted nursing diagnoses. A complete list of current approved nursing diagnoses can be found in most medical/surgical nursing textbooks.

Planning, the third step in the nursing process, includes setting priorities and writing the nursing care plan. The sample nursing care plan in Table 5-2 demonstrates how a nursing care plan should look. It can be developed in several ways. Either a professional nurse responsible for admitting patients to a particular unit or service or a primary nurse responsible for planning a particular patient's comprehensive care may develop a nursing care plan.

Another way the nursing care plan may be developed is through a formal patient care conference, which may consist only of nursing team members or may consist of multidisciplinary members. A multidisciplinary conference includes nurses, social workers, physicians, pharmacists, often the family, dietitians, physical and occupational therapists, and others who are involved in providing care for a particular patient. In either case, a meeting is held to develop a plan of care based on the patient's total needs.

Another way a nursing care plan may be developed is less formal than the previous two methods. Nurses contribute to the care plan and revise it as the patient's condition and needs change. In this situation, the care plan is written by those nursing team members who have information relative to the condition of the patient or who become aware of nursing measures that assist the patient to achieve maximum health.

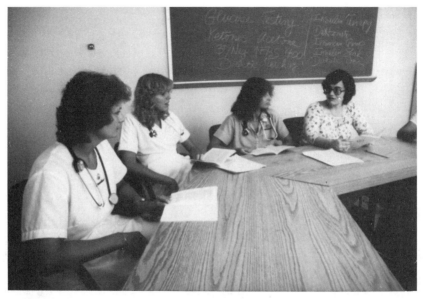

The nursing care plan is developed through patient care conferences.

TABLE 5-2 Sample Plan of Care According to Gordon's Functional Health Patterns

Assessment Data	Nursing Diagnosis/Collaborative Problem	Outcome	Nursing Orders	Evaluation

10/20
Health management/Health perception: Nonsmoker. Goes to aerobics 3× wk when well. States being ill and dependent on others is very difficult on her.
Nutrition/metabolic pattern: 20 lb overweight. Has had no appetite since illness started 10 days ago. Has had fever of 101° much of the time. Skin intact—no rashes.
Elimination pattern: BM q other day, usually. Now has diarrhea 10–15×/day. Has external hemorrhoids. Urine dark and concentrated.
Activity/exercise pattern: Has not been out of house for past 10 days. Feels she is too weak to go out.
Cognitive perception pattern: College graduate. Alert and appropriate in communication.
	10/20
	1. *Fluid Volume Deficit* R/T Fever, diarrhea, and loss of appetite as manifested by dark concentrated urine.
	
	2. *Diarrhea* R/T unknown etiology.
		Will maintain hydration by drinking at least 2000 mL per day every day.
		
		Will develop normal bowel movements by controlling diarrhea through medication and diet by 10/22.
			10/20
			1. Keep ginger ale with juice at bedside.
			2. Urge fluids (clear liq) to: 1000 mL (7–3)
			  750 mL (3–11)
			  250 mL (7–11)
			3. Assess fluid intake every 2 hours while awake.
			4. Both nurse and pt should keep a record of I/O.
			5. Monitor electrolyte studies.
			  J. Martin, RN
			
			10/20
			1. Maintain clear liquid diet.
			2. Assess BMs q 3° while awake and give Lomotil prn.
			  J. Martin, RN
				10/22
				Fluid intake only 1500 mL last 2 days. JM
				Discussed her need to push more. JM
				Electrolytes WNL Urine output 700 mL and concentrated. JM
				Keeping own I/O record JM
				
				10/22
				Diarrhea ↓ to 4 × day Clear liquids maintained. Taking Lomotil qid. JM

10/20 *Sleeps/rest pattern:* Sleeps much of the time, but disturbed by having to get up to BR for diarrhea. *Self-perception/self-concept pattern:* States she's an independent individual. *Role/relationship pattern:* Married. Has one child. Worried because she says husband is "not good" with daughter. *Sexual/reproductive pattern:* Married. Other data collection deferred. *Coping/stress pattern:* States she's a "doer": likes to be active doing things when she is depressed. *Value/belief pattern:* Catholic. Attends Mass most Sundays.	10/20 3. *High Risk for Altered Family Processes* R/T illness of mother. 4. *High Risk for Impaired Skin Integrity* (rectal area) R/T diarrhea and hemorrhoids.	She and her husband will discuss how family will cope with illness by 10/22. Rectal area will remain clean and without signs of irritation.	10/20 Spend time discussing with husband and wife, together and separately, to determine how the family is adapting to illness and to identify potential problems. J. Martin, RN Encourage warm sitz baths qid especially p BMs. J. Martin, RN	10/22 Husband has not been to visit for longer than 10 minutes, and I have missed him both times. Told her to ask him to call me when he can. JM 10/22 Taking sitz bath. Rectal area clean, not red. JM

From Alfaro-LeFevre R: Applying Nursing Process: A Step-By-Step Guide, Third Edition. Philadelphia: JB Lippincott, 1994.

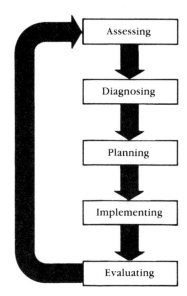

Steps of the nursing process.

Step 4, implementation, is the step in which the care plan is put into practice. From looking at the sample care plan, you can see that specific nursing orders are prescribed for this patient. Nursing team members should implement (put into practice) the recommendations made in the nursing care plan. Problems in implementing the care plan should be reported to the professional nurse responsible for the patient unit or department.

The fifth and last step in the nursing process is evaluating effectiveness of the care. At this point, the nurse is able to evaluate how well nursing interventions have worked in assisting the patient to achieve health goals. Evaluation of the care plan and how it is implemented is a continuous process and often results in reassessment of the patient, revision of some or all nursing diagnoses, and changes in the nursing care plan.

Planning patient care by using the nursing process helps you organize your approach to the patient. It requires you to integrate your knowledge of nursing, health, person, environment, and medicine to best serve the needs of the patient. It helps you communicate with other members of the nursing team and helps them communicate with you. Above all, the patient benefits from the quality of care that the nursing process encourages.

DISCUSSION QUESTIONS/LEARNING ACTIVITIES

1. Ask a nurse who graduated from nursing school 15 to 20 years ago to describe changes in nursing practice.

2. Discuss how nursing theory was used to develop your educational program.

3. What is your definition of health, and how does your definition differ from that of your classmates?

4. What are some of the ways you might handle a situation in which a patient refuses to accept nursing care or healthcare? How will you feel?

5. Read several actual nursing care plans for patients in your clinical facility. Can you provide the rationale (reasons) for the nursing orders?

READ MORE ABOUT IT

Alfaro-LeFevre R: Applying Nursing Process: A Step-By-Step Guide, Third Edition. Philadelphia: JB Lippincott, 1994.

Carpenito LJ: Nursing Diagnosis: Application to Clinical Practice, Sixth Edition. Philadelphia: JB Lippincott, 1995.

Fitzpatrick JJ, Whall AL: Conceptual Models of Nursing: Analysis and Application, Third Edition. East Norwalk, CT: Appleton & Lange, 1996.

Henderson V: Principles and Practices of Nursing, First Edition. New York: Macmillan, 1978.

Iyer PW, Taptich BJ, Bernocchi-Losey D: Nursing Process and Nursing Diagnosis, Third Edition. Philadelphia: WB Saunders, 1995.

Leininger MM: Culture, Care, Diversity, and Universality: A Theory of Nursing, First Edition. New York: National League for Nursing, 1991.

Neuman BN: The Neuman Systems Model: Application to Nursing Education and Practice, Third Edition. East Norwalk, CT: Appleton & Lange, 1995.

Nightingale F: Notes on Nursing: What It Is and What It Is Not, Commemorative Edition. Philadelphia: JB Lippincott, 1992. (Originally published in 1859.)

Orem DE: Nursing: Concepts of Practice, Fifth Edition. St. Louis: Mosby-Year Book, 1995.

Roy C: The Roy Adaptation Model: The Definitive Statement, Second Edition. East Norwalk, CT: Appleton & Lange, 1996.

6

The Healthcare System

OBJECTIVES

When you complete this chapter, you should be able to:

Define the terms "healthcare provider," "healthcare facility," "healthcare service," "healthcare regulation," "healthcare financing," and "healthcare system."

Describe the purpose of healthcare regulatory agencies.

Discuss the purpose of quality assurance programs.

List the two major sources of health insurance.

Explain how diagnosis-related groups are used to control the cost of healthcare.

Discuss the role of the U.S. government in healthcare.

Name the five divisions of the U.S. Department of Health and Human Services.

Outline the major functions of the Public Health Services division of the Department of Health and Human Services.

Give three examples of current events that are affecting the healthcare system.

A hot shower always changed Mary Kelly's outlook on life. The shower she took one Saturday morning saved her life. Mary was 31 years old. She was married and had a son, Erik. Her husband was a successful automobile dealer. The young family had a bright future.

As Mary lathered herself, she touched a small lump in her right breast. She had never noticed it before. She felt it again. She had two choices. She could assume the lump was not serious and do nothing, or she could make an immediate appointment with her doctor for a breast examination. For a moment Mary was undecided. Then she laughed nervously. "Oh, it's nothing," she said. She finished her shower and quickly dressed. By midmorning the lump was forgotten. But that afternoon Mary remembered a pamphlet sent by the American Cancer Society. It told her how to do a breast self-examination. She located the pamphlet and followed its instructions. This time she immediately called her doctor.

The discovery of the lump and taking appropriate action saved Mary's life. Her own and her family's future remain secure because she used the services of the healthcare system.

Obtaining healthcare in the United States is not often as simple as it may at first appear. Traditionally, the physician was the person who provided healthcare and the hospital was the place where patients went to be treated for illnesses that could not be managed in the doctor's office. Today, the healthcare system is far more complex, and there are many options and choices for healthcare. These recent changes in the healthcare system are sometimes confusing. This chapter will help you understand where and how healthcare is provided, regulated, and financed. Through this understanding, you will be better able to influence legislation regarding healthcare; answer your patient's questions about healthcare; participate in approval and accreditation procedures; and influence the future of healthcare in the United States.

THE HEALTHCARE SYSTEM

Some general descriptions will help you understand the present healthcare system and why Americans are so concerned about the future of the largest business in this country.

Healthcare providers, healthcare facilities, healthcare services, healthcare regulation, and healthcare financing together comprise the *healthcare system*. The healthcare system's goal is to improve the health of people in this society.

There are government and nongovernment (private) components of the healthcare system. Some of the government components of the healthcare system include veterans' hospitals and nursing homes, military hospitals, Medicare and Medicaid health insurance, and the Department of Health and Human Services.

Some of the nongovernment components of the healthcare system include private providers (physicians, optometrists, dietitians, psychologists, nurse practitioners, etc.), private for-profit healthcare facilities, private nonprofit healthcare facilities, health clinics, private health insurance companies, preferred providers organizations, health maintenance organizations, and managed care systems.

A variety of healthcare providers who provide a wide range of services in a multitude of healthcare facilities which function under an array of regulations makes it difficult for the public to know how to obtain the best treatment from the best provider at the least cost. An understanding of the components of the healthcare system will help you not only as a consumer but also as a patient advocate.

Healthcare Providers

Healthcare providers include people, institutions, and organizations that make healthcare services available to those who want or need them. Physicians, dentists, optometrists, nurse practitioners, and podiatrists are examples of people who provide healthcare.

Primary healthcare providers are those who people see first for health maintenance or treatment of illnesses. Primary care providers usually provide a person's initial contact with the healthcare system. Health care providers and members of the healthcare team will be reviewed in more detail in Chapter 7.

Institutions that provide healthcare include hospitals, long-term care facilities, ambulatory care facilities, walk-in clinics, community mental health centers, kidney dialysis centers, and state or local health department clinics. Institutions qualify as healthcare providers because they, through their employees, provide healthcare to their "customers."

Organizations such as health maintenance organizations (HMOs), preferred provider organizations (PPOs), managed care organizations, and health insurance companies qualify as healthcare providers. These organizations qualify as healthcare providers because they either hire or contract with individuals or groups of

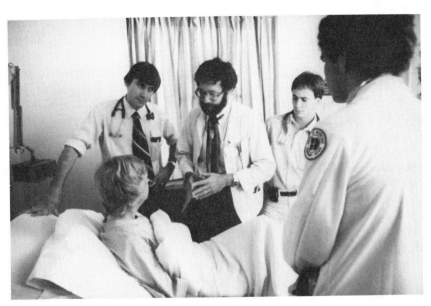

Individual healthcare providers often refer or admit patients to healthcare institutions.

individuals to provide healthcare. These organizations usually charge a fee that allows member access to all necessary medical and hospital services. This fee is not increased even for prolonged hospitalization, nor is it refunded if the member does not use any healthcare services.

Healthcare Facilities

Until the early part of the 1900s, the traditional healthcare facility for treating illness, injury, and dying was the patient's home. The healthcare "team" was the patient's family. If a patient could afford the services of a physician, these services were also provided in the patient's home.

The changes in hospitals and nursing begun by Florence Nightingale during the Crimean War (1854–1856) and by American reformers after the Civil War (1861–1865) started the trend toward improvement of healthcare facilities that is still going on today.

In 1993, there were more than 6500 hospitals, 26,000 long-term care facilities, and 5000 community health agencies in the United States. While the number of hospitals is declining, the number of long-term care facilities and community health agencies is increasing.

Hospitals

A hospital's primary role is to provide healthcare. In addition, hospitals are often medical education centers. They furnish training, seminars, and resources to physicians, nurses, technicians, social workers, dietitians, therapists, emergency medical technicians, and many other healthcare workers.

Some areas of education available at hospitals include disease prevention and treatment, health maintenance, pathological analysis, and rehabilitation. Hospitals also have clinics and laboratories for the treatment, analysis, and research of illness and injury.

Hospitals are classified by ownership, the kind of services they offer, their size, and the length of patient stay. Eligibility for funding, accrediting guidelines, staffing requirements, and allocation of medical equipment often depends on how a hospital is classified.

Ownership can be public or private. Public hospitals are those owned by federal, state, or local governments. Veterans Administration hospitals, U.S. Public Health Service hospitals, and military hospitals are examples of hospitals owned by the federal government.

State university hospitals, state mental institutions, and state prison hospitals are examples of state-owned hospitals. County and municipal hospitals are owned by local governments.

Private hospitals, also called voluntary hospitals, are owned and operated by individuals, partnerships, corporations, religious groups, and labor unions.

Hospitals operated as businesses are called proprietary, investor-owned, or for-profit hospitals. Hospitals operated as a service and not for profit are called nonprofit, nonproprietary, official, or not-for-profit hospitals. Public hospitals are not-for-profit hospitals. Private hospitals can be for-profit or not-for-profit hospitals, depending on their financial purpose.

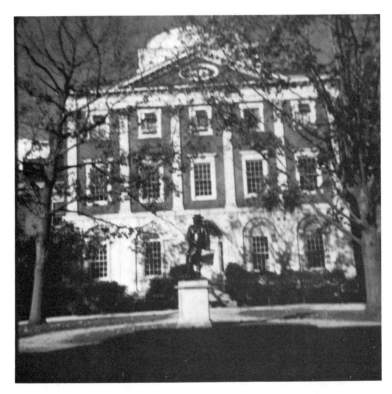

Pennsylvania Hospital, the nation's first hospital, is located in Philadelphia, Pennsylvania.

In the past, a for-profit hospital was often owned by a group of local investors. The current trend is toward investor-owned corporations, which may own 100 or more hospitals across the country.

In addition to ownership, hospitals can be classified by the kinds of services they provide. General hospitals provide healthcare for most kinds of disorders to patients of most ages. Specialty hospitals provide healthcare only for specific disorders or conditions or for limited age groups. Psychiatric hospitals, children's hospitals, and rehabilitation hospitals are examples of specialty hospitals.

Hospitals can also be classified according to their size: fewer than 25 beds, 25 to 49 beds, 50 to 99 beds, 100 to 199 beds, 200 to 299 beds, 300 to 399 beds, 400 to 499 beds, and 500 or more beds.

The fourth way that hospitals can be classified is by the average length of stay. Short-term care hospitals provide treatment for acute conditions requiring specialized personnel and sophisticated equipment and procedures for a short time. Short-term hospitals serve patients whose average stays are generally less than 30 days.

Long-term hospitals provide treatment, maintenance, and rehabilitation for patients with chronic conditions needing extended care. Long-term hospitals care for those with average stays of 30 or more days. Examples of long-term hospitals include mental and rehabilitation hospitals. A hospital may provide both short-term and long-term care.

Chapter 7 includes an explanation of how the administration of a typical general acute care hospital is organized.

Patient-Care Units

An acute-care general hospital serves a variety of patients with diverse medical and nursing needs. To provide competent and efficient care, a patient may be assigned to a patient-care unit according to his or her primary diagnosis or by the amount of care required.

Units that specialize in specific types of care include coronary care, pediatric, medical, surgical, obstetric, and psychiatric units. Depending on the size of the facility, these units may fill a portion of a floor, a whole floor, or even a wing.

Patients can also be assigned to nursing units in which all the patients require the same relative amount of care. The overall management of patients by the amount of care needed is called *progressive patient care*. Progressive patient-care units include intensive care, intermediate, self-care, and long-term care units.

Intensive Care Units. Intensive care units are reserved for patients who are seriously or critically ill, who require total care and monitoring by means of specialized techniques and knowledge, and who require equipment that is immediately available in the unit. Personnel working in these units are highly skilled in using all available resources to assist the patient to recover from serious injury, disease, or major surgery.

There are several types of intensive care units:

1. Coronary care unit
2. Surgical intensive care unit
3. Medical intensive care unit
4. Neonatal intensive care unit
5. Pediatric intensive care unit
6. Burn intensive care unit
7. Postanesthesia and recovery unit

Intermediate Care Units. Intermediate care units include the general medical and surgical units, the pediatric unit, the orthopedic unit, the newborn nursery, and the psychiatric unit. Some or all of these units are found in a general short-term (acute) care hospital. Patients in these units are admitted for diagnosis or treatment of illness that cannot be treated on an outpatient basis. Patients admitted to these units are not critically ill; however, they do need the specialized medical and nursing care available in a hospital. During the early stages of rehabilitation, teaching patients how to care for their own health is an important activity in an intermediate care unit.

Self-Care Units. Self-care units are for patients with no or minimal limits on what they can do for themselves but who still need extensive rehabilitation and healthcare teaching or specialized therapy. These units are as homelike as possible. Patients eat in dining rooms, wear their own clothes, use recreational facilities, and keep their own appointments at other departments within the hospital.

Long-Term Care Units. Some short-term care hospitals have designated wings or floors for use as long-term care units. Patients in these units have needs similar to those of patients who are admitted to nursing homes. Long-term care is that care provided to patients who have an illness that may not be curable but whose condition may be improved through medical and nursing care.

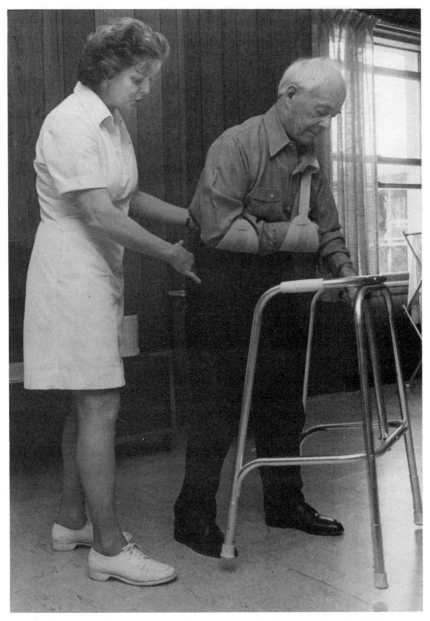

The rehabilitation center. (Courtesy of the Jewish Home for the Aged, Portland, Maine.)

Other Healthcare Facilities

Other types of healthcare facilities that provide health services include nursing homes, rehabilitation centers, freestanding surgical centers (surgi-centers), dialysis centers, doctor's offices, neighborhood health centers, local health departments, industrial health centers, and community health centers.

A nursing home is a facility that provides care, generally, to older people who cannot care for themselves. Nursing homes are classified as either skilled nursing facilities (SNFs) or intermediate care facilities (ICFs). SNFs provide skilled nursing services; residents in an SNF are too well to remain in a short-term care hospital but too ill to return to their home. Rehabilitation services are often an important part of an SNF. SNF residents often require the level of nursing service that is directed by registered nurses and licensed practical/vocational nurses.

ICFs are designed to provide long-term care, usually to people over the age of 65 years who cannot continue to live alone or with their families. Residents of ICFs often have chronic medical problems such as senility, Alzheimer's disease, paralysis resulting from a stroke, or a generalized weakness that makes it difficult for them to care for themselves or for their families to care for them. These residents often need assistance with activities of daily living such as bathing, dressing, eating, and walking.

Rehabilitation centers may be a division within a short-term care hospital, or they may be privately owned by physicians, physical therapists, or occupational therapists. These centers work with individual residents and their families to assist residents in attaining as much independence as possible.

Surgical centers (surgi-centers), usually not part of a hospital, provide minor surgical services for outpatients. The cost of procedures performed in these centers is less expensive than the same procedure performed in the hospital. Patients go home the same day as the surgery.

End-stage renal dialysis centers are often privately owned by physicians or other healthcare providers. They provide dialysis services to people whose kidney function is inadequate. People report to the dialysis center three or more times a week for renal dialysis. The cost of renal dialysis is often covered through one of the federal government health insurance programs.

Doctor's offices can also be considered healthcare facilities. The major portion of healthcare is provided through them. There are many arrangements of doctors' offices. Some offices have only one doctor; others have many. When several doctors share patients and space, the term *group practice* is used to describe the office.

Neighborhood or community health centers are usually found in low-income neighborhoods. These facilities provide a range of healthcare services to people of all ages. These centers depend on local, state, and federal funding to subsidize the cost of the medical care they provide.

Local health departments are also healthcare facilities. Larger cities are often divided into health districts, with each district served by an office that provides healthcare to residents of that particular district. In less populated areas, the county health department may provide the same services to all residents of the county.

Industrial healthcare facilities are found in businesses and industrial plants. These centers are staffed by a variety of healthcare personnel. Larger businesses and industries may employ physicians and nurses and offer a broad range of health screening and diagnostic services for their employees. Some of the health centers in larger businesses and industries offer fitness centers, counseling, and other health services.

Community mental health centers are generally organized as outpatient facilities for the diagnosis and treatment of mental and emotional disorders. These centers provide counseling services for patients who can continue to live in society but are in need of specialized treatment.

Healthcare Service

Healthcare service is a term used to describe the actual delivery of healthcare by healthcare workers. Healthcare service includes the prevention, diagnosis, and treatment of illnesses. It also includes providing care during an illness. Healthcare service can take many forms: a surgeon who performs an appendectomy; the nurse who provides home care; a dietitian who plans the week's menu for a nursing home; a hospital administrator who orders equipment for the physical therapy department; a public health nurse presenting information to a community group on cancer prevention; a volunteer in a hospice facility; and the licensed practical/vocational nurse bathing a patient. All are delivering healthcare service.

You will be a member of a team delivering healthcare services. Your contributions as a member of that team are vitally important to the success of the healthcare service. The Healthcare Team is the topic of Chapter 7.

Healthcare Regulation and Accreditation

Healthcare regulation is a term used to describe methods designed to control not only the quality of healthcare but also the cost of healthcare. The need to regulate the quality and cost of healthcare can be attributed, in part, to increasingly complex technology, social, and ethical issues and increasing costs. Regulations that affect the healthcare industry are usually developed by governmental bodies. These governmental bodies have the legal authority to close down those who do not comply.

Healthcare accreditation is a term used to describe a process in which an accrediting agency uses their written standards of excellence to examine the operation of a healthcare facility or organization. Accreditation lets the public know that the accredited organization exceeds the minimum regulatory standards for operation. In some cases, accreditation is voluntary. Accreditation of providers and facilities that receive Medicare and Medicaid funds or other federal or state government money for education and research is mandatory.

Regulations and Primary Healthcare Providers

You will recall that primary healthcare providers are usually those who are first to see the patient, such as a physician, a nurse practitioner, a dentist, or any one of a number of other healthcare providers. Primary healthcare providers must be licensed by the state in which they practice their profession.

Licensure is mandatory. This means that someone cannot say that he or she is a physician and use the initials MD (doctor of medicine) or DO (doctor of osteopathy) unless licensed to do so. A license is usually obtained after the candidate for licensure has met educational and practice requirements and has passed a licensing examination in that particular profession.

Agencies that directly regulate the practice of primary healthcare providers are the licensing boards of individual states. It is the responsibility of each state's board to protect the citizens of that state. Therefore, the board examines applicants for licensure and issues, renews, and revokes licenses. Although licensing boards have many other responsibilities, regulating the practice of licensees is their major responsibility.

Primary healthcare providers are also regulated by the ethical codes of their professions. Codes of ethics will be discussed in more detail in Chapter 10.

Regulation and Accreditation of Hospitals

Each state department of health regulates and evaluates the activities of hospitals. To accept patients and offer medical care, hospitals must be approved by the state department of health or a similar organization. Standards specific to hospitals are applied during the evaluation process. A hospital that meets these standards is then approved to operate in that state.

Most hospitals seek accreditation from the Joint Commission on the Accreditation of Healthcare Organizations (JCAHO) or the American Osteopathic Association. Accreditation is a voluntary process and indicates that the hospital has met the accrediting agency's specific standards and criteria for operating a healthcare facility. Accreditation of a hospital is mandatory if the hospital wants to sponsor medical educational programs and wants to receive payment from Medicare and several other health insurance plans.

Regulation and Accreditation of Nursing Homes

As is the case with hospitals, nursing homes are regulated by an appropriate organization in the state in which the nursing home is located. Nursing homes can also apply for accreditation by the JCAHO. State regulations and standards for accreditation are designed to evaluate the unique healthcare activities that occur in nursing homes.

Regulation and Accreditation of Home and
Community Healthcare Organizations

Home health and community health organizations are also required to comply with state regulations. Those who comply with state regulations are issued a license to operate within the state in which the organization is located.

Three organizations accredit home and community healthcare organizations. In 1992, the National League for Nursing's Community Health Accreditation Program (CHAP) became the first organization to receive government approval as a home health accrediting agency. CHAP also provides accrediting services for community and public health organizations.The JCAHO and the Health Care Financing Administration (HCFA) also accredit home health agencies.

Regulation of Other Healthcare Facilities

Other organizations and facilities that are regulated by the state department of health (or similar department) include boarding homes, residential treatment facilities, group homes, clinics, adult and child day care centers, and community mental health centers.

In fact, just about any organization or facility that offers healthcare must meet certain regulations in order to operate.

Regulation of Agencies That Receive Medicare and Medicaid Payments

The federal government pays, through the Medicare and Medicaid insurance programs, the healthcare costs of a tremendous number of its citizens. To ensure that adequate services are provided at a reasonable cost, the government has established regulations affecting those hospitals, nursing homes, physicians, and other providers of healthcare that receive reimbursement for services directly from one of these insurance plans. Many of the regulations originally established by the federal government are now being adapted for use by private insurance companies, such as Blue Cross and Blue Shield, as well as HMOs, PPOs, and other managed care organizations. Although many of the regulations developed by the government are complex, they are a step toward controlling the ever-increasing cost of healthcare in the United States.

Quality Assurance and Risk Management Programs

One aspect of regulation and accreditation of healthcare providers, paid for their services through Medicare or Medicaid or other government funds, is the requirement for developing a mechanism for assuring that patients receive quality care. Quality patient care is a goal shared by all members of the healthcare team, but providing quality in a complex healthcare system with many recent technological advances is not as easy as it may seem. The purpose of quality assurance programs in healthcare is to evaluate and improve the level of service to patients to ensure that at least minimally accepted levels of service are provided at the lowest cost possible.

Continuous quality improvement (CQI) through quality assurance (QA) and quality improvement (QI) programs are part of a continual evaluation process and are required by some accrediting agencies such as the JCAHO.

QA sets minimal standards of care. This is usually done by a committee of people who are experts in a particular area. For example, nurses who have an extensive educational background in maternity nursing and several years experience working with women in a maternity department meet together and define, in writing, standards of nursing care that would ensure safe care.

QI is intended to help an organization move beyond minimal standards to higher standards of care. This is often done through patient surveys, staff questionnaires, and patient chart reviews. The result of this evaluation process leads to changes in procedures, which leads to greater patient satisfaction and lower costs.

CQI program committees include healthcare workers who are experts in their specialty. Some of the things this group or committee reviews are patient charts, incident reports, patient surveys, and costs of care. They look for and implement ways to improve the quality of care provided in their facility.

The Utilization and Quality Control Peer Review Organization (shortened to PRO) was created by Congress in August 1982 to ensure that healthcare providers who are paid by Medicare provide care according to or above a predetermined standard. Defining standards of medical care and measuring how well healthcare providers meet those standards of care are far more complex than this simple explanation indicates.

Peer review can be described as the examination of someone's work by other people of equal standing. As a result of PRO, many expensive diagnostic and laboratory tests are no longer done and many surgeries are now performed on an outpatient basis. This has eased the financial burden of both the patient and the healthcare system.

Risk management is another QA program that is intended to prevent financial loss to the organization or facility. This is done by identifying those situations that result in longer lengths of stay in the facility, injury to patients, visitors, or staff, and incidents of patient care errors. Based on the findings of the risk manager, changes in policies and procedures are made to reduce the financial risk to the organization.

Because CQI, PRO, and risk management programs in healthcare facilities are the rule rather than the exception, you will most likely be employed in an agency that has these programs. Your employer will expect you to provide a certain standard of care; to keep accurate written records; probably to serve on special committees; and perhaps to participate in a peer review program. Your contributions will go a long way toward making yourself an important part of the healthcare team.

HEALTHCARE FINANCING

Healthcare financing is a term used to discuss payment of healthcare. The healthcare system in the United States is at a critical place in its history. Health care expenditures per person were $143 in 1960; $1068 in 1980; $2686 in 1990; and $3299 in 1993. Rapidly escalating costs are placing a heavy burden on the healthcare system, as well as on consumers. While health insurance pays much of the cost of healthcare, in 1993 there were 40 million people with no health insurance coverage.

Two major sources of health insurance are private health insurance and government health insurance. In 1993, just over 70% of the populations was covered by private health insurance and about 15% were covered by government insurance including Medicare. More than 15% of the population had no health insurance. Other sources of payment for healthcare are voluntary and private organizations and special foundations.

Private Insurance

Private medical insurance is the type a person buys as an individual or as a member of a group. This type of insurance is sold by commercial insurance companies and others in the same way that life, homeowner's, and automobile insurance is sold. There are two basic types of private medical insurance plans: indemnity insurance and prepaid insurance. It is estimated that there are more than 2600 health plans available to cover the costs of healthcare.

Indemnity insurance pays its policyholder or assignee (someone authorized to receive payment, such as a healthcare provider) the amount stated on the policy when an approved claim is made. This amount may pay for all or part of the claim, depending on the amount of coverage purchased. Cost of the policy will vary with the amount of coverage desired, deductible amount, the insured person's age and health, and other factors. Blue Cross and Blue Shield insurance are examples of indemnity insurance. Most indemnity insurance plans pay only for purchased services that result from a claim specifically covered in the policy. Usually the insured person may choose the care provider, as long as that provider or the services provided are not specifically excluded.

The second type of private insurance, prepaid insurance, often stresses the importance of disease prevention. These plans provide a range of prepaid services to their policyholders. HMOs, PPOs, and other managed care organizations are examples of prepaid insurance plans.

In an HMO or PPO, the policyholder pays a set monthly (or other period) charge. This payment entitles the policyholder to use the plans' services for routine healthcare and hospitalization as needed. Some plans include long-term care and other services. Cost of the plan varies according to services offered. The policyholder usually does not get to choose a healthcare provider. An HMO's or PPO's primary healthcare providers (eg, physicians, nurses) are usually salaried employees of the HMO or PPO or work under contract. HMO or PPO employee salaries may or may not be directly related to the profits (or losses) of the organization.

There are advantages and disadvantages to each type of insurance. With indemnity insurance, the insured person can choose a provider and health services facilities. The HMO or PPO subscriber must receive treatment by the HMO or PPO member providers. On the other hand, indemnity insurance does not generally pay for preventive care, as HMOs and PPOs do. This distinction is diminishing and will probably continue to do so as studies show that preventive measures actually reduce hospitalization and the accompanying costs.

Government Insurance

In 1965, the federal government passed legislation that made it a major healthcare insurance provider. The Social Security Act of 1965 included Titles XVIII and XIX, better known as Medicare and Medicaid. Medicare is a federally funded health insurance program, while Medicaid is a jointly funded federal-state health insurance program.

Medicare is a hospital and healthcare insurance plan for persons 65 years of age and older. Money for this program comes from Social Security taxes paid by workers and their employers to the federal government. Services provided under Medicare are the same nationwide.

Medicaid, a state-administered program, pays for healthcare services for the poor of any age with funds that come from both the state and federal governments.

Because Medicaid is administered by the state, services provided vary from state to state.

Medicare and Medicaid clients may choose their healthcare services and facilities from participating healthcare providers. Although not all healthcare providers accept Medicare and Medicaid insurance, the majority will accept these insurance plans as payment for services. Those who do not accept Medicare and Medicaid insurance cite smaller payments and slow payments as reasons for not accepting patients with these plans.

Diagnosis-Related Groups

From 1965 to 1983, the Medicare program paid healthcare providers (eg, physicians, hospitals, nursing homes) for services provided to people who were eligible for healthcare under the Medicare program. This system, called *retrospective payment*, meant that the healthcare provider ordered any and all medical care he or she believed was necessary or desirable without consideration of the cost. The providers were reimbursed by Medicare for their costs. As a consequence of rising healthcare costs, a new payment system was instituted in 1983. This system, called the *prospective payment method*, was developed by the federal government in an attempt to control healthcare costs associated with the Medicare program. The principle of prospective payment is to set rates for healthcare services in advance, rather than after the service has been delivered.

For example, under a prospective payment plan the cost for an appendectomy is calculated and fixed ahead of time. The calculated cost would allow for appropriate patient care and for an ordinary profit for the treating facility. If the hospital and physician delivered the treatment below the fixed rate, they would keep the difference, but if actual costs exceeded the allowable rate, they would have to bear the extra expenses themselves.

The government, to determine the costs of treatment in advance of that treatment, developed a system in which rates are based on a major diagnostic category (MDC). Within each MDC, there are groups of diagnoses, therefore, the term *diagnosis-related groups* (DRGs). Today, there nearly 500 DRGs.

Medicare or Medicaid patients are assigned an MDC diagnosis, and the DRG is based on age, complications, and several other factors. Each DRG has a set amount of money that will be paid by Medicare or Medicaid. By knowing the amount of reimbursement that will be received for services to patients with these types of insurance, healthcare facilities and other healthcare providers can control how much they will spend and thus ensure a profit while still providing necessary healthcare.

The prospective payment system has helped to control costs and for this reason, many private health insurance companies have begun using DRGs as the basis of payment for health insurance claims.

HEALTHCARE AND THE U.S. GOVERNMENT

The federal government became active in healthcare for citizens of the United States when medical care was authorized for American merchant seamen in 1798.

Since then the federal government has been involved with many health-related issues in areas of regulation, prevention, and control.

The U.S. Department of Health, Education, and Welfare was created in 1953 to address the health, education, and social concerns of Americans. This department was divided into the Department of Health and Human Services and the Department of Education in 1980. The Department of Health and Human Services (DHHS) has five divisions:

1. Office of Human Development Services (HDS)
2. Public Health Services (PHS)
3. Health Care Financing Administration (HCFA)
4. Social Security Administration (SSA)
5. Family Support Administration (FSA)

The Office of Human Development Services is concerned primarily with the health and welfare of elderly persons, children, youth and families, and Native Americans. PHS is that division of the DHHS concerned with diseases, their prevalence, and treatment. The HCFA administers Medicare and Medicaid programs. The SSA collects and disburses money under the Social Security Act. The FSA is concerned with ensuring support payments to single-parent families.

The division of the DHHS of particular interest to nursing is PHS. Figure 6-1 indicates that there are six separate agencies under Public Health Services: the Centers for Disease Control (CDC); the Food and Drug Administration (FDA); the Health Resources and Services Administration (HRSA); the National Institutes of Health (NIH); the Alcohol, Drug Abuse, and Mental Health Administration; the Agency for Toxic Substances and Diseases Registry; and Indian Health Services.

The CDC is concerned with prevention and control of diseases. It maintains statistics on diseases and their spread and supports research for controlling communicable diseases.

The FDA, through its various bureaus, protects the public from impure and unsafe foods, medications, and cosmetics; regulates the use and labeling of medicines and devices for preventing and treating diseases; sets food additive and labeling standards; conducts research; develops policy; and provides information.

The HRSA's emphasis is on healthcare resource problems in the areas of healthcare personnel, healthcare facilities, and healthcare delivery systems. This division is also concerned with providing leadership in planning and delivering health services.

The NIH comprises over a dozen separate agencies. The National Cancer Institute, the National Institute of General Medical Sciences, the National Institute on Aging, and the National Institute on Nursing are examples. Each agency is engaged in the research and treatment of specific problems.

The Alcohol, Drug Abuse, and Mental Health Administration directs its energies to research and treatment of health problems associated with drug and alcohol abuse and to the improvement of mental health through separate institutes.

The Agency for Toxic Substances and Diseases Registry is a recently created branch of the PHS. Its mission is to assess the prevalence and effects of environmental pollutants on the health of people in this country.

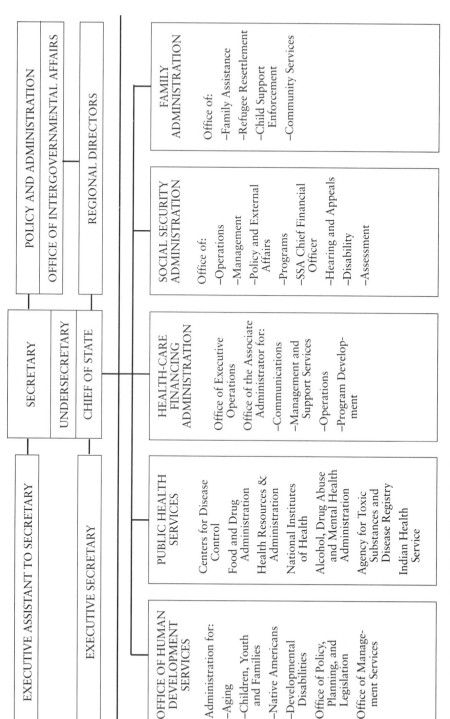

Figure 6-1. Department of Health and Human Services.

The Indian Health Services division of Public Health Services is primarily concerned with the health of Native Americans living on reservations. This branch of the government provides a variety of healthcare services on many reservations throughout the United States.

All of the divisions of the PHS routinely share information with other countries. Although the health of Americans is the primary concern, communicable diseases, toxic waste, and diseases, such as acquired immunodeficiency syndrome (AIDS) are international problems that are of concern to the PHS.

STATE AND LOCAL HEALTH DEPARTMENTS

State governments are also involved in the delivery of healthcare services. A commissioner of health, a secretary of health, or someone with a similar title is assigned the responsibility of overseeing state health programs. This office also administers the state Medicaid health insurance program for residents with low income.

State health department functions may also include the licensing of healthcare workers, hospitals, nursing homes, pharmaceutical manufacturers and distributors, and other healthcare agencies. State health departments also disseminate information and educational material, such as films, books, and pamphlets, on health matters to both the general public and healthcare agencies.

Divisions of the state health department may include public health, communicable diseases, vital statistics, maternal and child health, mental health, and other programs. State health departments in some areas have a direct relationship with local health departments.

Local health departments place their emphasis on healthcare needs of people living in specific geographic areas. Their jurisdiction may include a town, a city, a county, a borough, or some other clearly defined area. Functions of the local health department include reporting communicable diseases, keeping vital statistics, managing sanitation, providing a safe water supply, providing child and school health services, and managing other matters of local public health.

PRIVATE ORGANIZATIONS THAT SUPPORT THE HEALTHCARE SYSTEM

Many additional types of healthcare are provided through a variety of organizations. Although these services are not the typical ones we think of when we think of the healthcare system, they do contribute to the health of our society. Some of them include adult and child day care centers, Meals on Wheels, suicide and child abuse hotlines, family planning services, homemaker services, and specialized transportation services for ill and disabled persons.

Many groups are organized to provide emotional and psychological support for individuals and families with health related problems. A few examples include Alcoholics Anonymous, Women Organized Against Rape, Women

Against Abuse, Reach for Recovery (for patients recovering from mastectomies), Sudden Infant Death Syndrome Foundation, and the Zipper Club (for patients recovering from heart surgery).

Many Americans are using nontraditional approaches to maintain or improve health or to treat illness. Alternative types of healthcare includes using herbs, diets, vitamins, stress reduction techniques, acupuncture, behavior modification, and meditation. Some people are consulting with faith healers, chiropractors, nutritionists, naturopaths, masseurs, and exercise physiologists. While many traditional healthcare providers may dismiss some or all of these as a waste of time, the federal government is providing money to investigate the value of nontraditional approaches to healthcare.

The United States healthcare system also includes a large assortment of private organizations dedicated to meeting specific healthcare needs of the population. National organizations include the American Heart Association, the American Cancer Society, the March of Dimes Birth Defects Foundation, the United Way, and many more. Financial support for these organizations comes from fund drives, individual contributions, business and corporate gifts, and donations raised through radio and television marathons. Although these organizations do not generally provide healthcare, they do contribute millions of dollars to support research and treatment of specific diseases.

Private funding for healthcare services also includes community drives that raise money to help an identified individual or family cope with a catastrophic and expensive illness. You have probably been approached by a friend or neighbor and asked to contribute to a healthcare fund for a needy individual in your community. These people-to-people programs do a great deal to improve the health of this society.

Individuals and organizations contribute millions of dollars that otherwise would not be available to conduct research and to treat patients who have some of the more common diseases in this country. These contributions to the healthcare system must be recognized, supported, and appreciated by everyone.

ISSUES AND CONCERNS

Healthcare System

In the United States, a national healthcare system does not exist. Multiple organizations, a diversity of independent providers, a wide variety of facilities, cumbersome regulations, and poorly distributed financing all contribute to a confused public.

President Clinton's 1993 proposal to create a national healthcare system brought hope to many Americans. His plan emphasized providing healthcare for all Americans while at the same time controlling costs through various mechanisms including managed competition. While no national system of healthcare is yet in place, it is evident that people, through the political process, are making it known that adequate healthcare is of critical importance to them.

Healthcare Providers

A persistent concern has been the geographic concentration of a smaller number of primary care doctors and an overabundance of doctors specializing in areas such as anesthesiology, radiology, and emergency medicine. There are many areas of this country with no doctor available for hundreds of miles while large cities and major medical centers have a high physician-to-patient ratio.

Nurse practitioners and nurse-midwives have done much to alleviate the shortage of primary care doctors. Studies have shown that nurse practitioners and nurse-midwives provide quality primary and preventative care at a reasonable cost. They often provide this care to those who are poor or underserved by primary care physicians. In 1994, there were approximately 100,000 nurse practitioners. That number is expected to increase dramatically over the next few years.

The future role of the multipurpose worker and the cross training of current healthcare providers is also a concern. Multipurpose workers are those who are taught to perform the skills usually performed by workers in other job classifications. Cross training implies that a worker is trained to do not only his or her own job but the also the job of others. Issues related to these workers include concerns about their education preparation for the things they do, how their practice is regulated, and licensure.

Another concern is related to the financial security of the individuals who provide healthcare. Institutional providers are hiring part time and per diem employees to fill their staffing needs. This leaves many employees without access to health insurance and other benefits.

Healthcare Facilities

Healthcare is the largest industry in the United States and its future depends on its ability to operate as a big business. Healthcare facilities are already experiencing major changes. Integrated healthcare systems exist in almost every part of the country. These systems are conglomerates of smaller hospitals, nursing homes, home and community health agencies, and rehabilitation facilities, which have been built or purchased by investor-owned corporations. These large corporations make a profit for their investors by using the profits from one subsidiary to offset the losses from another. If losses are too great, the corporation may close the facility.

Another concern of healthcare facilities is related to unreimbursed care. Those patients who come to the hospital emergency room with a serious illness must be treated by that hospital. If the patient does not have insurance, the hospital must pay the cost of care. Hospitals that do not have sufficient funds to cover the cost of unreimbursed care will not survive.

In the past 15 years, more than 900 hospitals have closed. While hospitals are closing, the trend toward an increase in the number of nursing homes, home and community healthcare agencies, and other types of healthcare facilities is continuing.

Healthcare Services

One of the major concerns related to the United States healthcare system is access to healthcare services for all citizens. It is likely that we will see more services offered in community health centers. Healthcare services in school-based health clinics will become the rule rather than the exception. Incentives to primary care providers, including nurse practitioners, to practice in underserved geographic areas may help improve the public's access to healthcare.

Healthcare Regulation and Accreditation

As costs continue to rise and as patients continue to express dissatisfaction with the quality of healthcare they receive, more and more regulations will appear. These regulations will most likely be aimed at improving the quality of care through QA programs; containing the cost of care through extensive peer review; determining who healthcare insurance companies are permitted to include and exclude for coverage; and determining where primary care providers are permitted to practice.

The JCAHO, CHAP, HCFA, and other accrediting agencies are continually revising their standards for accreditation. Recent revisions of their accreditation guidelines include standards that show how an organization or facility coordinates and works together to provide efficiency in the care of their patients.

Healthcare Financing

Despite efforts by the federal government to reduce spending for healthcare, costs are continuing to increase. There are several reasons why this trend is difficult to change. One of the most significant reasons for this increase in healthcare costs is the increased number of elderly people in America. In 1994, 3 million people were age 85 or older. By the year 2050, the number of Americans age 85 and older is expected to be about 16 million. Increasing age does not necessarily mean illness, but many older people do have extensive and expensive healthcare needs. Because the primary source of health insurance for the older Americans is Medicare, many are concerned that Medicare funds will be depleted in the near future.

Another factor that is increasing healthcare costs is the increasing number of people with AIDS. In 1985, there were 8249 diagnosed cases of AIDS; in 1993, there were an estimated 1 million Americans harboring the human immunodeficiency virus (HIV). Patients who have AIDS generally require medical care for long periods of time. As the incidence of the disease increases, so too does the cost of caring for these patients. Many health insurance companies will not insure those who have AIDS or HIV, leaving the government responsible for paying for their care.

HMOs, PPOs, and other managed care organizations will continue to attract more and more members. These plans offer preventive and wellness programs which, by keeping people well, have reduced the cost of care for long or chronic illnesses. In 1980, more than 9 million people were enrolled in a HMO; in 1993, more than 45 million people were enrolled in an HMO. Because of lower insurance premiums, it is expected that more and more people will join HMOs, PPOs, and other managed care organizations.

Other factors that contribute to increasing the cost of healthcare include the treatment and care of those with chronic conditions (tuberculosis, kidney disease, heart disease, stroke, and cancer); increasing labor costs; increasing costs of lawsuits; the increasing cost of technology; and the cost of caring for those with no healthcare insurance.

It remains to be seen if the federal government will be able to create an organized healthcare system. It is predicted that without healthcare reform, the economy of the country will collapse under the weight of healthcare costs well before the year 2050.

No matter what direction healthcare reform takes, the goal of the healthcare system in the future will be to provide safe, efficient, and effective care at the least cost and to restore health in the shortest possible time. You will be in a position both to affect and to be affected by changes in the healthcare system. You will affect the healthcare system by the efficiency with which you provide care; you will be affected by what healthcare services you can afford for yourself and your family.

DISCUSSION QUESTIONS/LEARNING ACTIVITIES

1. List as many different facilities as you can where healthcare services are provided. (You might use the telephone directory for additional information.)

2. How is the practice of primary healthcare providers (physicians, nurse practitioners, and hospitals) regulated in your state?

3. Ask the librarian to direct you to the JCAHO guidelines for accreditation of hospitals or long-term care facilities. Briefly scan this document to determine the requirements for accreditation.

4. Try a short peer review after your next clinical day. Ask one of your classmates to evaluate your performance during the day. How does your classmate's assessment of your performance compare with facility standards and with your standards?

5. Ask some of your family, friends, or relatives to describe their healthcare insurance. Do they know what services are excluded? How much does their insurance cost, and does their employer pay any part of the cost?

6. Discuss the DRG method of payment for healthcare with your classmates. What are the advantages and disadvantages of this system to both the patient and the healthcare provider?

7. List some of the ways you can directly contribute to controlling healthcare costs, both as a nurse and as a consumer of healthcare.

READ MORE ABOUT IT

Best EJ: The Assurance of Quality in Health Care, First Edition. London: Pergamon Press, 1996.

Ellis JR, Hartley CL: Nursing in Today's World: Challenges, Issues, and Trends, Fifth Edition. Philadelphia: JB Lippincott, 1995.

Harrington N: Health Policy and Nursing: Crisis and Reform, First Edition. Boston: Jones-Bartlett, 1994.

Jonas S: An Introduction to the U.S. Health Care System, Third Edition. New York: Springer, 1991.

Kalisch PA, Kalisch BJ: The Advance of American Nursing, Third Edition. Philadelphia: JB Lippincott, 1995.

Kos-Munson B: Who Gets Health Care? An Arena for Nursing Action, First Edition. New York: Springer, 1993.

Lee DE: The Nation's Health, Fourth Edition. Boston: Jones and Bartlett, 1994.

Raffel MW, Raffel NK: The U.S. Health System: Origins and Functions, Fourth Edition. Albany: Delmar, 1994.

The Healthcare Team

OBJECTIVES

When you complete this chapter, you should be able to:

Describe the function of several healthcare team members.

Define the term "healthcare team" and describe the educational preparation of several of its members.

List the members of the nursing team and describe their major responsibilities related to patient care.

Explain and describe differences in case, functional, team, and primary nursing care delivery models.

Alice parked her car in the lot behind Riverview, the nursing home where her grandmother lived, and hurried inside.

As she approached her grandmother's room, she saw her sister, Jeanne, in the doorway. "They're taking Grandma to the hospital," Jeanne said in a worried voice. "She's having trouble breathing." The two women accompanied the stretcher to the waiting ambulance. The elderly woman's breathing was labored. Alice spoke to the emergency medical technician (EMT) as the stretcher was put into the ambulance. "I'm a licensed practical nurse," she said. "May I go along?" "Sure, get in," the EMT said.

The ambulance delivered Alice's grandmother directly to the emergency department of the hospital. Alice was soon joined by her sister, who had followed in her car. "What's going to happen?" Jeanne asked. She was clearly worried.

"Don't worry," Alice said reassuringly, as she patted Jeanne's shoulder. "Grandma will get the best of care here." The two women went to the admitting office, where a clerk took the necessary information about their grandmother. Then they returned to the emergency department.

"How is my grandmother?" Alice asked one of the nurses on duty.

The nurse smiled. "They took her up to the Coronary Care Unit. It's her heart. The doctor wants to change her medications and monitor her heart rate for a few days." Alice and Jeanne went upstairs. One of the staff nurses was speaking with their grandmother's physician. A lab technician stopped at the nurse's station. He spoke briefly with the unit secretary, who gave him a tray of freshly drawn blood samples. As they spoke, a nursing assistant appeared. He handed a package from the hospital pharmacy to the clerk, who read its label and made a notation on a chart. The doctor left the Unit.

An LPN emerged from a room down the hall carrying a tray of medications. A maintenance worker, pushing a repair cart, hurried by. Others moved through the halls, each with a task to do.

Jeanne watched all the activity in amazement. "Is it like this every day?" she asked.

Alice shook her head. "No," she said. "Some days it gets busy!" A week later the sisters met again at the hospital. This time they were taking their grandmother home. Not to Riverview, but to Alice's home. A home care plan had been arranged through the hospital's social service department.

"Is this something special they did because you're a licensed practical nurse?" Jeanne asked, as Alice poured tea for her sister and their grandmother.

Alice smiled. "No. It's all a part of a team effort that works inside the healthcare system," she said. She winked at her grandmother, who lay propped up on a rose-colored pillow in bed, and said, "And I'm proud to be a member of the healthcare team."

THE HEALTHCARE TEAM

The term *healthcare team* refers to all of the personnel in all of the departments of a healthcare facility. When we think of people who provide healthcare services, we immediately think of doctors, nurses, x-ray and lab technicians.

But it takes more than doctors and nurses and technicians to provide healthcare services. In fact, the Dictionary of Occupational Titles list over 230 job titles in healthcare. Many healthcare workers specialize in administration, medical records, social services, food services, purchasing, research, education, risk management, management information systems, finance, pharmaceuticals, and building maintenance.

All healthcare facilities, regardless of type, size, sophistication, or service, depend on the people who staff them to deliver healthcare services. The biggest, best-equipped healthcare facility is no better than the team that runs it and delivers care there because healthcare comes from people, not from the tools and technology used to provide it.

The primary function of a healthcare facility is to deliver healthcare services to its patients, clients, or residents. The patient, client, or resident has to be the "center of attention" of everyone who works in that facility. Healthcare workers are individuals who have personal problems and concerns just like everyone else but when they are at work the focus has to be on the patient and his or her needs.

Personal Qualities of Healthcare Workers

In addition to special skills, people who provide healthcare services must have special qualities. They must arrive for work on time and keep personal problems and concerns to themselves. They must like to work with and be able to get along with others. They must be willing to work holidays, weekends, evenings, and nights. Additional qualities are listed in Box 7-1.

A constant assessment of your personal qualities will help you make changes that will enhance your ability to provide the best healthcare possible.

ORGANIZATIONAL ARRANGEMENTS

Every facility has its own specific organizational arrangement. Depending on their size and the services provided, healthcare facilities may have a few or many separate departments. Administrators are responsible for the overall daily operation of the facility while departments provide specific services or functions for the facility. Each department has a manager or department head who is responsible for the operation of his or her department.

BOX 7-1. PERSONAL QUALITIES OF THE HEALTHCARE WORKER

Dependable
Empathetic
Effective communicator
Practices good personal hygiene
Reasonable moral standards
Keeps information confidential
Respects co-workers and patients
Organized
Problem solver
Uses critical thinking skills
Abides by rules and regulations
Honest

Uses good judgment
Concern for others
Patience
Good listening skills
Flexible
Kind
Considerate
Role model
Ethical
Creative
Energetic

An organizational chart shows how the administrator and departments in a healthcare facility relate to one another. Figure 7-1 is an example of how a typical hospital might be organized. To determine who reports to whom, start at the bottom of the organizational chart and work toward the top. This is known as the chain-of-command and it outlines of lines of authority and accountability.

Most healthcare administrators get their authority from a board of directors or a board of trustees. The board members are a group of responsible individuals

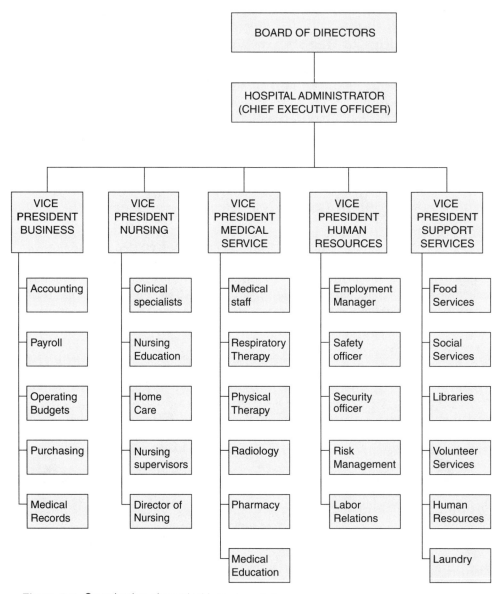

Figure 7-1. Organization of a typical large hospital.

who may or may not have day-to-day involvement with the facility's operation. They set the overall objectives and see that they are carried out. A board of directors has ultimate control of a facility. In some situations, the board of directors may be a group of local people while in the case of an integrated healthcare system, the board of directors may be hundreds or even thousands of miles away.

The administrator of a healthcare facility may have the title of chief executive officer, chief operating officer, director, or president, and is responsible to the board of directors for the facility's overall operation. Educational preparation for this position usually includes advanced degrees in business, management, and finances related to healthcare.

The activities of the healthcare facility are usually divided into several major areas of service. These areas of service include, but are not limited to, business, nursing, medical services, human resources, and support services. These departments are often headed by vice presidents.

Business matters are under the direction of a vice president for business. The person oversees offices that manage payroll, purchasing, accounts payable and receivable, and other areas of operation involving finances. Educational preparation for this position includes advanced degrees in business and accounting.

The nursing department is under the direction of a professional nurse who has advanced degrees in nursing, business, and management. Those who report to the vice president (or director) of nursing may include clinical nurse specialists, nursing supervisors, and nurse educators. Figure 7-2 outlines an organization chart for a typical nursing service department.

The medical services department is under the direction of a physician (or a group of staff physicians). The vice president for medical services oversees all departments that provide medical care in the facility. The heads of each medical specialty department are accountable to the medical director. Educational preparation for the position of medical director is completion of medical school plus several years of experience in practicing medicine.

Other services include human resources and support services. While this organization is typical, it is probably not identical to the organizational chart of the facility to which you are assigned for clinical experience or where you will work.

It is important to understand the organizational chart of the facility in which you work. As a worker, you are expected to follow the chain-of-command and discuss any work-related problems or concerns with the person to whom you report.

MEMBERS OF THE HEALTHCARE TEAM

A healthcare team at a typical facility might include the following (keep in mind that advances in technology continually generate the need for skilled personnel with new job titles):

> Administrator—a physician, nurse, or college graduate with a degree
> in business or hospital administration. This person is often the
> manager or director of one of the several departments in a
> healthcare facility.

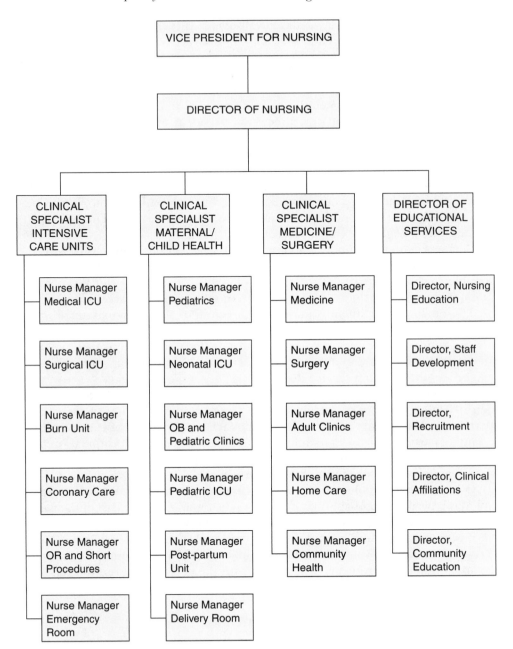

Figure 7-2. Typical organization of a large hospital nursing service department.

Case Managers—most often an experienced professional nurse with additional education related to financing of healthcare. The case manager's job is to monitor a patient's healthcare in an effort to provide safe and effective care and at the same time contain costs.

Case managers may specialize in fields such as geriatrics, pediatrics, obstetrics, or adult health.

Dentist (DDS)—a state-licensed practitioner of dentistry with a 4-year undergraduate degree plus 4 years of dental school. Dentistry is the treatment and prevention of disorders and diseases of the teeth and related structures of the mouth, including repair, replacement, and restoration of teeth.

Dietitian—a 4-year college graduate specializing in dietetics. Dietetics involves food, nutrition, and diet planning and preparation according to sound nutritional principles, especially as they relate to health and disease. A registered dietitian has passed the American Dietetic Association examination and is required to continue related education.

Electrocardiograph Technician—one who is trained in the use of an electrocardiograph (ECG), a device used to record heart muscle activity to detect cardiac (heart) problems or to monitor the heart activity of patients known to have cardiac problems.

Health unit coordinator—sometimes called unit secretaries, work under the supervision of the nurse manager or charge nurse. Their duty is to manage the clerical work at a nursing station.

Laboratory Assistant—one trained to perform simple laboratory tests and procedures; usually a high school graduate. Laboratory technicians and technologists may be required to have a college degree and, in some states, certification and licensure.

Licensed Practical/Vocational Nurse—a state-licensed graduate of an approved LP/VN program, which is approximately 1 year in length.

Medical Doctor (MD)—is a state licensed graduate of 4 years of college and 4 years of medical school. After an internship of 1 year and a residency of up to 5 years, the MD can enter practice. A general practitioner or primary care physician is a nonspecialist who provides general healthcare.

Medical Technologist (MT-ASCP)—a person trained and certified to work in a medical laboratory under a pathologist's supervision. A medical technologist has a minimum of 4 years of college education plus 1 year of training approved by the American Medical Association. MTs are certified by the Registry of Medical Technologists of the American Society of Clinical Pathologists (ASCP) after successfully passing the required exam.

Nurse Aide/Nurse Assistant—a person who receives instruction either on-the-job or in the classroom. Primary function is to assist the nursing team with patient care.

Nurse Practitioner (NP)—a registered nurse who has advanced education in a specialty such as geriatrics, obstetrics, pediatrics, oncology, school health, or adult health. Nurse practitioners may be primary care providers who work independently or with a physician. In about 20 states, NPs are permitted to write prescriptions and order diagnostic tests. NPs who pass a certification test such as those offered by the American Nurses Association are permitted to use the title, Registered Nurse, Certified (RN C) after their name.

Occupational Therapist—one who has a minimum of 4 years of college education and helps patients readapt to daily life after illness or injury.

Optometrist (OD)—a licensed specialist in eye examination and prescribing and fitting eyeglasses.

Osteopathic Physician, Osteopathic Surgeon (DO)—a physician trained and licensed in osteopathy, a practice of medicine that emphasizes the role of the body's organs, muscles, and skeletal system in treating disease.

Pathologist—a licensed physician who specializes in the nature and causes of disease.

Pharmacist—one who has a bachelor of science (BS) degree with several additional years of college, and who is a licensed and registered specialist in compounding and dispensing medications.

Physical Therapist—one who has a minimum of 4 years of college education and works with patients to regain full physical function through exercise, massage, and other techniques, after illness or injury.

Physician's Assistant (PA)—one who is specially trained to provide assistance to a physician under the physician's direction and supervision; also called physician's associate, medex, or medic. Most PAs practice primary healthcare.

Podiatrist (DSC, PODD)—a graduate (usually 6 years of college) licensed to specialize in the treatment of foot disorders.

Psychologist—a graduate (master's or doctoral degree) who specializes in diagnosis, treatment, and counseling of patients with mental, emotional, or emotionally caused physical problems.

Radiologic Technologist (RT)—one trained in the use of x-ray equipment, fluoroscopy, radiation therapy, and the administration of radioisotopes.

Registered Nurse (RN)—a graduate of a diploma, associate degree, or baccalaureate programs with a major in nursing. Graduates are qualified to apply for the licensing exam to become a registered nurse. The registered nurse is also known as the professional nurse.

Respiratory Care Practitioner (RCP)—a graduate of a 2-, 3-, or 4-year approved program that provides training in the use of gases, drugs, and equipment under medical supervision to restore normal pulmonary function in patients recovering from illness or injury. More than 45 states require licensure of RCPs.

Risk Manager—often an experienced professional nurse who has specialized training in how to identify and correct situations that may make the healthcare facility "at risk" for unnecessary or avoidable costs such as lawsuits from personal injury or malpractice.

Social Worker—one who has a minimum of 6 years of college education and helps patients and their families adjust to personal problems.

Unit manager—a person in charge of the clerical management of several units who works under the supervision of a hospital administrator.

Accountants, attorneys, human resources managers, and a variety of others fill out the staff of a large healthcare facility.

THE NURSING TEAM

A nursing team may have many or few members and varies from institution to institution. Regardless of the number of people on the team, each person is responsible for his or her own performance. It is each member's personal obligation to do the assigned work at or above accepted standards of practice for healthcare workers at his or her level of education and competence. Education should not be confused with competence. A job title or assignment to perform a specific task does not necessarily qualify that person to do it.

On the other hand, someone with the required skill to do a procedure does not automatically have the right to do it. Because you are personally and legally responsible for what you do at all times, for your own protection and the protection of your patient and employer, never perform nursing acts beyond your competencies.

How the nursing team is organized will vary from facility to facility. It will be your responsibility to learn the organization of the nursing department where you are employed and to conform to the lines of authority and responsibility it sets. An example of the organization of a nursing department is shown in Figure 7-3.

A typical nursing department is headed by a director of nursing (or vice president or administrator) who is in charge of all nursing services.

Clinical Nurse Specialists

Many larger healthcare facilities hire clinical nurse specialists who are specially trained and certified registered nurses to work with nurse managers to plan care and solve clinical problems related to their patients. There are nearly 30 organizations that offer certification in specialty areas for nurses. To be certified, a nurse must meet the certifying agency requirements for education, experience, and continuing education and must pass a competency examination.

The Society of Gastroenterostomal Assistants offers certification of licensed practical/vocational nurses in this specialty. The National Council of State Boards of Nursing in cooperation with the National Association for Practical Nurse Education and Service provides a certification exam for licensed practical/vocational nurses who want to demonstrate their competency in long-term care.

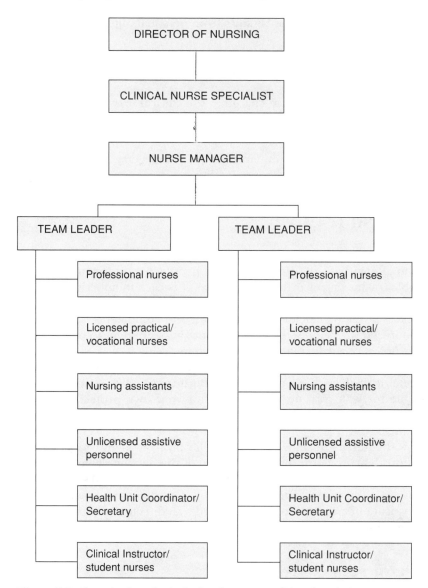

Figure 7-3. Organization of a typical patient care unit in a hospital.

Nurse Managers

Nurse managers (also know as head nurses or charge nurses) are registered nurses who are appointed to their job by the director of nursing and are responsible for directing those working under their authority.

Nurse managers generally have the responsibility for planning, supervising, and evaluating nursing care in a single patient-care unit, such as the emergency department, obstetrics, or the surgical unit. They are also responsible for managing their own budget, hiring staff, and work schedules. In large nursing units, assistant nurse managers or charge nurses may assume some of the responsibilities of the nurse manager.

Professional Nurses

Professional nurses, or staff nurses, are RNs who usually have direct responsibility for patient care. Typical functions of a staff nurse include assessing a patient's physical and psychological condition; administering medications; monitoring vital signs; providing personal hygiene; teaching patients and families; and carrying out treatment regimens. In addition, staff nurses develop nursing care plans based on nursing diagnoses and collaborate with physicians to resolve medical problems. Staff nurses collaborate with their nurse manager and clinical coordinator to solve nursing problems.

The staff nurse is a patient advocate and, as such, communicates with other hospital departments to meet the many needs of a person receiving services in the healthcare system.

Licensed Practical/Vocational Nurses

Under the supervision of other licensed personnel, LP/VNs provide nursing services for which they are licensed and qualified. The source of supervision is clearly defined in the nurse practice acts of the state in which each practical/vocational nurse works. Many state nurse practice acts require that LP/VNs work under the direct supervision of a licensed physician, professional nurse, or dentist.

LP/VNs working as a member of the nursing team are expected to be a contributing member of the team. Providing direct patient care and assisting the professional nurse in meeting the needs of the patients in a particular healthcare facility requires excellent communication and observation skills. The beginning skills of the LP/VN were discussed in detail in Chapter 4.

Nursing Assistants

Nursing assistants, as members of the nursing team, help RNs and LP/VNs by providing basic nursing care to patients. Nursing assistants may also be called aides, orderlies, or attendants. Their functions generally include making beds; assessing temperatures, pulses, respirations, and blood pressures; filling water carafes; distributing and collecting meal trays; and feeding some patients.

Nursing assistants who are employed in long-term care facilities that receive Medicare funds must complete a state-approved course of classroom and clinical instruction and must pass a written and performance examination. Those who pass the examination are listed on the nurse aide registry of the state in which they passed the examination.

Unlicensed Assistive Personnel

Unlicensed assistive personnel (UAP) are those who are taught to perform specific tasks associated with patient care. Some of their duties include making beds, taking vital signs, feeding patients who need assistance, and bathing patients. Licensed nurses are legally responsible for making sure that the UAP is capable of safely performing the tasks they are assigned. The delegation of duties to UAPs will be discussed in more detail in Chapter 13.

Health Unit Coordinators

Health unit coordinators or unit secretaries provide secretarial services for a particular nursing unit. Their duties include answering the telephone, preparing patient charts, accessing information through the computer network, ordering equipment and supplies, and serving as a receptionist. In some healthcare facilities, unit clerks transcribe doctor's orders.

Student Nurses

Student nurses, whether in a professional or a practical/vocational nursing education program, learn clinical skills under the instruction of a clinical instructor. The clinical instructor, in turn, works closely with the nurse manager and other members of the nursing team. Clinical instructors are legally responsible for the actions of their students and, for this reason, are careful to observe and evaluate student performance.

Student nurses do not replace staff nurses and LP/VNs on the nursing team, but they are a part of that team. As a part of that team, student nurses are expected to provide safe and competent patient care. Student nurses are expected to seek the assistance of their clinical instructor when questions regarding patient care arise.

Multiskilled Workers

This is a controversial concept that some healthcare administrators believe will reduce the cost of hiring additional staff and at the same time provide needed care.

A multiskilled worker is a person who has completed the educational and, if required, licensing requirements for a specific job. Through crosstraining, this person is given additional training in skills that are not a part of their basic job. For example, through crosstraining, a unit secretary may be taught to perform electrocardiograms, draw blood samples, and take and record vital signs.

What effect multiskilled workers will have on who provides healthcare remains to be seen. Issues related to these workers involve state licensure laws, definitions of scope of practice, and regulation of the length and content of crosstraining educational programs. For these reasons, nursing organizations, without exception, are opposed to the use of multiskilled workers in healthcare facilities.

MULTIDISCIPLINARY TEAM

As managed care continues to prove that this approach reduces the costs of healthcare, multidisciplinary teams are becoming the rule rather than the exception.

A multidisciplinary team includes a number of healthcare workers who work together to solve problems, increase efficiency, decrease the length of stay, and enhance the quality of care. This team provides a single point of contact for the patient. The team provides information to the patient on all of the treatment options for a particular illness, as well as rehabilitation and after care.

Which healthcare providers are included on this team depends on the patient's diagnosis, as well as on his or her other healthcare needs. Multidisciplinary team members may include physicians, clinical nurse specialists, social workers, physical therapists, dietitians, home health nurses, and hospice nurses,

NURSING CARE DELIVERY METHODS

Methods of providing nursing care can be divided into a number of different types or methods to ensure the highest level of care performed in the most efficient and economical manner. The method used by one facility may differ from that of another. Which method of nursing care an institution will use is based on the availability of staff and equipment, size and nature of the physical plant, and administrative and nursing philosophies.

As a student and later when you enter practice, you will most likely be assigned to a unit where one of the following general nursing care delivery methods is followed: (1) case method, (2) functional nursing, (3) team nursing, and (4) primary nursing.

Case Method

The case method is the oldest approach to nursing care delivery. In this method, the nurse is responsible for the entire care of one or more patients for one shift in a 24-hour period. This method is frequently used in intensive care units, home care nursing, and is always used in private duty nursing. It is often the method used with student nurses during their clinical experience.

Functional Nursing

Functional nursing is a system in which each nursing team member is assigned a specific function or task. For example, one team member takes the vital signs of all the patients on the unit, other team members make all the beds, and so forth. Functional nursing is sometimes efficient but it is a fragmented approach to patient care. Patients often have a difficult time establishing a relationship with the nursing team because so many members of the team are responsible for their care.

Team Nursing

Team nursing, instituted in the mid-1950s, was intended to minimize the fragmentation associated with the functional nursing method of patient care. The team consists of a team leader, who is usually a professional nurse, staff nurses, LP/VNs, and auxiliary personnel (such as aides and orderlies). A patient unit may have two or more teams, each having responsibility for the nursing care of 10 or more patients. The team members work together to combine their diverse educational preparation to benefit their group of patients. Team conferences are held to develop individual patient-care plans.

Primary Nursing

The most recently developed nursing care delivery method is called primary care. In primary nursing, a professional nurse has total responsibility for a particular patient or group of patients 24 hours a day, 7 days a week, for the entire time the patient is in the hospital through discharge. This model's purpose is to provide continuity and coordination of care.

When the primary nurse is not physically present in the healthcare facility, patient care is provided by an associate nurse. The associate nurse may be a professional nurse or a licensed practical/vocational nurse.

Functions of a primary nurse include an performing an admission assessment; developing, planning, implementing, and revising the nursing care plan; directing care in his or her absence; collaborating with physicians and families; making referrals; teaching health concepts; and making discharge plans.

DISCUSSION QUESTIONS/LEARNING ACTIVITIES

1. Using the hospital in which you will receive the primary portion of your medical and surgical clinical experience, find out how many different job titles there are.

2. Complete the same information requested in Question 1 for a local nursing home.

3. In addition to those members of the healthcare team discussed in this chapter, how many additional members can you list? Also list their educational preparation and their major function.

4. Obtain an organizational chart for the nursing service department in one of the healthcare facilities to which you are assigned. How do the job titles of the various members of the nursing department differ from those in Figure 7-2?

5. What nursing care delivery method is used in your clinical affiliation? Is this the same method used in all patient-care units in the facility?

READ MORE ABOUT IT

Ellis JR, Hartley CL: Nursing in Today's World: Challenges, Issues, and Trends, Fifth Edition. Philadelphia: JB Lippincott, 1995.

Fisher ML: Quick Reference to Redesigning the Nursing Organization, First Edition. Albany: Delmar, 1996.

Flarey DL: Redesigning Nursing Care Delivery: Transforming Our Future, First Edition. Philadelphia: JB Lippincott, 1995.

Kendrick K: Innovations in Nursing Practice, First Edition. San Diego: Singular, 1996.

8

Cultural Diversity

OBJECTIVES

When you complete this chapter, you should be able to:

Explain why an understanding of cultural and ethnic influences is important for nurses.

Give examples of cultural and ethnic characteristics that may influence individual or family healthcare practices.

Describe ways in which a nurse can communicate with someone who does not speak or understand the language well.

Discuss the possible influences of religious convictions on an individual or family's healthcare practices.

Identify some ways to incorporate cultural differences in your nursing care plan.

As Mr. Thompson walked into the classroom, the noise was so loud that he could hardly hear himself think. "What is all this noise about?" he shouted.

As the class quieted, he asked Kim Yoo to explain the reasons for the loud and noisy "discussion." Kim, a first generation immigrant from Vietnam, said "We were just talking about the classes we had this week on maternal-child health." "So why does that have everyone in such a turmoil?" asked Mr. Thompson.

"Well," said Kim, "I think it is all my fault. I started it." "Why is that, Kim?" "Remember when you said sexual intercourse was not harmful to the fetus? I said that my family believes that if people have sexual intercourse during pregnancy, the mother and the baby might die." Mr. Thompson, recognizing that there are many cultural and ethnic beliefs and customs associated with pregnancy, decided to ask the class to share some of their customs and beliefs with the rest of the class.

Reluctantly, Ruth Cordova, whose parents moved to the United States from Puerto Rico a few years ago spoke. "I don't know about sex being dangerous during pregnancy but when you explained cord care for the newborn—well, that's not how we do it." "How do you do it, Ruth?" asked Mr. Thompson. Ruth seemed hesitant but she finally explained that everyone she knows puts this special oil on the cord and wraps a belly binder around the baby's stomach. "Doing it this way is suppose to give the baby a nice belly button and keep it from getting a hernia," she said.

"Would anyone else like to add anything to this discussion?" asked Mr. Thompson.

Charles Freeman, who could trace his family to a 17th century Southern plantation, spoke. "My great grandmother, my grandmother, and my mother all had a special treatment for colic in newborn babies. They would feed the baby a mixture of 2 or 3 drops of turpentine in a bottle of water and just like magic, the colic stopped." "I sure am glad you started this discussion, Kim!" said Mr. Thompson. "When we talked about maternal-child health, we only talked about the dominate cultural practices in the United States. This discussion should help us all become more aware of cultural differences and their importance to our practice of nursing." Continuing the discussion, Mr. Thompson said, "Some practices, such as the one Charles described, are unsafe and could seriously harm the baby. The practice of putting oil on the baby's cord and covering it could lead to infection. And in the belief Kim described, the woman who did have sexual intercourse during pregnancy and lost the baby before term would probably suffer a great deal of guilt, remorse, and shame."

Mr. Thompson continued. "Whether we consider a patient's beliefs to be based on old wives tales, voodoo, magic, witchcraft, will of the spirits, or fate, we must first know what the patient believes. When we know what the patient believes, we can then work to use those beliefs as well as medical facts to find a way to respect cultural beliefs and practices and at the same time help the patient comply with treatments and procedures that will improve or at least not harm that person's health. This is what transcultural nursing is all about."

UNDERSTANDING YOUR PATIENTS

The United States is a country to which people from all over the world continue to immigrate. As a result, it is a country rich in diverse cultural and ethnic groups. It is estimated that there are more than 150 different ethnic groups and more than 500 tribes of Native Americans in the United States.

It is likely that you will be directly responsible for caring for patients from diverse cultural and ethnic backgrounds during your career as a nurse. One of the ways to fulfill that responsibility is to understand your patients as completely as you can.

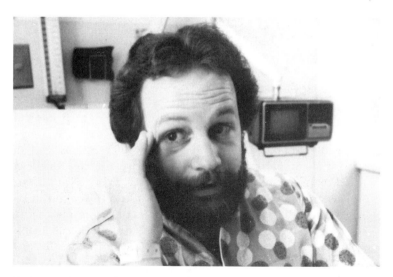

Understand your patients as completely as you can.

As a nurse, you will always have to be on the alert to treat each of your patients as an individual with individual needs, but an understanding of cultural and ethnic differences among groups of people will give you a foundation upon which to individualize your care.

Cultural Characteristics

Culture refers to values, beliefs, customs, attitudes, roles, and behaviors, that are shared by a large group of people and are passed from generation to generation. From the time a child is born, he begins to learn the culture of his family and as he grows older, the culture of his society. He learns to know what kinds of behaviors are right and what kinds of behaviors are wrong; he learns what attitudes are acceptable and what are not; he learns what is expected of him in his role as child, adult, parent, spouse and worker; and he learns acceptable social behaviors.

Unlike opinions, preferences, and attitudes, which change, cultural characteristics are deeply rooted and are difficult or impossible to alter. They are tightly woven into an individual's personality and character. Your patients reflect their cultural heritage each time they interact with the world around them. In a situation that is alien to them (eg, a healthcare setting), their differences may seem magnified because in stressful situations, most people cling more tightly to what they are familiar with to protect themselves against the unknown.

People's reactions to circumstances vary according to culturally learned behaviors. Customs and values reflect behavior that is correct within a culture. Therefore, behaviors that are correct or expected in one culture may be very different from those of another culture. This is particularly true in the American healthcare system. Many healthcare providers direct their treatment plans toward middle class white Americans. They tend to ignore the cultural diversity of their patients and then wonder why treatment regimes are not followed. Finding ways to incorporate cultural differences in healthcare will result in better healthcare for everyone.

Ethnic Characteristics

Ethnic refers to cultural subgroups. These subgroups, while part of the larger culture, have certain distinguishing characteristics.

An ethnic group shares, for example, food preferences, racial similarities, religious practices, a common ancestry, clothing preferences, language and linguistic styles, and mannerisms. While cultural characteristics vary little, there are wide variations in ethnic characteristics. These variations depend in part on the education of the group, their geographic location, and the number of members in the group. An example is the differences seen between an ethnic group found in the southern part of the United States and one found in the northern part of the United States. Both groups may share similar religious practices, racial characteristics, and mannerisms but they may have different language patterns and accents.

While cultural and ethnic distinctions can be made, they are often studied under the topic of culture. In the context of this book, the term culture includes both culture and ethnic behaviors.

Cultural Assessment

Many healthcare facilities have printed forms (tools) to use to complete a cultural assessment. Find out if your clinical affiliation has a cultural assessment tool and if so, begin using it to develop a better understanding of cultures other than your own. If your clinical facility does not have a cultural assessment tool, "Andrews/Boyle Transcultural Nursing Assessment Guide" (Appendix I) is excellent.

When collecting information for a cultural assessment, it is important to use common sense and good interviewing skills. Much of the information about a person's values and beliefs related to healthcare and religion can be obtained informally through conversation. Some information such as folk remedies that have been tried can only be obtained through a formal interview. Other information about a person's culture may be irrelevant to the situation and should not be requested.

It is impossible to completely know every cultural variation of the people for whom you will care. The best way to provide culturally appropriate healthcare is to use an assessment tool and to involve your patient and his or her family in determining the plan of care. If a treatment, medication, diet, or procedure is unacceptable, it will be necessary to work with that patient to find an alternative that will be acceptable.

Language

Language is common to everyone but not everyone shares the same language. Differences in language and how words are used can lead to misunderstanding. When a patient speaks a different language or English is not the native language, it does not mean the patient's needs are different, only that the language is different.

When a patient's language difference is enough to seriously limit communication and understanding, take the time to clarify that you understand what the patient is trying to communicate. In addition, give the patient an opportunity to let you know that you are being understood. If necessary, obtain an interpreter or family member to assist in communicating with the patient because not being understood and not understanding what is being done to you and why can be a very frightening experience.

Since much of our communication is nonverbal, you can provide reassurance and comfort without using the spoken language. A smile and a gentle touch will go a long way toward comforting those who do not understand the spoken language.

Race

The federal government defines five major racial groups: white, African-American, Asian/Pacific Islander, Hispanic, and American Indian/Alaska Native. Distinctions among races are physical, such as skin color, eye shape, hair color and texture, nose and lip shape, and stature.

While a person's race does predispose him or her to certain diseases, nurses must recognize that race is only a physical distinction. Knowing the race of a person will not assist you to better understand a person's cultural or ethnic background.

The Elderly

In about 4 years, approximately 6.5% of the population of the United States will be age 75 or older. As people grow older, they tend to have a more frequent need

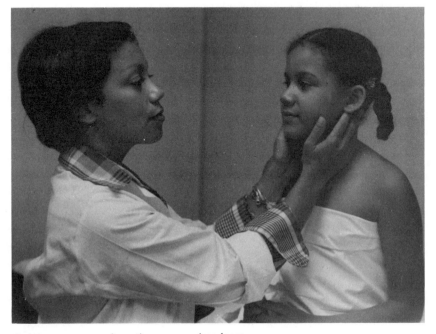

Quiet reassurance from the nurse calms fears.

to seek healthcare. Whether the ill elderly seek healthcare or not is often based on cultural values. Some believe that to get old is to get sick and that nothing can be done for them. Other cultures stress the value of healthcare and its members make every effort to maintain their health.

In some cultures, the elderly are respected for their age and wisdom. In others, the elderly are often treated with disrespect, ignored, and even abused. In some cultures, it is the absolute responsibility of the family to care for the ill elderly at home while members of other cultures do not feel the same sense of responsibility.

If the culture of the older family member requires that younger female family members care for them and the younger family members have their own families and job responsibilities, the potential for a conflict in cultural values is a real issue.

Recognizing the vast array of cultural variations in the role of the elderly person in the family will help you as you learn to work with families to solve these problems.

Childbearing

There are many cultural variations related to pregnancy and childbirth. To avoid deformities and even the death of a fetus, some cultures believe that certain foods should not be eaten during pregnancy; others believe that photographs should not be taken of the mother. Some believe that the mother should not witness any emotionally upsetting event; others believe that sexual intercourse should be avoided during pregnancy. The list of do's and don't's for the pregnant woman goes on and on and is as varied as the cultures in which the mothers live.

In many cultures, the anatomical position for delivery is squatting or sitting. In the Anglo-American culture, until very recently, the position for delivery was supine. In some cultures, the father is not expected nor even wanted during the delivery process; in others, the father is a part of that process. In many cultures, lay women or midwives deliver the baby at home; in others, the delivery occurs in a hospital or a birthing center.

How the infant is treated immediately after birth also depends on the cultural background of the parents. In some cultures, the infant is immediately given to the mother and in others the baby is placed in a bassinet and cared for by someone else. How the cord is cared for, how the episiotomy is managed, whether the baby is breast or bottle fed, and when the baby begins to eat foods all depend on the culture into which the child is born.

Behaviors surrounding pregnancy, birth, and childrearing are culturally learned and personal to the parents. If, in your practice as a nurse, you encounter people from cultural groups other than your own, you must learn as much as you can about their childbearing practices so that family's culture will be included in your plan of care.

Religion

Religion is an area of individual preference and a part of a person's culture that must be accommodated in any healthcare setting. It can be an especially sensitive issue because religious beliefs are among the most fundamental beliefs people have. People facing immediate questions of health, life, and death will frequently turn to their religion for answers. Circumstances in a hospital, nursing home, or other healthcare setting can make it difficult for patients to continue their religious practice. No one should stand between the patient and his or her beliefs. Patients should be given every opportunity possible to practice or express their religious beliefs and rituals. This includes extending an open mind and every courtesy to the patient's priest, minister, rabbi, or other religious representative.

The three major faiths by population in the United States are Catholicism, Protestantism, and Judaism. There are many other religions that are not as large in numbers but are just as significant to those who practice them. It is important to remember that to each of your patients, their religion is "the" religion. Remember, too, that many people do not belong to organized religious groups and may do not practice or acknowledge any established religion. This does not mean they are antireligion or not religious.

Although you cannot be expected to know all the differences among the more than 1200 religious organizations in the United States, it will be helpful to you to become acquainted with basic religious convictions of a few. Religious practices of the three major U.S. faiths, as well as some others, are described below. To facilitate the practice of lesser known religions, your patient will probably be the best source of information.

Catholicism

The basic tenet of the Catholic religion is that God, as Jesus Christ, lived and died as a human being so that all of humankind can attain eternal salvation. Various rites known as sacraments (sacred) are performed at appropriate times by Catholics priests. Among the sacraments you may encounter in a healthcare setting are Baptism, Anointing of the Sick, Eucharist, and Reconciliation.

Baptism is administered only once in a Catholic's life. The parents of a hospitalized infant who has not been baptized may request that a priest perform this sacrament in the hospital.

The Eucharist is also called the Holy Eucharist or Holy Communion. A patient preparing to take this sacrament is required to abstain from food or drink for an hour before the rite, although water and medications are allowed at any time. If a patient is unable to attend church or chapel, the Eucharist may be brought to him or her. Also, if a patient requests the Eucharist preceding surgery, inform your supervisor, the chaplain, or the patient's priest.

Reconciliation is a rite for the forgiveness of sins. The patient's confession is heard by a priest, who then pronounces absolution. It is a private matter and should be respected as such.

The Sacrament of the Sick, in which the patient is anointed with holy oil, is frequently misinterpreted as the "last rites" given to someone facing imminent death. This is not the case, and most Catholic families understand this. However, assurances to the patient's family and others that the sacrament is intended for restoration of physical and spiritual health and is not a preparation for death will help dispel fear and misunderstanding.

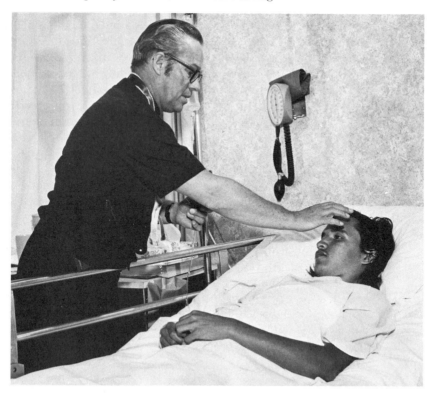

The sacrament for the sick, administered by a Catholic priest, provides comfort.

Protestantism

Hundreds of separate denominations and sects constitute the faith known as Protestantism. Some of these denominations include Baptists, Episcopalians, Lutherans, Methodists, Presbyterians, members of the United Church of Christ, Mennonites, and Seventh-Day Adventists. A number of their practices differ, although they share many others in common.

Baptists do not practice infant baptism. For them, baptism is a rite to be given only after a believer confesses his or her faith. They believe that this can be done only by someone who is old enough to understand the significance of baptism. Baptism is performed by full immersion in water rather than by sprinkling.

Episcopalians have a number of similarities with Catholics, including Reconciliation, Anointing the Sick, Holy Communion, and Baptism, although each differs somewhat. Anointing the Sick, for example, is more often given as a healing sacrament, although it is also administered to those facing death. Episcopalians believe that a dying infant should be baptized, following a ritual similar to that described for Catholics. The usual administration of these sacraments is by Episcopal priests.

Lutherans practice baptism of children and adults by sprinkling. They also celebrate Communion, at which they believe Christ is present in spirit. Personal faith plays an essential role in their religion, which holds that Christ is both God and man.

Methodists acknowledge the baptismal rites of other religions and practice both infant and adult baptism by sprinkling and by immersion in water. For them, religion is a matter of personal belief; they use conscience as a guide for living.

Communion (at which Christ is believed to be present in spirit) and baptism (generally by sprinkling) are also practiced by Presbyterians. Salvation is believed to be a gift from God.

Members of the United Church of Christ practice infant baptism and Communion.

Seventh-Day Adventists do not believe in infant baptism. They practice public and private worship, as well as private and group Bible reading. They are generally vegetarians, although some may eat meats that are specified in the Bible. This preference should be respected in the healthcare setting and notification given to your supervisor or to the dietary department.

Judaism

Judaism, which is the religion and a way of life for Jewish people, is based on the five books of Moses called the *Torah*. Culture and religion are deeply intertwined in the Jewish faith. As a result, ritual, tradition, ceremony, religious and social laws, and the observance of holy days (holidays) are often major influences in Jewish daily life.

There are three groups in Judaism: Orthodox, Conservative, and Reform. Although all share the fundamental teachings of Judaism, they vary in how strictly they follow the traditions. Orthodox Jews are the strictest in following Jewish tradition. The Conservative group is less strict, and the Reform group even less rigid. The rabbi is the spiritual head of a Jewish congregation and is the representative to inform when a patient of the Jewish faith requests it.

Because there are wide differences among Jews in the observance of customs, rituals, and laws of Judaism, ask your Jewish patients what their preferences are. When you show a genuine interest and willingness to personally care for the physical, emotional, and spiritual needs of any patient regardless of their religion, beliefs, or background, most patients will respond.

The Jewish Sabbath, a day devoted to prayer, study, and rest, begins at sunset on each Friday and lasts until sunset Saturday. The Sabbath meal is an important occasion.

Circumcision, a religious custom in Judaism, is performed on male infants 8 days after birth by a pediatrician or a rabbi. In some instances, the procedure is done by Jewish religious representatives specially trained for the ritual. Jewish boys receive their name at this ceremony. Jewish girls receive theirs at their parents' synagogue (house of worship).

Dietary practices vary among the three Jewish groups. These practices are derived from traditional observances dating from early Jewish history. Kosher, meaning clean or fit to be eaten, restrictions apply to meats, fish, and dairy products and to the utensils they are prepared and served in. The dietary department in healthcare facilities will observe these restrictions for your patients when they are informed to do so.

Various procedures regarding death are observed in Judaism, though not all by each of the three groups. Generally, all believe that a dying person should not be left alone. Autopsies and embalming are not allowed by Orthodox and Conservative Jews. Funerals are held on the day after the person dies, before sundown, but burial on the Sabbath and some holidays is not permitted.

Other Religions

Members of other religious groups that you may provide care for include those belonging to the Church of Jesus Christ of Latter Day Saints (Mormons), Jehovah's Witnesses, Islam (Muslims and Black Muslims), Christian Scientists, and Buddhists.

Mormons do not believe in baptizing infants or in the use of tea, coffee, cola drinks, alcohol, or tobacco. Baptism occurs at age 8 when it is believed the child has reached the age of reasoning. Mormons who are worthy to enter the temple wear a special type of underclothing called a garment. Mormons are permitted to remove this garment when necessary healthcare procedures require it.

The Mormon blessing of the sick is performed by two elders. One elder anoints the person with oil while the other elder offers a prayer for healing. During this blessing, both elders place their hands on the head of the patient.

Members of the Mormon Church usually have a number of visitors who represent the church. These visitors are important and you should provide as much privacy as possible.

Jehovah's Witnesses are prohibited from receiving any blood or blood products or from coming in contact with any equipment that has been in contact with the blood of someone else. They also believe that Jesus Christ is King. For that reason, they do not participate in any political activities such as voting, pledging allegiance, or serving in the military.

The religion of Muslims (also, Moslems) is Islam. Islam holds that Allah is the supreme deity and that Mohammed, the founder of Islam, is the chief prophet. Moslems are forbidden to eat pork in any form or to use alcoholic beverages.

Black Muslims are members of the World Community of Al-Islam, a predominantly black religious group. They have strict dietary, dress, and personal relationship codes.

Christian Scientists belong to the Church of Christ, Scientist. There are no ordained or appointed leaders of the church. Many larger cities have Christian Science reading rooms where literature is available to the public.

The basic premise of the Church of Christ, Scientist is that healing, both spiritual and physical, is a result of drawing closer to God in how one lives and thinks. Christian Science practitioners are available to pray with those who are ill for their healing. Christian Science nurses provide the physical care that may be needed for people who are unable to meet their own needs. Most Christian Scientists do not use medications and do not accept blood or blood products. In general, any measures that interfere with the natural progression of life are avoided.

Buddhists believe in Buddha or the "Enlightened One." There are a number of Buddhists sects in the United States, each having some differences from the others. The primary emphasis of Buddhism is for each individual to find what is right and through that discovery, achieve Nirvana or supreme tranquility.

In all religions, the patient's religious representative should always be informed that the patient has entered your healthcare facility when requested by the patient and when circumstances suggest that spiritual counseling is required. The best way to ensure that this important need is not overlooked is to ask the patient what his or her wishes are. It's perfectly appropriate to ask, and it also shows your concern for the whole person beyond his or her immediate physical and medical needs.

Pain

In your experience as a nursing student or as a nurse, you know that people express pain in different ways. There are those who say nothing and refuse medication and those who moan and groan loudly and beg for medication. How one responds to pain is often as much a result of one's culture as it is of one's personality and emotional state at the time.

You will no doubt care for many patients who are in pain. As a nurse, you must be careful to avoid expecting your patients to express their pain in the same way you do. In some cultures, it is considered a weakness to cry when in pain and in others, crying is permitted and even encouraged for even mild pain.

For these reasons, it is important for nurses to consider more than physical expressions to assess pain. A patient may physically appear to be in excruciating pain, however a careful assessment may indicate that a change of position reduced the pain to the point where medication was not needed. On the other hand, a patient who you believe should have some complaints of pain may be lying quietly in the bed. A careful assessment of this patient may reveal rather intense pain.

A good rule of thumb is to ask the patient if he or she is in pain. If the answer is yes, make an assessment and recommend an action. If the patient is not comfortable with your recommendation, it is appropriate to ask what measures he or she would prefer to use to relieve the pain. Narcotics, barbiturates, biofeedback, acupuncture, herbs, guided imagery, religious rituals, and therapeutic touch are just a few of the measures that can be used to alleviate pain.

Nutrition

The *Food Guide Pyramid* published by the United States government identifies the number of servings that should be eaten from each group of food each day. While these guidelines may work well for Anglo-Americans, they are not guidelines that are incorporated by many other cultures.

People in some cultures use various foods to cure illnesses or ward off evil spirits. In some cultures, men and women eat separately and in others, it is unheard of to eat alone.

People in some cultures eat diets high in rice or beans. Some make no distinction between breakfast and dinner foods. Some eat five or six times a day, and others eat every other day.

To assess a patient's diet, it is more appropriate for the nurse to ask what the patient ate and when rather than what he or she ate for breakfast, lunch, and dinner.

Adequate nutrition is important to the healing process. If your patient is not eating, it is necessary to find the reasons. If it is a dislike of the types of foods being served, you might suggest that the dietitian work with the patient and family to find a more agreeable diet.

Death and Mourning

Death is viewed in different ways by different cultures. For some cultures, death is a natural extension of life; for others, it is a time of great loss. Regardless of how death is perceived, all cultures prefer that people who are dying do so with dignity.

Nurses are in a unique position to provide dignity in the last moments of a person's life. Respecting the wishes of the patient and family for privacy; permitting the family to carry out religious or cultural rituals; limiting interruptions; and providing gentle and compassionate care are just a few things nurses can do to help the patient die with dignity.

But not all deaths can be anticipated. In those situations where death is a result of an accident or violence and family members have not had time to prepare, not having a chance to say goodbye to their loved ones is particularly difficult regardless of the cultural background. The nurse can provide support to the family in this situation by providing a private area and offering to contact those who would be able to support the family during a time of crisis.

Care of the body after death is deeply rooted in cultural and religious traditions. In some cultures, there is a ritualistic washing of the body; in others, certain clothing is required for burial; and in others the body is quickly buried. If you are uncertain of how to handle the body after death, ask a family member or a religious representative before doing anything.

Mourning is the cultural expression of grief and all cultures have rituals associated with mourning. The nurse must recognize that his or her own personal ways of mourning are not the only way people mourn the loss of a loved one. Understanding that there are wide variations in how different cultures cope with death and how mourning rituals vary widely within cultures and ethnic groups will help the nurse provide support for the relatives and friends of the deceased.

TRANSCULTURAL NURSING CARE

According to Madeleine Leininger, the goal of transcultural nursing care is to preserve, accommodate, or repattern the culture of the patient. When cultural beliefs and values do not have an effect on care, nurses must make every effort to help the patient preserve his or her culture. For example, a Jewish patient who follows a Kosher diet must have that aspect of his culture preserved.

In some situations, it may be necessary to make accommodations to preserve the culture of the patient and the family. For example, in a culture where the male has no role in homemaking or child care and the female is unable to carry out her duties in the home, a homemaker may provide an accommodation that permits the male and female roles of the culture to be preserved.

Repatterning the culture of the patient requires the patient to essentially change his or her way of life. For example, in a culture where foods high in cholesterol and fat are routinely eaten, the nurse must provide detailed information on how continuing this diet will affect the cardiovascular system. Working with the patient who needs to make such drastic changes requires patience and under-

TABLE 8-1. **Guide for the Assessment of Cultural Manifestations**

I. Brief history of the origins of the cultural group, including location
II. Value orientations
    A. World view
    B. Code of ethics
    C. Norms and standards of behavior (authority, responsibility, dependability, competition)
    D. Attitudes toward:
        1. Time
        2. Work vs. play/leisure
        3. Money
        4. Education
        5. Physical standards of beauty, strength
        6. Change
III. Interpersonal relationships
    A. Family
        1. Courtship and marriage patterns
        2. Kinship patterns
        3. Childrearing patterns
        4. Family function
            a. Organization
            b. Roles and activities (sex roles, division of labor)
            c. Special traditions, customs, ceremonies
            d. Authority and decision making
        5. Relationship to community
    B. Demeanor
        1. Respect and courtesy
        2. Politeness, kindness
        3. Caring
        4. Assertivenesss vs. submissiveness
        5. Independence vs. dependence
    C. Roles and relationships
        1. Number and types
        2. Functions
IV. Communication
    A. Language patterns
        1. Verbal
        2. Nonverbal
        3. Use of time
        4. Use of space
        5. Special usage: titles and epithets, forms of courtesy in speech, formality of greetings, degree of volubility versus reticence, proper subjects of conversation, impolite speech
    B. Arts and music
    C. Literature
V. Religion and magic
    A. Type (modern vs. traditional)
    B. Tenets and practices
    C. Rituals and taboos (eg, fertility, birth, death)

(continued)

TABLE 8-1. (Continued)

VI. Social systems
    A. Economics
        1. Occupational status and esteem
        2.. Measures of success
        3. Value and use of material goods
    B. Politics
        1. Type of system
        2. Degree of influence in daily lives of populace
        3. Level of individual/group participation
    C. Education
        1. Structure
        2. Subjects
        3. Policies
VII. Diet and food habits
    A. Values (symbolism) and beliefs about foods
    B. Rituals and practices
VIII. Health and illness belief systems
    A. Values, attitudes, and beliefs
    B. Use of health facilities (popular vs. folk vs. professional sectors)
    C. Effects of illness on the family
    D. Health/illness behaviors and decision making
    E. Relationships with health practitioners
    F. Biologic variations

From Boyle JS, Andrews MM: Transcultural Concepts in Nursing Care, Second Edition. Philadelphia: JB Lippincott, 1995.

standing on the part of the nurse. As mentioned previously, changing a part of one's culture is not easily done.

Whether preserving, accommodating, or repatterning the culture of a patient, it is essential that the patient be involved in making decisions about his or her healthcare. Nurses who respect cultural differences are more likely to succeed in getting their patients to practice healthier lifestyles. Table 8-1 provides a guide that is useful in assessing a person's cultural characteristics.

SUMMARY

Working with culturally diverse people provides you with great opportunities to grow not only as a person but as a nurse. Learning about the values, traditions, and beliefs of others, finding ways to communicate with people who may not fully understand the language you speak, and helping people retain their culture and at the same time benefit from all of the technology and treatment available in the U.S. healthcare system can be as challenging as it is rewarding.

DISCUSSION QUESTIONS/LEARNING ACTIVITIES

1. Cultural and ethnic differences exist in almost every group. What are some of the cultural and ethnic food and clothing differences of students in your class?

2. How many different religious organizations are there in your community? You might begin by using the telephone directory.

3. Make a list of your beliefs about the things a pregnant woman should and should not do during pregnancy. Then ask someone from a different cultural background than yours to do the same. What are the similarities and what are the differences? Are any of the practices considered unhealthy or dangerous to the baby?

4. Attend a social event being held by a cultural or ethnic group different from yours. What were you able to learn from the experience?

5. Develop a plan to teach a diabetic diet to a person who is not a member of your cultural group. Where can you find resources to help you and the patient select foods that are culturally acceptable and at the same time meet the requirements of the prescribed diet?

6. Practice using the Transcultural Nursing Assessment tool found in Appendix I.

READ MORE ABOUT IT

Barkauskas VH: Quick Reference to Cultural Assessment, First Edition. St. Louis: Mosby, 1994.

Barnum BS: Spirituality in Nursing: From Traditional to New Age, First Edition. New York: Springer, 1996.

Boyle JS, Andrews MM: Transcultural Concepts in Nursing Care, Second Edition. Philadelphia: JB Lippincott, 1995.

Ellis JR, Nowlis EA: Nursing: A Human Needs Approach, Fifth Edition. Philadelphia: JB Lippincott, 1994.

Geissler EM: Pocket Guide to Cultural Assessment, First Edition. St. Louis: Mosby, 1994.

Giger JN, Davidhizar RE: Transcultural Nursing: Assessment and Intervention, Second Edition. St. Louis: Mosby, 1995.

Leininger M: Culture, Care, Diversity, and Universality: A Theory of Nursing, First Edition. New York: National League for Nursing, 1991.

Lindberg JB, et al: Introduction to Nursing: Concepts, Issues, and Opportunities, Second Edition. Philadelphia: JB Lippincott, 1994.

Murray RB, Zentner JP: Nursing Assessment and Health Promotion Strategies Through the Life Span, Fifth Edition. East Norwalk, CT: Appleton & Lange, 1995.

Spector RE: Cultural Diversity in Health and Illness, Fourth Edition. East Norwalk, CT: Appleton & Lange, 1996.

The Patient: Focus of Nursing Care

9

OBJECTIVES

When you complete this chapter, you should be able to:

Illustrate with examples how nurses can create a positive relationship with their patients.

State the purpose and value of visitors in the healthcare facility.

List some of the precautions that must be taken to maintain a safe environment.

Explain the purpose of learning to understand the general needs of various groups of patients.

Identify ways in which nurses can meet the group-specific needs of their patients.

Gwen was aware of the butterflies in her stomach as soon as she opened her eyes that morning. It was her first day on her new job as a licensed vocational nurse, and she had a case of the jitters at the thought of putting into practice all she'd been learning this past year. What if she forgot something? "Maybe if I walk to work it will help calm me down," thought Gwen. "Central Memorial Hospital is only 20 minutes away, and it's a lovely day." Steve Jamison was at his usual spot, watching the neighborhood activity. His wheelchair was drawn up next to his first-floor window so that he could see clearly up and down the street. The disabled man waved to Gwen as she passed. "On your way to school?" he asked.

Gwen smiled. "I graduated last week," she said proudly. "Today's my first day on the job." "Good luck," Steve called after her.

Gwen heard the shouts of children playing as she approached the playground. She stopped for a minute to watch the lively ball game before she continued on.

A dirty, disheveled woman in a ragged coat and floppy sneakers several sizes too large for her was pawing through a trash can on the corner. "That poor woman could certainly use a bath and some tender loving care," thought Gwen. It seemed she saw more and more such people every day, pushing their shopping carts filled with the castoffs of the city, shouting and mumbling in turn to exorcise their particular demons.

Gwen spotted a small crowd outside the Hill Street Clinic, a small neighborhood health facility. A man was handing out flyers to anyone who would accept them. A young woman attempted to enter the building.

"Abortion is wrong," said the pro-life demonstrator, trying to block the clinic door.

The woman shook her head and quickly slipped past the man into the building. Pro-life demonstrations outside the clinic were a daily occurrence.

Further down the street a volunteer sat at a table collecting signatures of passersby. "Please sign the petition to the Governor asking for additional funds for AIDS research. We need more money to help find a cure." The man's words sent a chill down Gwen's spine. "AIDS," she thought, "the twentieth-century plague."

"Excuse me," a wistful voice said. "I'm looking for the day care center." It was a young girl with her small child.

Gwen put her hand on the girl's shoulder. "It's across the street," the young nurse said, pointing to a storefront with a simple sign in the window. The girl thanked Gwen and hurried across the street with the child in tow.

In the next block, softly ringing church bells sounded a counterpoint to the traffic noise. Two elderly women reverently entered St. Mary's Church. On the next corner, a bearded young man wearing a skullcap was sweeping the walk in front of the synagogue. He paused to exchange greetings in Hebrew with another man.

As she reached the entrance to Central Memorial Hospital, Gwen thought, "I wonder who my first patient will be?" She recalled each of the people she had seen as she walked to work. She smiled. "It could be anybody."

NURSE-PATIENT INTERACTION

Medicine has been traditionally involved with the diagnoses and treatment of disease or, in other words, with *curing* disease. Nursing is involved with *caring* for people who have healthcare needs. To care for people or patients in a variety of healthcare settings means many things. It includes the obvious such as performing treatments and procedures, giving medications, assisting with activities of daily living, meeting nutrition and elimination needs, and teaching about self-care. But caring for people or patients goes beyond these technical skills.

A nurse is there when a baby is born; a nurse is there when a diagnosis of terminal illness is given to the patient; a nurse is there when the patient is dying; a nurse is there as the patient regains health. Being involved with people who are experiencing life-altering events creates a special relationship between the nurse and the patient.

Being able to let a patient know that you care about him and how these events are affecting him and his family requires energy, self-understanding, and self-confidence. Without confidence in your ability and a good understanding of yourself, you may be reluctant to use the technical skills you have learned.

Your confidence in yourself and your understanding of yourself will be what cements your relationships with your patients. You will be able to draw on your own feelings of caring and understanding as you relate to your patient as another human being. The nurse who is shy, insecure, self-serving, or more concerned with meeting personal needs than patient needs will not be able to provide the "caring" part of nursing. Your obligation as a nurse is to get the best education you can and to develop a self-awareness that will allow you to interact with your patients as a skilled, empathetic, sensitive, and caring human being.

Sympathy and empathy are distinctly different. Effectively relating to your patients requires that you have a clear understanding of the difference. Empathy is the ability to understand, be aware of, and sensitive to another person's feelings without having those feelings yourself. Sympathy means to share the feelings of others. A nurse who shares feelings of sympathy for patients all of the time will quickly become emotionally exhausted. A nurse who feels empathy will be able to convey sensitivity without the emotional involvement that sympathy requires.

The interpersonal relationships you establish between yourself and your patient can provide great rewards to you in your career as a nurse. Almost anyone can be taught to perform the technical skills your patients will need. But not everyone, and unfortunately not every nurse, will be skilled in providing caring and compassionate nursing care. Work on your caring skills and try to remember that you may be the only person in the healthcare system who is in a position to provide both physical and emotional care.

VISITORS

Most patients in a healthcare facility welcome visitors, but some have no visitors. For those without visitors, you and your co-workers become substitutes for the family, relatives, and friends who might otherwise stop in to see them.

The presence of visitors can have a major effect on the patient's recovery. The effect can be positive or negative. As an objective but concerned party to the patient's welfare, you can influence what that effect will be by creating a positive relationship with your patient's visitors. By being open, friendly, courteous, kind, and otherwise responsive to the visitor's concerns, you will instill a feeling of trust.

Being friendly does not mean that you give up your authority when the patient's best interest is in question. You must remain firm and persuasive when visiting hours are over, when a distraught visitor would do more harm than good, if a scheduled procedure requires visitors to leave the room, and in other situations where your duties supersede visitors' wishes. Yet you must demonstrate your authority in a pleasant way, even when the visitor resorts to unpleasantness.

Always respect your patient's privacy. If your duties can wait until visitors leave, avoid disturbing them. On the other hand, if nursing care is required, you may have to ask the visitors to leave the room. When it is necessary to ask visitors to leave, tell them how long you will be and suggest to them a comfortable place where they can wait. When you are finished, you can let the visitors know that they can return to the patient's room.

Consult with your instructor or facility guidelines regarding policies on visiting hours, when a patient can receive visitors, how many visitors are allowed, and other restrictions.

SAFETY

An irony of a healthcare facility is that people may be in danger by being there. Healthcare facilities are complex. They are filled with people in constant activity and are equipped with machines and electronic devices. A wide variety of combustible materials, including flammable liquids and gases, are everywhere. The potential for an accident or a fire is never far away. Patients, dependent on you and others for their physical safety, are in the middle of it all.

Learn the fire and safety regulations of the facility you serve. Know the locations of all exits. Personally check where fire extinguishers are kept so that you know where to get one if needed. Mention any safety problem, no matter how small, to your team leader. A loose wire, a lamp that sputters, a peculiar smell, a loose bed rail, a slippery spot on the floor, or a machine that feels hot but shouldn't are all significant enough to report.

If you do smell smoke or see flames, immediately follow the procedure set by your facility's regulations. Don't attempt to put out a fire without first informing the appropriate person or giving the required alarm. Don't panic. Your patients will need you in the event an evacuation is necessary.

Other aspects of patient safety may be less apparent but just as important. Be sure the patient has an identification bracelet on the wrist. Check the name on the bracelet to be sure you are administering medications or treatments to the right patient. Be sure that medical supplies are removed after treatments or procedures are completed. A needle or other potentially dangerous piece of equipment left in the patient's bed or room can cause serious injury.

Know whether it is required that bed rails be up for a particular patient. If they are to be up, be sure you leave them up when you leave the patient's room. This is especially true for children in cribs. If the height of the bed is adjustable, be sure it is in the low position before you leave the patient. If restraints are ordered to prevent a patient from injuring himself, be sure they are snug but not too tight. Check the patient frequently to be sure restraints have not constricted circulation.

Clean up spills when they occur. Not only might a spill cause a patient to slip and fall, but nurses and others may also fall. Close doors and drawers when you are finished. Many an injury has been caused by tripping over open cabinet doors or bumping into the corner of an open door.

There are many opportunities in the healthcare facility for accidents to occur. Use common sense, look around you, and accept personal responsibility for correcting situations that could lead to accidents and injury. Don't wait to be told to take action. If a situation is beyond your ability to correct (eg, a frayed electrical cord), be sure you report it to your instructor or other appropriate person. Then be persistent so that the situation that needs correcting is not forgotten.

SOCIAL DIVERSITY

There are a number of groups in our society that have special needs and concerns. The emphasis of Chapter 8 was cultural differences; the emphasis of the remainder of this chapter is differences in social or quasi-social groups.

The Child

Children may experience a lot of fear in their lives because so much of what they do is new to them. Not all fear is registered as open-eyed trembling. In a hospital or other healthcare setting, children may appear to be perfectly normal—sitting quietly or doing just what they've been told to do. Or they may scream and fight any efforts to hold them, especially when facing a procedure that might hurt, such

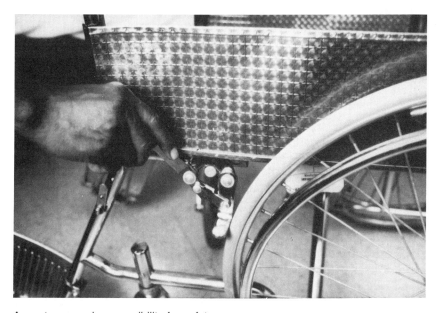

Accept personal responsibility for safety.

as having blood drawn. Whether quiet or screaming, chances are good that children in healthcare settings are generally afraid.

Talking to a child to determine whether he or she is afraid may not work because a young child, or one who is very frightened may not be able to communicate effectively. A nod or a shake of the head from the child will not provide enough information if you have to make a clinical judgment about the child's physical and mental condition.

It is better to assume that a child is afraid and treat the child accordingly than to neglect the possibility. If it turns out the child is not afraid, no harm has been done. If the child is afraid, your actions will help the child deal with his or her fear.

To help children deal with fear, you must try to make them feel secure by being warm, open, friendly, and honest. Although you are not a relative or even a family friend, you may be in an excellent position to help a child ward off or calm fears. Holding, touching, and praising a child, and attempting to reduce fear by quiet reassurance, are the kinds of behaviors a child should get from a parent. When a parent is not present, those needs remain. You may be able to meet at least some of them to a certain extent.

You can be equally important to the child's well-being by establishing good relationships with parents and other family members. A smile, an answered question, reassurance, and a willingness to listen to parents' concerns can help the child learn to trust you.

The Child Who Is Abused

At some time you may find yourself caring for a child who has been abused. Abused children who are hospitalized need more love and attention than any others. They may have an induced fear of adults that could be overwhelming when combined with the normal fear some children have of hospitals and other healthcare facilities. Most states have laws that mandate that physicians, nurses, teachers, and others report suspected child abuse. Consult with your instructor or supervisor when you suspect that a child has been abused. Also learn whether you, when you become licensed, will be obliged to report child abuse.

The Patient Who Is Elderly

An older person is not an old child. And it is inaccurate to use words such as hopeless, obstinate, demanding, confused, irrational, slow, or stubborn to describe older people. While older people are as different from one another as are younger people, there are some physical and social changes that generally tend to affect older people as a group.

It is important to understand that as a consequence of a long life, many changes occur. The older one gets, the more losses one experiences. A partial loss of hearing or reduced vision affects many older people. The incidence of arthritis, osteoporosis, and cardiopulmonary diseases increases with increasing age and can lead to loss of mobility. Other losses may include the loss of a home, driver's license, and the loss of a spouse through death. In general, most elderly people have suffered some losses. Therefore, it is more important than ever for you to

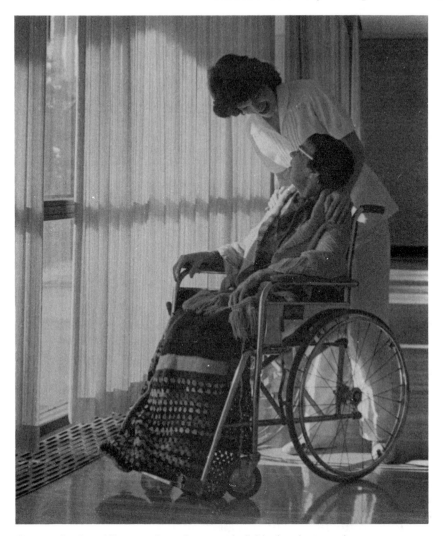

Communication skills are adapted to meet individual patient needs.

treat your older patients in a manner that will reduce further loss. Simple things such as the loss of privacy may not affect a younger patient, but an older patient who loses privacy may be losing one of the few important things he or she has left.

Independence is a strong characteristic of people in a free society. Institutionalization (being hospitalized or confined to a healthcare facility such as a nursing home), by its nature, reduces one's independence. To limit elderly patients' independence further by treating them as though they're unable to do anything for themselves is a serious blow. An older patient may need help, and your responsibility is to provide it. But don't make the assumption that because a patient has gray hair or walks slower than you that that patient is totally dependent. Learn by observing and by asking your older patients what you can do to help them.

For many reasons, the elderly persons you meet in a healthcare facility may show more than average loneliness, depression, confusion, and a sense of being rejected. In many cases, these symptoms have medical causes that can be alleviated. For example, it is not uncommon for elderly persons to neglect their diet. Certain dietary deficiencies can produce depression. Careful assessment may provide clues to the causes of depression.

Elderly persons constitute a highly visible population in healthcare settings and especially in long-term and extended care facilities. The elderly population is growing very rapidly, and the likelihood is that you will encounter more older patients than young ones in your nursing practice. It will be to your benefit to closely study aging and its associated factors.

Greater understanding and knowledge will help improve your relationships with older patients, assist you in making clinical decisions in helping older patients, and increase your career opportunities.

The Patient Who Is Having an Abortion

Abortions are a combination of a physical event (the abortion itself) and the postabortion period that follows. They are often emotionally charged events in a woman's life and can be very upsetting. A nurse caring for an abortion patient should provide extraordinary understanding along with the routine nursing care required.

There are many facets associated with abortion, including legal, medical, religious, social, emotional, family, and other concerns. You are not expected to be a specialist in these areas, but compassionate understanding in all of them is important.

Regardless of your personal feelings about abortion, it is legal in the United States. Although, as a nurse, you are required to provide nursing care, you may be exempt from assisting with this procedure. There are differences in state abortion laws. You can learn what they are in your state by asking your instructor or the legal representative of your healthcare facility after you are employed.

The Patient Who Is an Unmarried Mother

Pregnancies outside of marriage have increased significantly, particularly among adolescents. The phrase "children having children" reflects a real situation. The problems and concerns associated with pregnancy are much greater for young, unwed mothers than for adult women. Not all pregnancies of unmarried girls and women are unwanted, but the majority are.

There are many social implications of unwanted pregnancies, whether they are terminated by abortion or brought to term. The mother, especially the young mother, undergoes a considerable amount of emotional stress. She may face social, family, and personal scrutiny and criticism that can be overwhelming.

Regardless of whether an unwed pregnancy is accepted by the mother (and others) or not, it should be assumed that there may be underlying emotions that the mother, her family, and others associated with her may be feeling but not expressing. You should treat this situation delicately and be prepared to provide understanding and a willingness to listen at any time. Be certain that your instructor is informed of any behavior changes you see in your patient, and if the situation develops beyond your experience or capacity to manage, be sure that a qualified professional is notified.

The Patient Who Is Homosexual

For many years, homosexuality was so carefully hidden that virtually no one could say with certainty who was homosexual and who was not. With the openness that is now common, male and female homosexuals are less likely to hide their sexual preference, although many still do.

A patient may tell you he or she is homosexual, or you may learn it through other sources. The important thing to keep in mind when you are caring for a homosexual patient is that your obligation is to the patient as a person who requires healthcare.

If you have a patient who tells you that he or she is homosexual, acknowledge it and discuss it freely. Let the patient be the guide as to how much discussion is permissible because privacy is a right of all patients. It is particularly important to protect the patient's right to privacy by keeping this information confidential if so requested.

To the homosexual patient, the partner is the significant person in his or her life. You should recognize this relationship and handle it as you would for all of your patients and their families.

The issue of homosexuality has taken on new dimensions as a result of acquired immunodeficiency syndrome (AIDS). Many AIDS patients are homosexual. However, it must be underscored that a patient with this disease is not always homosexual. Heterosexuals, children, hemophilia patients, and intravenous drug users are also AIDS victims. There are no medical or legal distinctions to categorize homosexuals, and you owe it to your patient not to make any of your own.

The Patient Who Is Mentally Ill

Everyone has an emotional and a physical side. When both are in relative balance, a person is considered well. When either one or both are not balanced, a person is ill. Emotional or mental illness is a disease and must be treated as such. There is no place in a healthcare setting for terms such as "crazy," "loony," or "nuts," when one is describing behavior.

There are many healthcare facilities in the United States devoted exclusively to the care and treatment of mentally ill patients. In addition, many hospitals have psychiatric units especially designed to care for those who have mental illnesses.

Even if you don't work in a psychiatric setting, as a nurse, you will surely encounter emotionally disturbed patients. A healthcare facility often has an effect on people's emotional states. For example, someone who is facing a life-threatening situation but who is otherwise emotionally stable may become depressed. A patient who is anticipating major surgery may become extremely anxious. While waiting for test results with lifelong implications, a patient may become withdrawn and uncommunicative. And patients with known psychiatric conditions may get worse, for example, a depression may deepen to thoughts of suicide.

Not all expressions of extreme emotion are clinical, that is, with psychiatrically verifiable pathology (causes). An elderly patient with no relatives, who has no visitors, and spends the day wistfully in her room, may say, "I might as well be dead." Such statements do not always represent feelings of suicide, but they should always be reported to your instructor. Often they are cries for attention. You should not be the one to judge whether a patient's expressions of wanting to die are suicidal or are statements of loneliness.

Sometimes quietly listening to someone who is emotionally distraught is sufficient. Sometimes a gentle touch on the shoulder lets the patient know that there is someone who cares. Sometimes providing the privacy to cry alone is what the patient needs. Sometimes the suggestion of a visit by a clergyperson is helpful to the patient. If these usual nursing measures do not help the patient who is dealing with intense emotions, a psychiatric evaluation may be needed. Again, your instructor or team leader must be informed of your observations and assessments so that appropriate measures can be taken to benefit the patient.

The Patient Who Is Withdrawn

Some patients in a healthcare facility may ask for little or nothing from the nursing staff. But it is a disservice to overlook any patient who isn't clamoring for attention or mentioning a need. For example, an elderly patient who is lying on a painful pressure sore may suffer in silence rather than "impose" on you, or a patient who has soiled the bed may be too embarrassed to ask for help.

To avoid these and other situations in which nursing care is needed but may not be requested by the patient, you must make them understand that you want to help them meet their needs. Let them know that it is okay to tell you what is going on with them, what they need, and what they would like. If you're open and direct with your patients, those who might otherwise go unnoticed will get the full benefit of your care.

The Patient Who Is Hostile

There is another group of patients in healthcare facilities who are anything but unnoticed. They are the opposite of the shy, undemanding patient and may be disruptive as well. The disruption may be merely vocal, or it may also be physical. The solution is not to avoid the demanding shouts, grumbling complaints, or overt physical acts that are meant to get your attention, but to deal with the patient calmly. Avoid either fueling the situation by collapsing to the demands or fanning it hotter by becoming angry yourself.

Disruptive, complaining behavior is often a cry for attention. If you and your instructor can determine the underlying cause and satisfy the need, the patient will probably calm down. Seriously disruptive behavior should be reported because it may indicate deeper problems than just a lack of attention.

When behavior becomes truly abusive or hostile, and you, other patients or staff, or the patient himself is threatened with harm, the matter should be reported immediately to your supervisor. If the behavior is violent, as in the case of someone who is mentally disturbed or who is reacting to alcohol or drug abuse, protect yourself and other patients and call for help at once. Don't attempt to restrain a patient who is violent or threatening violence without qualified assistance.

The Patient Who Abuses Alcohol or Drugs

The substance-abusing patient may have psychological, medical, and legal problems all at the same time. People do not become addicted to drugs for pleasure or because they're thrilled with how their lives are going. They have underlying needs that are being inappropriately met through chemical interventions that eventually become addictive.

Your duty as a nurse is to provide care for any patient regardless of what caused them to need your care. Most people have strong feelings about substance abuse. Yours may be even greater because you know the dangers of substance abuse and you see the end result of years of abuse. You must not let those feelings come between you and your patient, as difficult as this may be.

Substance abuse is a disease and must be treated as such. Sometimes the consequences of a substance abuser's acts may cause outrage, for example, a drunk driver may run over and injure or kill a child. It will take an exceptionally strong commitment on your part, but you cannot turn your back on the abuser, any more than you could turn your back on the injured child.

Any person with a diagnosis of substance abuse needs more care than you alone can give. If your patient is not already under special care for substance abuse, see that such care is given by informing your instructor of the need and by providing information to the patient or the patient's family about where such care can be obtained.

The Patient Who Is Dying

A goal of healthcare is to save lives, but dying and death are facts that cannot be overlooked by healthcare personnel. The number of dying patients that you will care for will depend on the type of work you do after you enter practice. In some fields, death is remote, whereas in others it is a regular occurrence. You may never get used to working with dying patients, but there are ways to make the situation more comfortable for your patients, their families, and yourself.

When you are caring for someone who is dying, the most important thing you can do is to be secure with your own feelings. You must confront your own feelings about death before you can be of much help to others. As difficult as it may be for some of us to accept, death is inevitable. Whenever it occurs, it is usually an emotionally wrenching experience.

Death in a healthcare setting comes in two general ways: expected, as in the case of terminally ill patients, and unexpected, as in the case of accident victims, heart attack victims, and others who, except for the immediate cause, would not have died. The latter group includes patients who die suddenly during an otherwise positive recovery.

Little can be done to prepare for unexpected deaths except to know they will happen, and when they do, to get past your own shock and disbelief so that you can continue to care for your other patients and also provide solace for the deceased's family and friends.

A patient who is known to be dying—as in the case of someone with a long-term illness—will pass through a series of stages that, if completed, will prepare them for death. Dr. Elizabeth Kübler-Ross distinguished five stages of dying in her book *Questions and Answers On Death and Dying.* These stages are denial, anger, bargaining, depression, and acceptance.

The first stage, denial, may last a short or a long time. It expresses the patient's unwillingness to accept a serious illness and its likely consequences.

When the reality of what is happening can no longer be denied, the patient will become angry. This anger may be expressed by being demanding, difficult, critical, and unpleasant. This second stage may be difficult for you to deal with because one reaction to someone who is being objectionable is to respond in the same way. You must not. It is here that your objectivity will get you through. The patient's behavior toward you is not personal, though it may sound that way. Realize that the patient must express this anger to progress toward full acceptance of events he or she cannot control.

As the patient understands more fully that death is inevitable, bargaining for time is a common behavior. This can take the form of making promises to society, to God, to a church, or to someone on the healthcare facility staff. These promises can take any form, but the offer is usually to exchange something (eg, a donation to a cause, a promise to be good) for more life.

When it is even more clear that nothing can be done to change what is happening, the patient may become depressed. This may be expressed through crying, through silence, or by mourning past life events—things that the patient feels should have been done differently or losses already experienced. This kind of depression is similar to that which everyone experiences from time to time. As time passes, the nature of the patient's depression changes as he begins to mourn his own death. It is a grief that cannot be shared, because the dying patient is grieving over the impending loss of everyone, and only someone who is dying can know what that must be like. However, the patient must be allowed to express this grief. You can encourage this expression by making it okay to cry or to talk about this grief if the patient desires.

If the preceding stages are allowed to be completed by the patient, and when denial, anger, bargaining, and grief are finished, the patient may reach the stage of acceptance. Acceptance of death does not mean willingness to die but it does mean the patient is in some way ready.

Dr. Kübler-Ross believes that all patients sense they are terminally ill, even if they have not been told. It is not your responsibility to inform a patient that he or she is dying. However, knowing what the patient has been told about his or her condition will improve your ability to help the patient through the dying process. Ask your instructor or supervisor whether your patient has been told if he or she is dying. If so, you can deal with the situation openly.

In the course of a terminally ill patient's care, you will also get to know family, friends, and other regular visitors. They may rely on you for information, for trust, and as someone to whom they can express their feelings. Your best preparation is to have a thorough understanding of your own feelings and the knowledge that you can interact with compassion and empathy while maintaining the required objectivity that allows you to function efficiently.

SUMMARY

This chapter has provided the foundation upon which you can individualize patient care. Understanding the needs of these groups helps you focus on general needs but you must never overlook the individuality of each patient. Not all unmarried expectant mothers are unhappy, not all substance abusers want help, and not all withdrawn patients will ask for assistance just because you encourage them to do so.

You will be more effective and feel better about the nursing care you provide when you take the time to approach each person under your care as a unique human being with his or her own special needs.

DISCUSSION QUESTIONS/LEARNING ACTIVITIES

1. What are some of the things you could do to make a healthcare facility stay more pleasant for a patient who has no visitors?

2. You see an employee who is waiting for the elevator spill some water on the floor. The employee realizes what she did but the elevator doors open and she gets on the elevator. What should you do?

3. Think about the following situation: A 35-year-old man is admitted to the emergency room of a short-term (acute) care hospital after an automobile accident. He was alone in the car, his family and home are in a city 100 miles away, and he has never been in the hospital before. His most serious injury appears to be a broken leg; however, the doctors are considering the possibility of internal injuries. What do you think some of his thoughts and feelings might be while he is waiting for their diagnosis? How might you as a student nurse help this patient during this crisis?

4. Several special groups of patients were discussed in this chapter. Think of a group not discussed and outline some of the more significant characteristics of that group. What are some of the special nursing considerations for this group?

READ MORE ABOUT IT

Arnold E, Boggs KV: Interpersonal Relationships: Professional Communication Skills for Nurses, Second Edition. Philadelphia: WB Saunders, 1994.
Balzer-Riley J: Communication in Nursing, Third Edition. St. Louis: Mosby, 1995.
Ellis JR, Nowlis EA: Nursing: A Human Needs Approach, Fifth Edition. Philadelphia: JB Lippincott, 1994.
Kübler-Ross E: Questions and Answers on Death and Dying. New York: Macmillan, 1974.
Kübler-Ross E: Living With Death and Dying. New York: Macmillan, 1981.

Lipkin GB, Cohen RG: Effective Approaches to Patient's Behavior, Fourth Edition. New York: Springer, 1992.

Milliken ME: Understanding Human Behavior, Fifth Edition. Albany, NY: Delmar, 1993.

Purtilo R, Haddad A: Health Professional and Patient Interaction, Fifth Edition. Philadelphia: WB Saunders, 1996.

Sundeen SJ, et al: Nurse-Client Interaction, Fifth Edition, St. Louis: Mosby, 1994.

Tamparo CD, Lindh W: Therapeutic Communications for Allied Health Professionals, First Edition. Albany: Delmar, 1993.

10

Ethical Issues in Healthcare

OBJECTIVES

When you complete this chapter, you should be able to:

Define the word "ethical."

Describe what is meant by individual, societal, and situational ethics.

Explain why a study of ethics and ethical behavior is important in nursing.

State the purposes of a code of ethics.

Paraphrase the NFLPN and the NAPNES statements regarding ethical behavior of practical/vocational nurses.

Explain personal responsibility and accountability as it relates to ethical behavior.

Outline the process for making decisions related to ethical dilemmas.

Debate the pros and cons of a contemporary ethical issue in healthcare.

> Jim and Jeannie started practical nursing school 2 months ago. They were already good friends, and they often studied together. Jim was doing very well. His lowest grade was a 92. Jeannie was a different story. Her grades were generally poor. In fact, if she did not pass the upcoming exams, she would be terminated from the program.

Jim was concerned for his friend. "The exam is next week," he said. "I'll help you study this weekend, if you like." "Oh, that's very nice of you, Jim," Jeannie said as they chatted over coffee after their last class on Friday. "I just don't think I'll have time. I have some shopping to do tomorrow. And I've got a date tomorrow night." She thought for a moment. "But Sunday would be fine. Can you call me then to set up a time?" "I sure will," Jim said. "One day of study is better than none. Especially for you, Jeannie. It could mean your whole nursing career." Jeannie nodded. "I know," she said. She was very serious.

On Sunday morning, Jim called Jeannie. "What time do you want to meet me?" he asked.

There was silence for a moment. Then Jeannie spoke. "For what?" she said.

"We were going to study for the exam today," Jim said.

"Oh, I can't," Jeannie said. "I didn't get in until early this morning. I'm so tired I can't even think of studying." "Do you want me to come by later this afternoon?" Jim asked, unwilling to let his friend miss her last opportunity to prepare for the exam.

"Sure," Jeannie said. "That's a good idea." When Jim went to Jeannie's that afternoon, there was a note on the door. It said: "Jim. I forgot I had to go to my mother's for dinner. See you in class tomorrow. J." The next day, Jim met Jeannie in the hall. "I left a set of my notes under your door," he said. "Did you get a chance to read them?" Jeannie smiled. "That was so sweet, Jim. But, I just couldn't find the time. It was late and to be perfectly honest, I'm not really worried about this exam." "Well, I am," Jim said. "And I'm only trying to keep my average up. Not keep from getting terminated from the program." Jeannie squeezed his hand. "You worry too much," she said.

Later, when the class was assembled for the exam, Jim nodded to Jeannie. "Good luck," he said.

"Thanks," she whispered back.

The instructor distributed the exam papers. Jim glanced through it to familiarize himself with its content and to estimate how much time he would need to complete it. Other students did the same, although some started writing their answers immediately.

About halfway through the exam, Jim glanced across the aisle at Jeannie. He was astonished by what he saw. In her hand was a 3- by 5-inch index card. She looked at it and then slipped it out of sight before answering a test question. She did this a number of times during the exam. She was still writing when Jim turned in his paper and left the room.

Jeannie joined him a few minutes later. "That wasn't so hard after all, was it?" she said.

"You didn't think so?" Jim asked in surprise. "Maybe it wasn't the hardest exam we've had, but it sure wasn't the easiest. I know I couldn't have winged it." Jeannie said nothing.

"Did you get a chance to go over the notes I left?" Jim asked. Jeannie's hand shot up. "Oh, there's Diana," she said, waving her arm. "I have to talk to her about something. Diana! Wait up!" She turned to Jim. "See you tomorrow." The hall emptied as the last of the students left the exam room. Soon it was very quiet. Jim was deeply concerned. A flurry of questions raced through his mind. "Did Jeannie cheat on the exam? What should I do? Should I tell her what I saw? Should I ask her if she used notes? Should I report her? Is it my business to snitch on someone if I think she cheated? Is it my business to report someone if I know they cheated? What if we were on duty and I saw Jeannie do something dishonest that would harm a patient, like writing on a chart that she did something but really didn't? Would I be responsible?" Jim shook his head sharply. "I'll have to make Jeannie talk to me about this," he said to himself.

Jim's decision was guided by what he and his class were discussing at great length: the ethical issues that are the concern of everyone who accepts the responsibility of caring for others.

ETHICS

For many years now you have been developing personal standards of conduct and making decisions based on your personal beliefs and values. Before you entered nursing school, your personal standards of conduct, your beliefs, your values, and your prejudices probably had little influence on others. Perhaps those who did not agree with your opinions were not your friends; those who did not approve of the way you conducted yourself did not associate with you.

But now that you have decided to become a nurse, you must examine yourself, your heart and your soul, closely. By becoming a nurse, you agree to provide certain services to human beings, and human beings have certain rights that are absolute. That means that these rights apply equally to every human being. Human rights are absolute privileges that people have and that they have a right to expect because they are human. There are many human rights. Some are specific to individuals; others are specific to groups.

People are neither more nor less human because of their income, their occupation, their sex, their race, or any of an infinite number of factors that make people different. Although people are different in what they think, how they behave, the language they speak, and the clothes they wear, certain characteristics are common to all. All humans bleed when they are cut, and all need air, food, and water. All are born, and all die. All have hearts and lungs and livers. In other words, there are certain attributes that are fundamental to all humans.

The fundamental characteristics common to all humans raise certain philosophical questions that have been debated for centuries. What rights does a human being have just by being human, and what responsibilities are associated with these rights? Ethical questions are directly related to these philosophical questions. The word *ethical* comes from the Greek amethikos and means knowledge of right and wrong related to human conduct. Decisions based on this knowledge of right and wrong may be related to the individual, the society, or the situation.

An individual makes many decisions on the basis of what he or she personally believes is right or wrong. These beliefs begin developing early in life and generally evolve from what a child is taught by parents, friends, culture, religion, school, and society in general. This is a personal value system. A healthy individual changes his or her value system over a lifetime. What an individual believes about relationships with, and responsibilities to, other people changes as he or she learns and lives in society.

Decisions regarding what is right and what is wrong are also made by society. These decisions may be carried out through changes in customs and behaviors, or they may be written as laws. There are many examples of how society continually redefines the rights of its people. Abolition of slavery, the right to vote, women's rights, the rights of the disabled, and the right to die with dignity are just a few examples of how our society has redefined human rights over time. Laws that govern the conduct of societies are written statements that define right and wrong. Laws relating to healthcare will be discussed in Chapter 11.

Decisions about what is right and what is wrong can also be situational. That is, what is right in one situation may be wrong in another. As you become more involved in providing nursing care, you will be confronted with many situations in which there is no clear right or wrong action. Incredible advances in technology, complex social issues, and complicated work environments force us to ask questions about what is right and wrong more often than we might realize.

This is by no means an exhaustive discussion of ethics or ethical decisions. You should realize that human beings have fundamental rights, and that society gives nurses a responsibility for protecting those rights. Many of your nursing responsibilities to society will involve ethical decisions.

NURSING AND ETHICS

A study of ethical behavior and making decisions regarding ethical issues in nursing and healthcare is one of the most important aspects of your nursing education. Society has, through nurse licensing laws, given nurses "permission" to nurse other human beings. People who become nurses promise or agree to help all those human beings who need their services. Nurses, by virtue of their education, have the ability, the responsibility, and the obligation to help patients. The public trusts nurses to have the knowledge necessary to be a nurse, as well as the ethical commitment to fulfill the obligation of nursing.

Anyone can learn the knowledge and perform the skills assigned to nursing. But not everyone who has this knowledge and these skills can be called a nurse. A nurse is someone who has internalized the concept of what it means to be a human being and accepts personal responsibility for relationships with other human beings. A nurse has an obligation to do good and not harm anyone and makes a commitment to provide the same high quality and level of nursing service to all human beings.

Your interpretation of what it means to be human, your belief in what rights humans have, and your ideas of what is right and what is wrong are what make you the person you are. And you cannot separate these values from the nurse you hope to become. A strong belief in the right of people to be treated and respected as human beings must be the foundation of your relationships and interactions with your patients, with your fellow nurses, and with members of the healthcare team.

The National Federation for Licensed Practical Nurses (NFLPN) and the National Association for Practical Nurse Education and Services (NAPNES) have each developed a code of ethics for practical/vocational nurses. A code of ethics is a list of rules of good conduct for members of a particular group. Although laws establish the minimum behaviors of a group, ethical statements attempt to describe the ideals of that group.

The legal/ethical status section of the "Nursing Practice Standards for the Licensed Practical/Vocational Nurse," published by the National Federation of Licensed Practical Nurses (Appendix E), indicates that practical/vocational nurses "shall recognize and have a commitment to meet the ethical and moral obligations of the practice of nursing." NAPNES has also issued a statement regarding ethical behavior and the practical/vocational nurse. The full NAPNES statement also appears in Appendix F. Both of these statements identify those standards of behavior that reflect the high ideals of the practical/vocational nurse.

You will be provided with many opportunities during your educational program to acquire the knowledge, skills, and ethical behaviors expected of practical/vocational nurses. Your faculty will assist you in reaching your goal of becoming a nurse and learning the ethical behaviors that are expected. It is through their instruction and guidance that you will learn not only how to bathe a patient but how to accept personal responsibility for what you do. You will learn to recognize that with responsibility comes accountability.

A desire to help others and a commitment to be responsible and accountable for your actions is the ethical foundation of your career as a licensed practical/vocational nurse.

PERSONAL ACCOUNTABILITY

Being responsible means to accept being the cause of an action. For example, saying "I broke the window" indicates the acceptance of personal responsibility. Being accountable means to accept the consequences of the action, for example, paying for the broken window. Being held accountable for what you do and how you do it can be the most rewarding part of your career in nursing. You can be proud of how you perform your nursing skills, you can feel great personal satisfaction about the knowledge you gain as you accumulate experiences in nursing, and you can accept the admiration of your peers because of your high ethical standards. Your patients will feel your concern for them as individual human beings, and they will remember the kind, caring nurse who helped them through a difficult time in their life.

UNETHICAL BEHAVIOR

Unfortunately, not all nurses adhere to their code of ethics or practice nursing based on high ethical standards. You may see situations in which there is blatant disregard for basic human rights. You may hear patients referred to as the gallbladder in Room 212 or the appendectomy in Room 324. You may see members of the healthcare team ignoring a patient's questions or generally treating them without respect. You may find yourself working with people who chart procedures that were not done, don't wash their hands properly, or ignore body substance isolation guidelines.

In addition, the chemically impaired nurse; working in situations where the shortage of nursing staff compromises the quality of patient care; poor performance by peers; medication and patient care errors; theft of supplies and equipment; breaching confidentiality of patient information; and disregard for the rights of individual patients to make their own decisions regarding healthcare can create conflict for you. All of these situations are difficult for you as a person and also as a nurse.

ETHICAL DILEMMAS

These are just a few examples of situations that can lead to an ethical dilemma. An *ethical dilemma* is a situation in which there is conflict or opposition between personal values, moral principles, laws, personal and professional obligations, and the rights of the individual and society. When you feel conflict or opposition with what is being done or being planned, you are confronted with the need to make a decision about your concerns.

What you choose to do is a difficult decision. If the majority of the people you work with frequently ignore the human rights of patients, your best decision may be to resign from that position. If the problem is limited to just a few people or one person, your nurse manager may also be concerned. Together, with tact and courage, you may be able to help that nurse perform his or her responsibilities at a level that reflects positively not only on the nurse but on all of nursing.

In most situations involving ethics, there is no one right or wrong answer and the best course of action may vary from situation to situation. To help you evaluate what, if any action to take, general guidelines for dealing with ethical dilemmas can provide a framework for ethical decision making.

GUIDELINES FOR MAKING ETHICAL DECISIONS

Ethical dilemmas of contemporary nurses are varied. They may be related to the more dramatic bioethical issues that will be discussed later in this chapter, but they also include the daily practice of nursing as previously discussed.

Before taking any action, you need to decide whether the problem is a legal one or an ethical one. To do this, you need to have a good understanding of the code of ethics, the nurse practice acts of the state in which you are working, and the policies and procedures of the healthcare facility in which you are employed. This will help you separate ethical issues from legal issues. For example, a nurse who is administering medications that have not been prescribed is breaking the law; a nurse who is giving substandard care is creating an ethical dilemma.

Some ethical dilemmas may have legal implications. For example, the nurse who is stealing drugs is not only breaking the law but also creating an ethical dilemma for the people with whom he or she works. Is your best course of action to report what you saw to your nurse manager, your state board of nursing, or to a local law enforcement agency? Once you have decided that ethics is involved in the situation, there are several guidelines that will help you decide on a course of action.

Your first guideline in thinking about a specific ethical dilemma is to collect the facts. Did you directly observe the situation or did you get the information from someone else? Did the situation happen once or does it happen frequently? Was someone's life in danger? Was the quality of patient care compromised? Is the question one of what is right and what is wrong in relation to human beings, or is it a question of what you would personally prefer? These are questions you must answer clearly and factually for yourself.

The second guideline is to ask yourself what would happen if everyone acted or behaved in the manner in question. Your answer to this question may make the right course of action clear to you.

If your ethical dilemma is not resolved, a third guideline may provide further direction. In this step, you discuss your concerns with an authority. The authority is someone with extensive experience and knowledge who can help you separate the facts from the emotional components of ethical dilemmas. The discussion process may provide you with new insights, an appreciation of differing points of view, and perhaps even a better understanding of your own values.

After collecting the facts, asking yourself what would happen if everyone behaved in a certain manner, and consulting an authority, you have to choose a course of action. You may decide to do nothing or you may decide to pursue your concerns.

If you decide to pursue your concerns, often the best course of action is to discuss the issue with your immediate supervisor. This person is often in a position to deal effectively and positively with an ethical dilemma. If, after a reasonable time, you believe that your immediate supervisor has not taken the necessary action, you may decide to report your concerns to an authority higher up. Almost all organizations have lines of authority that you should follow in pursuing your concerns.

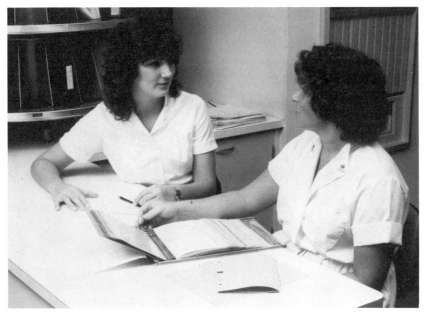

When you are faced with an ethical dilemma, it may help to discuss your concerns with someone with extensive experience and knowledge.

Because ethical behavior is difficult to define, particularly when specific situations may justify certain behaviors, an effective way to present your concerns may be through established institutional committees. The policy and procedures committee, the quality assurance committee, the peer review committee, the patient relations committee, and similar committees may share your concerns. Volunteering to serve on one of these committees or telling your concerns to a member of that committee may be the most effective approach to dealing with your ethical dilemmas.

Figure 10-1 provides an overview of the process involved in making decisions regarding ethical dilemmas. Each person brings the components of ethical decision making to the situation. The dilemma occurs when there is conflict or opposition within the components. It is essential in the decision making process to separate the facts from hearsay, gossip, rumors, and the emotional components of the situation. All possible courses of actions, with advantages and disadvantages of each, are considered. An analysis of your findings can help you make the best decision possible.

When you make a decision to pursue an ethical dilemma, you must be prepared to accept the consequences of your action. It is possible that other people will not see the situation the same way you see it. You may be labeled a "do-gooder," a "perfectionist," or a "spoiler." Or you may earn the respect of other people. Be sure of your facts and avoid making personal judgments about other people's behavior.

COMPONENTS OF ETHICAL DECISION MAKING	THE SITUATION	THE DILEMMA	SORT INFORMATION	LIST ALL POSSIBLE COURSES OF ACTION	DECISION
Religious beliefs	Describe the situation	Describe the dilemma based on conflicts or opposition between one or more of the components of ethical decision making	Facts	Advantages of action A disadvantages of action A	Using components of ethical decision making, facts, and advantanges and disadvantages associated with each fact, make a decision
Personal values					
Personal moral principles				Advantages of action B disadvantages of action B	
Laws					
Society's beliefs and expectations					
Individual and group rights				Advantages of action C disadvantages of action C	
Profession's code of ethics					
Professional obligations				Advantages of action D disadvantages of action D	
The obligation to not cause harm to anyone			Hearsay Rumors		
The obligation to do good for everyone			Emotional components of the situation	Action based on hearsay, rumors, or emotions would be inappropriate	

Figure 10-1. The process of ethical decision making.

Your motivation in pursuing ethical concerns has to be your desire to protect your patients' human rights.

CONTEMPORARY BIOETHICAL DILEMMAS

Inherent in being human is the right to make choices. Not that many years ago, choices related to healthcare were limited. But advances in science and technology in the past 40 years have created many more choices. Organ transplant and organ donation, advanced life support systems, and alternative methods of conception and contraception are examples of some of the bioethical dilemmas confronting people today. There is no doubt that the future will present us with bioethical dilemmas even more complex than those discussed in this chapter.

While you may not be directly involved in making decisions about who gets an organ transplant or asking a grieving family to donate the organs of a deceased family member, you will probably be directly involved in caring for patients and families who make these decisions.

If you have strong personal values associated with particular issues such as abortion, genetic engineering, organ transplants, or other medical procedures, you should not accept a position in a department or a healthcare facility in which these procedures are routinely performed. The stress created between your personal values and what you are expected to do will most certainly affect your health, as well as your nursing practice. For example, if your personal values oppose abortion, you should not accept a position in a doctor's office or clinic that provides abortions.

While you do have the right as a nurse to refuse to assist with a procedure you believe to be morally wrong, you do not have the right to refuse to provide nursing care for the patient. For example, you may believe abortion is wrong and you have a right to refuse to assist with an abortion. You do not, however, have the right to deny nursing care to the patient who has had an abortion. How you personally feel about the patient's decision can in no way affect the quality of nursing care you provide. You have, as a nurse, an obligation to provide nursing care.

Bioethics Committees

To attempt to make the best decision in situations where there is no clearly right or wrong action related to a bioethical dilemma, many healthcare facilities have created an Ethics Committee. Members of this committee may include doctors, clergy, community members, judges, lawyers, nurses, patients and their families, administrators, social workers, philosophers, and ethicists (people who study ethics). The work of this committee is to bring all available information and as many points of view as possible to a situation that presents a bioethical dilemma. The task of this committee is to make a decision about what action should be taken.

For example, a patient is in a persistent vegetative state. The family wants the doctor to "pull the plug" but she refuses. She also refuses to turn the care of the patient over to a physician who will do what the family wants. The family may decide to present their concerns to the healthcare facility's Ethics Committee.

The following bioethical dilemmas are common in our society. Many of these are discussed in newspapers, on the radio, and in television dramas.

Birth Control

Birth control is the general term used to describe methods of controlling conception. The ethical issue over birth control is whether or not individuals have the right to control conception, and if so, what limitations, if any, should be imposed on them.

Limitations include questions regarding which methods are best, what age is appropriate, if methods should be available to married and unmarried people, whether parental consent for minors is needed, and if methods and information should be available through schools or public-supported clinics. Methods of birth control include contraception, sterilization, and elective abortion.

Contraception prevents fertilization by blocking the union of sperm and egg by means of various devices such as spermatocides or oral contraceptives on a regular basis. When contraception ends, fertilization is again possible. Should taxpayer money be used to supply contraceptive devices to the poor, children, or anyone who asks? Sterilization is a surgical procedure that can be performed on men (vasectomy) or women (tubal ligation) to prevent reproduction. It is virtually permanent because neither procedure can be reversed with certainty. Should those who are institutionalized for mental illness be subject to mandatory sterilization? Abortion is the termination of pregnancy. Spontaneous abortion results from abnormalities in the fetus or in the maternal environment and occurs naturally. Therapeutic abortions are performed to protect the mother's life. An elective abortion is intentional, performed at the mother's request, and for personal reasons.

Although abortion is legal, it raises numerous ethical issues. There is major controversy regarding the right of women to have control of their own bodies, whether and when a fetus is a human being, and whether a fetus has rights. The U.S. Supreme Court decided the legality of abortion in 1973, but the ethical and moral issues continue. Your personal views will determine whether and to what extent you can comfortably assist in matters relating to abortion.

Alternative Fertilization

For women who cannot conceive, medical techniques now give them the ability to bear children. In addition, men whose fertility was marginal can now father children, and couples can have children through the services of others (surrogates, meaning substitutes). These techniques involve artificial insemination, in vitro or "test tube" conception, and surrogate motherhood. All raise legal and ethical questions that remain unanswered.

Artificial insemination is the medical implantation of donor sperm into a woman's uterus to fertilize her own egg and thereby conceive a child. The sperm can be that of the husband or another donor.

Test tube conception is a procedure in which sperm and egg are mixed outside the body in a laboratory dish and the fertilized egg is then implanted into a woman's uterus. The egg and sperm can be from husband and wife or from donors.

When a fertilized egg is implanted into the uterus of a woman who is not the wife but who will carry the conceived child to term, or when a woman agrees to undergo artificial insemination for another couple, the woman is called a *surrogate mother*.

Some of the legal and ethical questions raised by these methods include the legitimacy of the child, maternal and paternal rights, and adultery. None of them have been fully settled. Your own views will be the basis for your decisions to participate in healthcare situations in which these issues are raised.

Genetic Screening

Procedures for studying genes and for probing the uterus to learn the status of a developing embryo or fetus in order to give physicians, researchers, and parents options and choices that never existed before are methods of genetic screening.

Amniocentesis is a procedure in which a long needle is used to draw amniotic fluid from the sac surrounding the developing child. The fluid can be studied in the laboratory for indications of Down's syndrome, hemophilia, Tay-Sachs disease, Duchenne's muscular dystrophy, sickle cell disease, and other diseases. It can also be used to determine the unborn infant's sex. When diseases or genetic abnormalities become known, the parents can be informed and counseled, after which they can decide what to do.

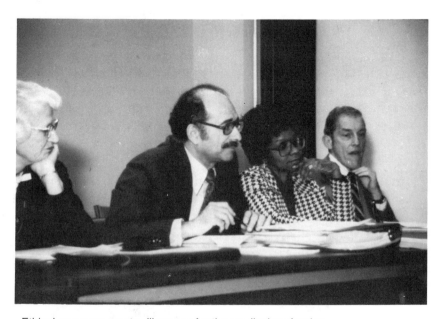

Ethical concerns create dilemmas for the medical profession.

Organ Transplants

The marvel of organ transplantation has become commonplace. Heart and/or lung, liver, pancreas, and kidney transplants are being done with more and more frequency. In 1981, there were no lung transplants; in 1994, there were 713 lung transplants. It is estimated that about 35,000 people were waiting for transplants in 1994. Cornea, bone, and skin grafts, which are forms of transplants, are also adding quality to the life of those who need them.

While there is no doubt that organ transplants and grafts save and improve the quality of life, there are those who are opposed to these procedures and research. These people raise questions about the cost of such procedures related to the benefit for society, sacrificing animals for their transplantable organs, and the potential to buy and sell human organs to the highest bidder. Others oppose organ transplants and grafts for religious reasons.

Living donors, such as those who give one of their kidneys, have the satisfaction of knowing that their act has improved someone else's chances for a normal life. What happens if the donor's other kidney stops functioning or is damaged in an accident? Most organs used for transplant come from deceased persons. Some donors make arrangements for organ donation before death through an act of consent in their will, on a special donor card, or by authorization on their driver's license. Other donations are made with the permission of next of kin immediately after the donor's death. Because the decision to donate organs must be made during a time of extreme distress, what happens a week or month or year later when the next of kin who signed for the organ donation has second thoughts?

Death

Determining when death occurs has been complicated by lifesaving devices and procedures. Respirators, heart and lung machines, and other assistive devices are able to keep patients alive who a few years ago would have died.

When death is in question, it is now defined on the basis of an electroencephalogram when it indicates the absence of brain wave activity. *Death* is legally defined as the irreversible cessation of brain function for a given period.

Although criteria have been established so that a person can be declared legally dead, it is now possible to continue a deceased patient's biological functions. Therefore, the question of whether the patient is alive or dead is still at issue, especially in situations where the removal of the life support system is requested by a next of kin.

Euthanasia

Sometimes called "mercy killing," *euthanasia* is the deliberate causing of someone's death by active or passive means. Active euthanasia is to cause someone's death by intentionally administering an agent that would bring about death. Passive euthanasia is to cause someone's death by withholding efforts to sustain life.

For example, in a healthcare facility, an act of active euthanasia could be the administration of a lethal dose of medication, whereas an act of passive euthanasia could be the withholding of a medication that the patient needs to stay alive. Active euthanasia is an unquestionably illegal act (murder) punishable by law. Passive euthanasia is not as well defined, but it is no less controversial. At what point in time is a decision made to discontinue feeding a patient? Who makes this decision?

Living Wills

In some instances, patients anticipate their death and make an allowance to let it happen naturally by signing a living will. A living will is a document that testifies that the patient does not want heroic lifesaving measures instituted to maintain life when death would otherwise be likely. Living wills are not universally recognized as legal documents, but they do express the wishes, at the time of signing, of those who sign them. What happens if a living will was signed 10 years before a person's illness? Is treatment available now that may provide a cure for what was considered a terminal illness when the living will was signed?

SUMMARY

In summary, learning to be a nurse requires more than passing written examinations and performing procedures correctly. It requires you to develop an ethical and moral commitment to provide the best nursing services you are capable of providing to every human being in your care. This commitment lives within you and cannot be turned on as you begin your nursing duties nor turned off when you leave your patients at the end of your workday. This commitment pervades your life and influences all your decisions. And the longer you are employed as a nurse, the stronger this commitment will become. Nurses who make this personal commitment to their fellow human beings are rewarded by great personal satisfaction; patients who receive nursing services from these nurses are rewarded by compassionate, personal, and competent care.

DISCUSSION QUESTIONS/LEARNING ACTIVITIES

1. Construct a list of what you believe to be basic human rights. Compare your list with that of one or two of your classmates. Do you agree or disagree on what constitutes basic human rights? Can you develop a list of basic human rights on which you both agree?

2. Think about your recent experiences in school or in your clinical facility and try to identify an ethical dilemma. How did you handle the dilemma, and what do you think you might do if the situation happens again? Indicate why you believe your concern is an ethical one and not a matter of personal values.

   If you cannot think of your own situation, you may use one of these: cheating on tests; discussing confidential patient information in an elevator; observing an employee taking a scrub suit for personal use at home.

3. Compare and contrast the NAPNES and NFLPN code of ethics. How are they similar? How are they different?

4. Talk with your classmates to determine their position on some of the ethical issues presented in this chapter. Listen to their points of view and compare them with your own. After this discussion, write a brief summary of why you think it is often difficult to find answers to ethical issues.

5. Create your own situations or use the following list of situations to describe your personal values/moral beliefs about each:

> Do Not Resuscitate (DNR) orders
> AIDS
> Abortion
> Living wills

In what ways might your personal values and moral beliefs affect your ability to provide nursing care? If you think your values and beliefs might contribute to denying care, what do you think you should do?

READ MORE ABOUT IT

Aiken TD: Legal, Ethical and Political Issues in Nursing, First Edition. Philadelphia: FA Davis, 1994.

American Nurses Association: Suggested State Legislation: Nursing Practice Act, Nursing Disciplinary Diversion Act, Prescriptive Authority Act, Pamphlet NP-78:1Ä46. American Nurses Association Publications, 1990.

Catalano JT, Springhouse Notes: Ethical & Legal Aspects of Nursing, Second Edition. Springhouse, PA: Springhouse, 1995

Davis A, Aroskar M: Ethical Dilemmas in Nursing Practice, Third Edition. East Norwalk, CT: Appleton & Lange, 1991.

Edge R: The Ethics of Health Care: A Guide for Clinical Practice, First Edition. Albany, NY: Delmar, 1994.

Fowler M: Nursing Ethics, First Edition. Philadelphia: JB Lippincott, 1990.

Husted GL: Ethical Decision Making in Nursing, Second Edition. St. Louis: CV Mosby, 1995.

Lipman M: Medical Law and Ethics, First Edition. New York: Brady, 1994.

Purtilo R: Ethical Dimensions in the Health Professions, Second Edition. Philadelphia: WB Saunders, 1993.

Springhouse: Nurses's Handbook of Law and Ethics, First Edition. Springhouse, PA: Springhouse Corporation, 1992.

White WE: Ethical Dilemmas in Contemporary Nursing Practice, First Edition. Washington, DC: American Nurses Association, 1992.

11

Legally Responsible Nursing Practice

OBJECTIVES

When you complete this chapter, you should be able to:

Discuss the purpose of Good Samaritan Laws.

List the two sources of laws and give examples of each.

Discuss the relationship between the nurse practice acts and the state boards of nursing.

Explain the association among responsibility, accountability, and legal liability.

Define the term "respondeat superior."

Define the term "breach of contract."

Define the term "tort" and give two examples of torts.

Illustrate the difference between a tort and a crime.

Differentiate negligence and gross negligence.

Discuss how nurses can assist in preventing malpractice claims.

Explain the purpose of malpractice insurance.

Give examples of crimes that may involve nurses.

Larry's phone rang a third time. He groped for the receiver.

"Hello?" he said drowsily.

"Larry?" a small voice asked. "Please help me. I'm sick." "Mrs. Thompson, is that you? I'll be right down," Larry said. He raced downstairs to his landlady's apartment.

Mrs. Thompson was lying on the floor next to her bed. Her eyes were closed. Larry dropped to his knees and put his fingertips on the pulse point on the side of her neck. "Mrs. Thompson? Can you hear me?" The sick woman's eyes opened weakly. Her mouth moved, but there was no sound before she lapsed into unconsciousness again. Larry quickly dialed the phone.

A shadow appeared in the open doorway as he waited for the call to go through. "What happened?" It was Milo Davis, the other tenant in Mrs. Thompson's building.

"I don't know, but she's unconscious," Larry said.

"I bet she didn't take her shot," Milo said, hurrying to the kitchen. He took a small bottle from the refrigerator and returned to the room where Larry was still holding the receiver.

"I'm calling an ambulance," Larry said.

"That's not necessary," Milo said. "She just needs her shot." He held up the bottle. It was a medicine bottle, but the label was smeared and unreadable. "She keeps the whatchamacallits in that drawer." He took a disposable syringe from the drawer and handed it to Larry. "Here. You do it." Larry shook his head. "No," he said without explaining further. He did not take the syringe.

"It's easy," Milo said. "I did it last year when this happened. Mrs. Thompson said you have lots of experience from the hospital, so you do it." "I'm a licensed practical nurse," Larry stated.

The man thrust the syringe at Larry. "Then do it!" he shouted angrily. "She might die." At that moment Larry's call went through. He said there was an emergency and requested that an ambulance be sent immediately. Larry made Mrs. Thompson as comfortable as possible and waited. He monitored her breathing and pulse from time to time. Milo Davis glared at him but didn't say another word. He also didn't administer the medication in the bottle.

When the ambulance was gone, Milo finally spoke. "How dare you call yourself a nurse if you'll risk an old woman's life like that?" he snapped, brandishing the syringe like an accusing finger at Larry. "You're not a good neighbor, and you're certainly not a Good Samaritan. I don't know what you call yourself." With that he stalked out of the apartment.

Larry picked up the bottle and looked at the label. It was unreadable, but an expiration date was still legible. The date was over 2 years old. He held the bottle to the light. A suspiciously cloudy mass swirled inside the bottle.

After the ambulance took Mrs. Thompson to the hospital, Larry smiled as he remembered what Milo had said. "What I call myself is a good neighbor, a Good Samaritan, and a very good nurse," he said as if the man were still there. "And do you know why I'm a good nurse? I'll tell you. It's because I know what to do and when to do it, what I can do within the law, and when to ask for help."

Contemporary practical/vocational nursing is an active process in which you will interact with your patients to provide care in a one-to-one relationship that is based on their trust and your competency. Your duty is to do good and to avoid harm in accordance with the law.

Laws are rules of conduct derived from cultural values, moral practices, and ethical beliefs. In a democracy, they are made and enforced by the authority of the group to whom they apply.

GOOD SAMARITAN STATUTES

The story of the Good Samaritan tells of a man who was beaten and robbed and then left to die at the side of the road. People walking by ignored him. But one man, a Samaritan, did not. He dressed the injured man's wounds and took him to safe lodging, without being asked and without being paid. Today, Good Samaritan laws protect people from prosecution who voluntarily go to the aid of others in an emergency if the person providing emergency care did not act recklessly or did not intentionally harm the victim. Good Samaritan laws have been passed by virtually every state.

They vary from state to state, and you are responsible to find out what the statute in your state says. Generally, such laws require that people who render aid are expected to act as any reasonable, prudent person would in that situation. Nurses and other healthcare providers are expected to render care equal to that of another provider with the same level of skill, training, and experience. The intention of Good Samaritan laws is to encourage the giving of emergency care outside the hospital or healthcare facility.

However, it is important to note that nobody, whether healthcare provider or layperson, is obligated by law to give emergency care outside the healthcare setting. To act or not is an ethical decision you must make when faced with an emergency situation in a noninstitutional setting.

SOURCES OF LAWS

Laws come from two general sources. The first source is the government (either federal, state, or local) and the second source is private. Laws that come from the government are termed *public laws.* One type of public law includes laws based on the Constitution of either the United States, an individual state, or a subdivision within a state. Federal constitutional laws are based on the U.S. Constitution and its amendments. State constitutional laws, among other things, identify the legal relationship between the state and its counties, cities, townships, boroughs, municipalities, and villages. Municipal (city) constitutional law prescribes the form of government through which the city will operate and conduct its business.

Another type of public law (administrative law) creates federal, state, and local administrative agencies that have the power to make and enforce rules and regulations. Nurse practice acts are laws that are passed by state governments to control the practice of nursing in that state. A nurse practice act is an example of an administrative law and will be discussed in more detail later in this chapter.

The last type of public law, criminal law, deals with offenses against the welfare or safety of the public. Criminal law includes minor offenses, misdemeanors, and felonies. An example of a minor offense is a traffic ticket. A misdemeanor applies to offenses that include fines of less than $1000 and less than 1 year in prison. A felony is a more serious crime than a misdemeanor. A conviction for a felony may make a person liable for the death sentence or for a life sentence in a federal or state prison. The federal government determines what constitutes a federal crime, and each state has the power to determine what it considers a crime.

Private law focuses on the enforcement of rights, duties, and other legal relations between private citizens. Laws related to enforcing contracts and laws related to torts, which are legal wrongs not included under contract law, are two divisions of private laws that are of particular interest to nurses.

Table 11-1 summarizes the major divisions within public law and private law. The examples included in this table are intended to help you understand the differences between public law and private law.

TABLE 11-1 **Sources of Law**

Public Law (Also Known as Statutory Law)

Constitutional Law

Federal government (the U.S. Constitution and the Amendments)

State government (the constitution of a state: many similarities to the U.S. Constitution)

Local government (the constitution or similarly titled document that identifies the political structure and social responsibilities of local governing bodies)

Administrative Law

Federal (Occupational Safety and Health Administration)

State (state boards of nursing)

Local (city department of licenses and inspection)

Criminal Law

Federal (transporting drugs between states)

State (murder of a citizen of the state)

Local (violation of a parking law)

Private Law (Also Known as Civil or Common Law)

Contract Law (implied, oral, written)

Written contracts (such as school loans)

Verbal contracts ("I will babysit for you on Saturday from 7 PM to 1 AM")

Law of Torts (legal wrong not included under contract laws)

Negligence

False imprisonment

Confidentiality

Defamation of character

Consent

Assault and battery

Fraud

NURSING PRACTICE AND THE LAW

The basic law governing your practice as a practical/vocational nurse is the nurse practice act (an administrative law) that was passed by your state legislature. You will recall that after a bill is passed, it becomes law, and that law is known as an act. A nurse practice act usually defines the legal functions, powers, and duties of the state board of nursing. It also identifies the membership of the board and how people become board members. A nurse practice act also defines terms such as *nursing* and the duties of the nurse practitioner, registered nurse, and practical or vocational nurse. Laws governing licensure and legal titles are also included in nurse practice acts. Any changes in the nurse practice act must be made through the state legislature and must follow the same process as any other proposed law.

Nurse practice acts are administered by state boards of nursing or committees with a similar title. Members of the state board of nursing are registered nurses, practical/vocational nurses, consumers, and others interested in the health and welfare of the citizens of the state. Such a board may be appointed by the governor of the state or elected by the people, and the majority of its members are usually registered nurses. Other members may include consumer representatives and licensed practical/vocational nurses. The board is headed by a salaried executive director, usually a registered nurse, who, with a paid staff, manages daily matters related to nursing in that state.

State boards have legal authority to interpret, implement, and enforce the laws governing nursing practice, nursing education, and licensure. The state board of nursing issues rules and regulations, which are interpretations of the nurse practice act.

Disciplinary hearings for licensees and prosecution of violations of nurse practice acts are conducted by the boards. Keep in mind that the law of the state in which you practice nursing is the law that applies to you and that ignorance of the law is not an excuse for illegal acts. You must know the law and practice within it, and you are held responsible for your own acts as a nurse.

Responsibility and Liability

Responsibility is the condition of being accountable for your actions. Whether you are a student or an employee, many of your responsibilities will be well-defined in the written or verbal contract you enter into with your school or employer. But because nurses have a relationship with patients that includes touching, treating, collecting information, and providing personal services, you will have a number of other responsibilities that are not written and are not easily defined. These are responsibilities that come with the job.

Accepting responsibility for one's actions means that the individual who commits an act is the one who must explain the act and accept any consequences that follow. A student who borrows a library book and then loses it is responsible for what happened to the book and accountable for its replacement.

Liability is the legal obligation a person has to make good for the loss of, or damage to, something for which he or she is responsible. In the case of the library book, the student who lost it would be liable (obligated) to replace or pay for it.

A person is always responsible and liable for his or her actions. As a nurse, you are legally responsible for the care you give or neglect to give your patients, as well as for your professional and personal conduct. Your best protection against charges regarding the performance of your duties, whether a legal action or a personal criticism, is to carry out your duties at or above the standards expected from someone with your education, ability, and experience. Even then, it is possible that a charge could be made against you, particularly in a social climate that fosters lawsuits.

Legal Relationships Between the Employer and the Employee

The legal relationship between employer and employee is fairly well-defined. The employer has the right to direct and control the performance of work. An employee is a person who accepts wages as a result of services provided to the employer.

A legal term, *respondeat superior,* is used to describe the legal responsibility of an employer for acts of an employee. In other words, both the nurse who injures a patient and the nurse's employer can be held liable for the nurse's acts.

To protect themselves and their employees from potential legal problems, employers and institutions develop guidelines governing their operations. These guidelines are not laws; they are policies that state what action is expected in specific situations. They are often more explicit than laws in that they provide detailed procedures and clear directions. Thus, it is imperative that you become thoroughly familiar with these guidelines.

Because institutional and employer guidelines must reflect current conditions to be effective, they are changed periodically. Your duties will put you in daily contact with your employer's policies and procedures. You will be in an excellent position to know whether these guidelines are meeting the needs for which they were written and to suggest changes when they are not.

Standards of Care

Standards of care are guidelines developed to identify appropriate levels of professional care. Nursing standards of care define the average degree of skill, care, and diligence that other nurses would provide under the same or similar circumstances.

A nurse practice act is the state law that governs the practice of nursing. The rules and regulations issued by a state board of nursing is based on a legal interpretation of the nurse practice act. These rules and regulations define standards of care expected of professional and practical/vocational nurses.

There are a number of other sources for standards of care. The Joint Commission on the Accreditation of Health Care Organizations, the National League for Nursing's Community Health Accreditation Program, and the American Osteopathic Association all include standards for nursing care. Many nursing specialty organizations such as the American Nurses Association, the American College of Nurse Midwives, and the American Association of Critical Care Nurses also publish standards of care.

The National Association for Practical Nurse Education and Service and the National Federation of Licensed Practical Nurses both publish standards of care affecting practical/vocational nurses. See Appendices E and F for the full text of these documents.

The policy and procedure manuals developed by healthcare facilities (the employer) identify acceptable standards of care and cover a wide range of topics from safety to specific nursing procedures.

It is important to be familiar with all laws, rules, and regulations; accrediting agency and professional organization standards for nursing care; and your employer's policies and procedures regarding standards of care. Failure to provide the standard of care expected of a nurse in the same or similar circumstance can result in a malpractice suit or disciplinary action.

PRIVATE LAW AND NURSING

Contracts

You will recall that private law deals with contracts and torts. A contract is an agreement between two or more parties. Contracts are either written or verbal promises in which something of value is exchanged. A verbal agreement to meet a friend is a social obligation and is not classified as a contract. A nurse who accepts employment, offered by either an institution, a healthcare provider, or a patient, is entering into a contract. The value exchanged in this type of contract is money (from the employer) for services (nursing).

When entering into an employment contract, you should have a written agreement that defines hours and wages, length of the contract, fringe benefits, vacation periods and lengths, length of sick leave, hours of work each week, insurance coverage, and job responsibilities expected by the employer. The employer, in turn, expects you to provide the services for which you will receive these benefits. These services are often understood to be those which are expected of anyone with the same education and license that you have.

Breach of contract is the term used to describe failure of one party to fulfill any or all parts of a contractual obligation. Breach-of-contract suits against nurses are most often suits in which damages are claimed. Damages are awarded to the complaining person if it can be shown that the plaintiff (complaining person) has suffered a financial loss. For example, suppose you agree to provide practical/vocational nursing services to one patient for 8 hours for $90. If you do not keep this contract, and the patient has to employ a practical/vocational nurse for $120 for that 8-hour period, the patient (plaintiff) may have a cause to act against you.

Torts

A *tort* is an injury or wrong committed by one person against another. There are two types of torts. The first is unintentional and includes negligence and the second is intentional. Both can include medical malpractice.

Nurses who provide nursing service frequently find themselves in situations where their behavior could result in a lawsuit claiming negligence. *Negligence* is the general term describing neglect by a physician or nurse to apply the education and skills, in caring for a patient, that other physicians or nurses customarily apply in caring for similar patients in similar circumstances. When a patient sues a licensed healthcare worker for negligence, it is termed a *malpractice suit.*

Negligence

Negligence is a tort under private law. Negligence includes professional misconduct, lack of skill in performing duties, and illegal or immoral conduct. If an act is so atrocious and human life has been endangered or even lost, the action is usually called *gross negligence.* A charge against the person may be filed in criminal courts and criminal charges brought against the defendant. Crimes related to nurses will be discussed in more detail later in the chapter.

Negligence also includes errors of omission and errors of commission. For negligence to be claimed, the nurse must have failed to do something that any reasonable and prudent nurse would have done in the same situation. In addition, some injury must result from the nurse's failure to act. Typical acts of negligence by nurses include failure to protect patients from burns caused by water bottles, bath water, or compresses; failure to ensure that bed rails are in place so that patients do not fall; failure to make sure that wrong dosages or medications are not given; and failure to properly identify patients before performing treatments.

Nurses commit acts of gross negligence when they perform duties beyond their education, experience, or legally defined limits. For example, if you administer a prescription medication without a physician's order and the patient dies as a result of your action, you may be guilty of gross negligence. You may be tried under private laws (tort) as well as under criminal law. Nurses must perform their duties as any ordinary, reasonable, and prudent nurse would in similar circumstances. Prudent nurses do not administer prescription medications without a physician's order.

False Imprisonment

A nurse cannot confine or restrict a patient to a place against his or her will except in situations specified by law (for example, when a physician orders it, or in an emergency situation where the patient might harm himself or others). Physical or verbal constraint without the consent of the patient or appropriate authority is false imprisonment.

Constraint means the prevention of free movement by any means. To keep a patient confined anywhere by threat of reprisal ("I'll take away your television privileges"), by removing clothes, or by actual physical constraint (tying a patient to the bed) can all be acts of false imprisonment unless appropriate measures are followed, even when done in the patient's best interest.

Always record your efforts to inform a patient why restriction is being used. If the patient refuses, notify your instructor.

Patients with psychiatric problems are more likely to bring charges of false imprisonment but any patient might do so, particularly if confused or uninformed of the reason for constraint.

Confidentiality

Even though the principle of confidentiality in nurse-patient relationships has not been clearly settled in the courts and is not recognized in some states, you are ethically obligated to treat certain information about your patients as confidential. Your intimate relationship with the lives of your patients gives you access to matters and information that in ordinary circumstances would be private. When the information you get is of a personal nature and when it has no direct bearing on the patient's treatment or well-being, this information is confidential and should be treated as such.

Unless the information you have suggests that harm would come to the patient or to others if it is withheld, you should respect its private nature. Normal exchanges of information with your supervisor and other members of the patient's healthcare team in the performance of your duties are not subject to this restraint. However, discussing a patient in public, whether confidential information is mentioned or not, may place a nurse in danger of being accused of breaking the principle of confidentiality. So-called shoptalk (idly discussing or gossiping about patients with co-workers and others) should be avoided for this reason alone.

The release of information to anyone other than those persons directly associated with caring for the patient, without permission, is a violation of the patient's right to privacy. It is generally outside the nurse's responsibility to provide information about patients to anyone, including the police, media, relatives, or visitors. Familiarize yourself with your program's, and later your employer's, standards on how patient information is to be handled and follow them.

Defamation of Character

Making false or malicious (intentionally harmful) statements to someone that may harm another person's character or reputation is defamation, or defamation of character. When statements are made orally, they constitute slander; when written, they are called libel. Both are violations of law and ethics, and they can be causes for lawsuits.

You can protect yourself against accusations of slander or libel by restricting your verbal or written comments about patients (or anyone else) to nonjudgmental, objective statements of fact. Limit discussion about patients to the appropriate time and place, and make statements in terms that can be documented. Avoid idle comments and gossip, and when charting, limit your written remarks to accurate, objective statements.

Informed Consent

A fundamental right of patients is to make decisions regarding their own healthcare. This right means that patients can accept or reject healthcare. A patient who accepts healthcare is said to give consent. For consent to be legal, it must be both voluntary (freely given) and informed (the patient clearly understands the alternatives).

Voluntary, informed consent by the patient to treatment is required by law. The right to informed consent is also specified in the AHA's "Patient's Bill of Rights" (Appendix J). Consent is obtained from a patient either verbally or in writing, with written consent preferred. The physician is responsible for getting a patient's consent for certain procedures; the nurse is responsible for getting a patient's consent for nursing care.

If a patient seems unclear or poorly informed about a particular treatment, tell your instructor, so that the patient's physician or nurse manager can provide additional clarification. Once given, consent can be withdrawn by the patient. Withdrawal of consent may occur at the most unexpected times. Technically, you should ask for and receive consent from your patients before administering every nursing procedure. This isn't as cumbersome as it sounds because patients are expected to have a reasonable awareness of the nature of nursing care.

Nevertheless, you should always inform your patients about what you are doing and ask their permission to do it. The request and the response don't have to be direct; they can be implied. For example, if you tell a patient you are there to give a bath, and the patient says, "Yes, I'm ready for a bath," or words to that effect, direct consent has been given. If the patient does not say anything, but nods or otherwise indicates by actions that the procedure is acceptable, implied consent has been given. In both cases you have consent to act. Conversely, if the patient says, "No bath today," or shakes his head, consent has been denied.

Obtaining direct or implied consent is always easier when the patient understands what is going on and why. Explain beforehand what you are doing and why it's necessary so that your patient can make an informed decision.

Consent for providing care for minor children is obtained from the minor's parent or legal guardian. It's a good idea to get the minor's consent as well, whenever possible. If care has been authorized by a legal guardian and a minor refuses it, inform your instructor before proceeding with treatment or before withholding it. Consent for providing care for mentally incompetent patients must also come from a legal guardian.

In some instances, a person may be unable to make an informed decision but is not legally incompetent. Intoxicated, unconscious, or confused patients are examples. It is not your responsibility to determine by whose authority consent can be given in such cases, but it's wise to know what the laws in your state are and what specific policy your employer or institution has regarding it.

Assault and Battery

One of the most common acts of nursing care, touching a patient, requires the patient's consent, whether the reason for touching is in his or her best interest or not. When direct or implied consent is not given, the potential for a charge of battery—touching another person without permission—is possible.

Permission to touch in a nursing care situation is generally implied but you should always inform your patients about what you are doing. If permission to touch is refused and explaining the reason for touching fails to change the patient's mind, inform your instructor. Don't continue with the procedure.

Assault is the threat to touch without permission. A charge of assault can be brought even if the threat could not be carried out but the patient fears that it could. For example, telling a patient to take a prescribed medication or be faced with getting it by injection may get the patient to do as asked, but a charge of assault could be lodged.

Fraud

Fraud is intentional deception to prevent a person from receiving what is lawfully his or hers. In a healthcare setting, a patient who has been charged for a service that was not performed has been defrauded. A nurse who falsely tells a patient that a medication has no side effects so that the patient will take it could be charged with fraud. It would be fraudulent to change a chart to cover up an error that, if discovered, could result in an action against the person who made the entry.

Malpractice Claims

Charges of poor care, patient harm, and patient dissatisfaction do not usually end in malpractice claims and lawsuits. But when they do, they are often influenced by factors you should recognize.

The public is increasingly sensitive to the real or imagined impersonality of the American healthcare system. When healthcare is seen as a big and profitable business, patients within the system are more apt to enter a lawsuit for an alleged wrong. The fact that healthcare employers and providers carry liability insurance is used by people to justify claims against them. This is especially true of large claims against healthcare providers, since many people believe that "insurance companies pay them anyway, and they [the insurance companies] can afford it." Also, frequent news stories of enormous judgments awarded in lawsuits may encourage some patients to initiate one to offset high medical care costs or even to solve financial woes.

Some patients are more likely to claim malpractice and bring a lawsuit than others. Called "suit prone," they are quick to sue for damages whether or not the damages are real or the suit is justified. Some of the traits they exhibit include high levels of criticism, faultfinding, hostility, uncooperativeness, and sensitivity to being offended. Success in earlier lawsuits in which they have been awarded damages (payment) may also encourage some patients to try again.

Use moderation when dealing with such patients. Work to meet their needs, rather than turn defensive or confrontational. Nurses who fail to respond to their patients' needs, who are insensitive and uncaring, or who exceed their own limits in providing care may encourage a lawsuit. Table 11-2 summarizes guidelines for avoiding malpractice claims.

Not all malpractice claims can be prevented but many can be discouraged by strict personal and institutional adherence to high standards of care. In addition to providing high standards of care, attention to accurate documentation and being aware of areas in which nurses are often found negligent may help you avoid having to defend yourself in court.

Documentation

Documenting your actions on your patient's chart contributes to a legal record of the events that occurred. The importance of chart accuracy, not only as an ongoing record of events, but as a lasting document that can be referred to later if the need arises, cannot be overstated. The care by which a chart is kept protects the patient while under medical care and can be used to protect those who administered care in the event of a lawsuit later. In both cases, the level of protection is

TABLE 11-2 Guidelines for Avoiding Malpractice Claims

- Maintain a healthy self-awareness of your competence to practice.
- Avoid allowing what you do to become so routine and unthinking that you perform your duties automatically.
- Find out what your strengths and weaknesses are and deal with each according to its need.
- Capitalize on what you do well and seek to improve those areas that need help through education, experience, or guidance from others.
- Don't hesitate to ask for advice from competent advisers.
- Don't accept assignments or perform duties that you are unsure of or for which you lack education, training, or experience.
- Evaluate assignments and establish priorities.
- Do not accept the role or duties of healthcare providers whose qualifications exceed yours.
- Don't "practice medicine" for friends and neighbors.
- Stay informed of you employer's procedures and policies.
- You have the right to refuse to do anything you are not qualified to do, that is unclear to you, or that is against stated policies, laws, nurse practice acts, and other legal restrictions.
- When you see a policy that is outdated, ineffective, or wrong, bring it to the attention of your instructor or appropriate authority so that the policy can be changed.
- Maintain accurate, legible, consistent, and complete records in strict accordance with your employer's policies.
- Continuously observe the safety rules and regulations set by your employer.
- Be aware that some practices in one's personal life—use of alcohol or drugs, for example—or other behavior that reflects poorly on one's character may be used against one in a malpractice suit.
- Accurately document pertinent information.
- Avoid "shop talk" and any breach of confidentiality.
- Always inform the patient and get his or her consent for nursing care.

determined by how well the chart is kept. Anything that is not recorded on a patient's chart is presumed not to have happened, even if it did.

Entries on the patient's chart should be factual, to the point, accurate, and related to the patient's needs or plan of treatment. Personal opinions and feelings should never appear on the chart. Saying that a patient is stubborn, uncooperative, and dirty and won't allow the staff to bathe him may be true, but the appropriate statement on the chart would be to say that the patient refuses to allow the nursing staff to bathe him.

When charting, it is also important to avoid including or implying reasons for errors in care. For example, it would be unwise to chart that "the patient received 60 milligrams of codeine at 10 AM and 60 milligrams of codeine at 10:15 AM because the staff was very busy and the nurse who gave the medication at 10:00 AM had not had time to record on the chart that she had given the medication." Recording the fact that the patient received two doses of medication within 15 minutes is appropriate; including or implying the reason is inappropriate.

Charts and charting procedures will be described to you by your instructor. Later, when you are employed, you will find that charting systems and procedures vary from one institution to another. Learn what is required and conform to that.

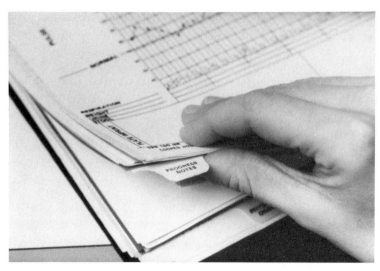

Patient charts are legal records of medical and nursing care.

Employers will expect you to be familiar with the charting process, but they will also recognize your need for time to learn the specifics of their system.

Be consistent when charting and use only agency-approved abbreviations and charting correction procedures, so that any given entry always means the same thing whenever it is written and errors will always be corrected properly. Keep in mind that if the patient claims malpractice, the entries on the patient's chart will be examined closely in court.

If you document your nursing actions on a computer, be sure that you do not leave the patient chart on the screen so that others can read confidential information. Also be certain that your access code remains secure with you and that you do not share that code with anyone else for any reason.

Areas of Frequent Claims of Negligence

The area in which nurses are most often found liable for negligence is related to patient falls. Other areas of negligence include medication errors, using improper techniques when performing procedures, not monitoring a patient's status frequently enough, not providing a safe environment, and not responding to a patient's request for care.

Unlicensed Assistive Personnel

Another area of increasing concern for nurses and one in which a claim of negligence is possible is the delegation of nursing tasks to unlicensed assistive personnel. The National Council of State Boards of Nursing in November 1995 issued a document that provides some guidelines on the licensed nurse's role in delegating nursing tasks. This document clearly indicates that the licensed nurse is accountable for the appropriateness of delegated nursing tasks. Inappropriate delegation by the licensed nurse to unlicensed assistive personnel may lead to legal action against the nurse. The full text of this document is included in Appendix K.

The best way for a nurse to avoid being sued for negligence is to constantly look for and correct situations in which a patient may suffer an injury. The nurse may be able to correct the situation immediately or it may require the revision of a policy or procedure or even a law. Providing high standards of safe care requires nurses to be constantly involved in suggesting methods to improve the quality of care provided by healthcare facilities.

Malpractice Insurance

Malpractice insurance for nurses is becoming increasingly important in a society that has become suit conscious. Paying for the defense of a lawsuit and paying any judgment that might be rendered are beyond the ability of most people. To protect their employees and themselves against any legal and financial consequences that could arise from provision of services, institutional employers carry malpractice liability insurance. However, because individuals are responsible for own their actions, it is still possible for an employee (eg, you as a nurse) to be sued personally. This is true even in states where "charitable immunity," the protection of non-profit hospitals from legal liability, applies.

A separate, personal malpractice liability insurance policy over and above your employer's policy is a wise investment that some would consider essential. There are at least three reasons why nurses should carry their own liability insurance policy. First, if you and your employer are co-defendants and found liable and the cost of the settlement exceeds your employer's policy limits, you may be required to pay the excess out of your own pocket.

Second, your employer's insurance company may sue you if they believe they incurred a loss because of your actions.

Third, many employer policies are claims-based rather than occurrence-based. A claims-based policy covers claims made while the policy is in effect. If your employer discontinues this policy and a claim is made later (which often happens), you would not be covered. An occurrence-based policy provides coverage if the incident occurs within the policy period. If the policy is allowed to lapse and a suit is filed for an incident that occurred during the policy period, coverage would be in place.

For your personal protection against claims against you, make certain your employer carries a policy of liability insurance that covers you. Find out the exact nature and limits of the coverage it gives you. Then, with a knowledgeable expert, determine what additional amount (dollar value) and type (occurrence- or claims-based) of personal coverage you should carry and purchase a policy accordingly.

Wills

A *will* is a legal statement of a person's wishes regarding the disposition of property after death. There may be times when patients ask you to help them prepare their wills. You should not accept the responsibility but should refer the matter to your instructor. An attorney is the appropriate person to help someone write a will, and the patient should be assisted to find one if so requested.

On occasion, you may be asked to witness a patient's will. Not all institutions allow nurses to witness wills. Abide by the guidelines set by yours. If witnessing a will is permitted, more than one witness will be required, which means that signing a will should be done only when other witnesses and the person whose will it is are present. Be sure the act of signing is accurately entered on the patient's chart, with particular attention to the time and date of signing.

Gifts

As a nurse, you should make it clear to patients and families that you do not accept gifts. It is legal to do so, but it is not ethical to accept gifts and it is certainly not ethical to solicit them.

However, there may be times when a patient may wish to give personal possessions as gifts to various people, including members of the healthcare team. This may be out of gratitude for care the patient has received or because he or she realizes that death is near. If the patient owns or has the right to dispose of the gift, and if the recipient accepts the gift, the act is valid within the law as long as the patient understands what he or she is doing and has not been coerced or deceived by anyone. Courteous refusal to accept the gift is the more appropriate response.

If a refusal is not accepted by the patient, particularly in times when the emotional climate is high, you should always protect yourself from any question about accepting a gift by having a witness present, informing your instructor or supervisor, and recording the patient's condition at the time.

CRIMINAL LAW AND NURSING

A *crime* is an offense committed against the public welfare and/or safety. You will recall that a tort is a legal wrong claimed by one person against another. Therefore, if you injure someone, the injured person is the one who prosecutes you. If you commit a crime, however, it is the state that seeks to prosecute you.

Criminal acts can be classified as minor offenses, misdemeanors, or felonies. Felonies are the most serious grade of criminal act and includes murder. A felony conviction can be grounds for denying, suspending, or revoking a nurse's license.

In many states with mandatory nursing licensure laws, practicing without a license is a felony punishable under public law. Those who may be arrested and tried include people who are practicing as nurses who were never licensed and nurses who have failed to renew their license.

Grossly negligent acts are considered crimes by many states. A nurse who restrains a patient against his or her will and without proper authorization may be charged with false imprisonment and prosecuted for committing a tort. However, if the same nurse became angry with a patient's behavior and restrains the patient with such force that circulation was impaired for a prolonged period causing the patient's hand to be amputated, the nurse would most likely be charged with a crime. To convict a nurse of a crime, the court would have to prove both a criminal act and a criminal intent.

In addition, other crimes in which nurses may become directly or indirectly involved include situations related to the right-to-die; violations of federal and state narcotic and controlled substance laws; fraud related to falsifying patient bills; robbery related to a patient's belongings; death because of lack of or incorrect nursing care; murder; and patient abuse.

Patient abuse is of great concern particularly in long-term care facilities. Governmental regulations related to criminal background checks of long-term care workers and a national registry of those convicted of abusing the elderly are currently being developed. Criminal abuse of the elderly includes physical abuse such as withholding food and water, hitting, slapping and punching, and restraining with intent to imprison. Other abuses of the elderly such as sexual abuse, failure to provide a safe environment, and failure of a healthcare facility to provide care may lead to criminal charges.

Whether the crime is a misdemeanor or a felony depends on the seriousness of the offense. In your nursing practice, you must practice within the law. You must be certain that your actions are based on your education, experience, standards of practice, and employer guidelines and not on emotional responses to sometimes difficult situations. You must think about what you are doing, why you are doing it, and whether a nurse with your similar education and experience would take the same or similar action that you intend to take.

DISCUSSION QUESTIONS/LEARNING ACTIVITIES

1. Read the 14th Amendment to the Constitution of the United States. Do you find in this amendment the basis for any present laws?

2. Obtain a job description for licensed practical/vocational nurses from your affiliating agency. Analyze how clearly the duties of the LP/VN are written.

3. Read your malpractice insurance policy if you have one. What acts are included and what acts are excluded? Is your policy claims-based or occurrence-based?

4. Ask your librarian to refer you to books that present summaries of malpractice suits. What similarities do you find in cases of negligence?

5. In addition to the suggestions presented in the chapter, what other actions by a nurse may reduce the possibility of a claim of malpractice?

6. Obtain and review the policy and procedures manual compiled by your affiliating agency. How do these documents define the standards of practice expected of this agency?

7. Imagine that you are driving to school and an automobile accident occurs in front of you. When you stop, you see that the driver of the car has hit his head on the windshield. What will you do and why?

8. Obtain a copy of the nurse practice act for your state. Analyze how these laws affect your practice of nursing.

READ MORE ABOUT IT

Aiken T, Catalano J: Legal, Ethical, and Political Issues in Nursing, First Edition. Philadelphia: FA Davis, 1994.

Bernzweig EP: The Nurse's Liability for Malpractice: A Programmed Curse, Sixth Edition. St. Louis: CV Mosby, 1995.

Catalano JT: Springhouse Notes: Ethical & Legal Aspects of Nursing, Second Edition, Springhouse, PA: Springhouse Corporation, 1995.

Goldstein A, Pruitt S: The Nurse's Legal Advisor: Your Guide to Legally Safe Practice. Philadelphia: JB Lippincott, 1989.

Hall JK: Nursing Ethics and Law, First Edition. Philadelphia: WB Saunders, 1996.

Lipman M: Medical Law and Ethics, First Edition. New York: Brady, 1994.

Springhouse: Nurses's Legal Handbook, Third Edition. Springhouse: Springhouse, 1996.

12

Leadership Skills

OBJECTIVES

When you complete this chapter, you should be able to:

Compare and contrast three styles of leadership.

Describe at least one situation where each style of leadership is appropriate.

List at least 10 qualities of effective leaders.

Describe in a paragraph the characteristics of effective followers.

Given a fictitious situation, discuss possible solutions to resolving conflict.

Assess your leadership and followership style.

"I never expected to feel the way I do today," Jane said to her best friend Cindy. Cindy looked at Jane and saw the tiredness in Jane's eyes.

"What are you talking about? What has made you feel and look so bad?" Cindy asked. "Remember," Jane said, "I told you I was scheduled for my 1-week team leadership experience this week." "Now I remember," said Cindy, instantly feeling that she should have recognized the symptoms. She had just finished her leadership rotation 3 weeks ago, and the experience was still fresh in her mind.

"How do you feel about being a team leader?" Cindy asked. "I always thought I was a leader until this week," Jane replied. "Why is that?" asked Cindy. "Well, Cindy, a number of things happened, and I don't think I acted like a leader. Everything seemed so disorganized, and I just couldn't get all the problems resolved.

Some of the team members complained about the assignments I gave them, and then two of them switched their assignments and didn't even tell me. I just feel as though I wasn't in control. I was really looking forward to being 'the boss' but it wasn't at all what I expected." "What did you expect?" asked Cindy. "Well," replied Jane, "I read all the assignments and even went to the special seminar on developing leadership skills. I expected..." At that point, Ms. Jones, their clinical instructor walked up to Jane and Cindy.

"How are you both doing?" asked Ms. Jones. "It seems to me that Jane is trying to recover from her team leadership experience," Cindy said. Ms. Jones shared with them that in her many years of teaching experience, the team leadership assignment is often very difficult for students.

"Why is that?" they both asked simultaneously. "I think it is because 1 week doesn't give you enough time to profit from the mistakes that you make. The team leader assignment gave you an opportunity to explore the role and responsibilities of a nursing team leader. You are now more aware, as a result of your experience, of the skills that a good leader needs," said Ms. Jones. As Ms. Jones walked away, Cindy and Jane looked at each other, and they both realized that if they ever wanted to be "in charge," they would need more preparation for that role.

A number of trends over the years have contributed to changing the roles and responsibilities of licensed practical/vocational nurses. The passage of Medicare and Medicaid legislation in 1965 and changes in the accreditation standards for hospitals, home healthcare agencies, long-term care facilities, and other healthcare agencies have created an overall rise in the demand for nursing service. The result is an increasing use of LP/VNs as team leaders, charge nurses, or patient care managers. This relatively new responsibility for specialized licensed practical/vocational nursing practice is reflected in the 1991 NFLPN "Nursing Practice Standards for the Licensed Practical/Vocational Nurse" (Appendix E). The LP/VN who is considering a leadership position is expected to have at least 1 year of experience at the staff level; have personal qualifications that will contribute to successful performance; and complete a program or course of study designed to prepare for the position.

The LP/VN in a leadership position in long-term care should complete the Certification Examination for Practical Nurses in Long-Term Care (CEPN-LTC). Those LP/VNs who successfully pass the certification examination will be authorized by NAPNES to use the credential CLTC (Certified, Long-Term Care) after their name.

Although it is still very early in your career, now is the time to begin developing the leadership qualities and management skills that will contribute to your opportunities for advancement in practical/vocational nursing. This chapter and Chapter 13 will provide an introduction to leadership and management in nursing.

LEADER AND LEADERSHIP DEFINED

A *leader* is a person who has specific goals and is able, through leadership skills, to get others to follow. Leadership is the process that helps a group of people achieve established goals.

The person responsible for leading the nursing team is called the nurse manager, the head nurse, the charge nurse, or the team leader.

Some of the specific goals of a nursing team leader could include:

Providing a safe environment for staff and patients.
Providing excellent nursing care.
Working as a team.
Minimizing nursing errors.
Establishing pleasant working relationships between nurses, patients, families, physicians, and other members of the healthcare team.
Sharing knowledge and experience.
Communicating accurately and effectively.
Motivating each team member to achieve his or her maximum potential.
Promoting an interest in incorporating new nursing skills in nursing practice.

While there are many other goals that a team leader might have, the above list provides an overview of some goals that can be accomplished through leadership and the efforts of the team members.

A job title does not make a person a leader. You have probably known or will know someone who has been a supervisor, nurse manager, or team leader, yet you would not identify that person as a leader.

Researchers have studied leaders and leadership skills extensively and have generally found that effective leaders use various styles, have diverse personalities and personal qualities, and handle people in dissimilar ways.

LEADER STYLE

The autocratic or authoritarian leader is one who is primarily concerned that tasks are accomplished. This type of leader has little concern for people and rarely involves staff in the decision-making process. The authoritarian leader often uses techniques such as coercion, threats, punishments, and constant observation to keep team members under control. An authoritarian leader issues directives and orders, determines rules for workers, and independently makes decisions that affect the entire team.

The permissive or laissez-faire leader provides little or no direction or control for the team. This type of leader assumes that the staff is self-directed and will do what needs to be done correctly and efficiently without supervision or direction. The permissive leader often has a personal need to be liked by everyone and, for this reason, avoids blame for team actions by giving responsibility to individual team members.

The democratic leader encourages staff participation and often consults and collaborates with staff. This type of leader believes that team members have knowledge and skills that can contribute to better decisions for the team and the organization. The democratic leader respects team members, and interactions between team members and the leader are open and trusting. Democratic leaders accept responsibility for the actions of team members and consider themselves an integral part of the team.

It should be evident that one style will not work in every situation. It is often necessary to use different styles in different situations. During an emergency such as a fire in a patient's room, the authoritarian style of leadership is most effective and most appropriate.

A democratic style would probably be the most appropriate style to use in the day-to-day operation of a nursing unit. A leader using this style would incorporate the opinions and expertise of his or her staff when making decisions affecting policies and the operation of the patient unit.

A permissive style would be most appropriate in a situation where all team members are experienced, skilled, self-directed, conscientious, and trustworthy. A group of professionals working on research projects might effectively work with a permissive leader.

As you can see, different situations require different leadership styles. This is called *situational leadership*. Situational leadership theorists believe that effective leadership occurs when the leader's style matches the overall situation. The overall situation includes the leader (style and expectations), the followers (knowledge and skills), and the events (work requirements) that are occurring. The leader is expected to take all three into account when selecting a style or combination of styles of leader behavior.

Caution should be exercised when changing your prevailing style as a leader. Everyone agrees that certain situations demand certain styles, however, frequent changes in leader style are detrimental. Leaders who are democratic one day, permissive the next, and authoritarian the third day create an environment of chaos and confusion for their team. Your prevailing style should be one that fits your personality and the personality of your team.

The diagram below illustrates that the most effective leadership style, for most situations, falls within the shaded area. The situation plus staff skills, knowledge, capabilities, and personalities, may require the leader to add some of the characteristics of the permissive or authoritarian leadership styles to his or her democratic style.

For example, all staff members are skilled in performing their duties and they have personalities that work well together. But almost all of the team members arrive 10 to 15 minutes late for work almost every day. This causes the previous shift to have to wait for them to arrive. Facility policies are very clear on the requirement to arrive for work on time. This situation has been discussed individually and with the team as a whole on several occasions but the problem was

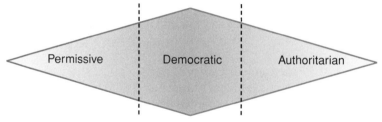

Democratic leaders occasionally display permissive and authoritarian behaviors to some degree.

not resolved. At this point, the democratic leader may decide to incorporate some authoritarian style and clearly outline to his or her staff the requirement of being on time and the actions that will be taken for continued lateness.

Regardless of the style or combination of styles that is most appropriate and comfortable for you, the hectic pace of the nursing unit offers many opportunities for you to experience tension and emotional stress. How you respond to this tension and stress will be evident in your behavior.

PASSIVE, AGGRESSIVE, AND ASSERTIVE BEHAVIOR

The word *passive* means to not take part in something. A person exhibiting passive behaviors avoids conflict and does nothing in situations in which an action is required. This person does not contribute ideas and suggestions to improve the work of the nursing team, does not encourage patients to participate in their care, and rarely, if ever, expresses how he or she feels about a situation.

Those who are passive often blame others, say "Yes" when they mean "No," and work extra shifts when they are physically unable to do so. The passive person who is scheduled to work on a requested weekend off will work. He or she will never confront the situation nor express his or her feelings to the person responsible. Over time, the passive person becomes angry and hostile because he or she feels hurt, used, and abused by others. The price one pays for not expressing feelings, needs, and wants is high.

Aggressive behavior is almost opposite of passive behavior. Other words that mean the same are pushy, forceful, hostile, and combative. People who are behaving aggressively ignore the rights and feelings of others. They are focused only on their own needs and feelings and often act and speak before thinking.

Those who use aggressive behaviors often get their own way at the expense of others. They, like those who are passive, are ineffective nursing team members. They make statements like "My way or no way," "I refuse to take care of Mr. Doe," and "You are incompetent." When assigned to work on a weekend they requested to be off, the aggressive person might say, "Before I'll work next weekend, I'll quit. Then you'll see."

Assertive behaviors are those behaviors in which you express your needs and feelings without attacking someone else. An assertive person uses statements that begin with "I" to describe his or her own feelings or needs. An example of assertive behavior with a supervisor is as follows: "I requested next weekend off over 2 months ago and I see on the schedule that I am assigned to work. I cannot work that weekend." The response may not be what you want but you did openly and honestly express your feelings. It is possible in this situation that the supervisor made an error, apologized, and corrected the situation, or the supervisor explained the reasons why you were scheduled or offered other solutions to resolving the problem. The assertive approach allows discussion and compromise; the aggressive approach leaves no options for the person making the statement. The passive response is actually no response and by avoiding any response at all, the person has no options but to work as scheduled.

Assertive statements such as "I do not want to hear gossip about others," "I do not share your views about (related to prejudices or people) and I expect you to respect my right to not hear yours," or "I find it very distressing when you criticize me in front of others. If you have something critical to say, please say it in a private place" will help you avoid accumulating the anger, hostility, and resentment that passive and aggressive behaviors encourage.

Learning to be assertive rather than passive or aggressive takes a conscious effort. Being assertive means:

Asking for your rights but not at the expense of others.
Expressing needs and feelings that are of significant importance to you.
Being honest and truthful with yourself and others.
Not deliberately hurting others.
Making statements that begin with "I."
Being sure that what you ask for is what you want.
Taking responsibility for your request.
Not being self-centered and selfish.

Learning to incorporate assertive behaviors with sensitivity, honesty, and flexibility will go a long way toward making your working relationships productive and pleasant.

In addition to effective style and behavior, there are other several other qualities that effective leaders possess.

QUALITIES OF EFFECTIVE LEADERS

An effective leader is much easier to recognize than to describe. From your own experiences, you can no doubt identify team leaders, nurse managers, and supervisors who are effective leaders and others who are not. Becoming an effective leader doesn't happen naturally; it takes study, experience, and work to develop a number of personal qualities.

Now is the time, early in your career, to begin studying and practicing the personal and interpersonal qualities of an effective leader.

Effective leaders are emotionally mature. They do not have temper tantrums, pout, complain, or find fault. They do not speak loudly or joke inappropriately in the presence of patients or their visitors. An emotionally mature leader is even-tempered, tolerant, and patient, and maintains a businesslike atmosphere everywhere, especially in patient care areas.

An effective leader is open-minded: willing to listen to the suggestions of others. The open-minded leader looks for better methods and safer procedures and frequently asks for others' opinions.

Effective leaders are fair. This means that a leader does not allow personal friendships and favoritism to cloud relationships with staff. He or she respects each member of the nursing team and expects everyone to make a maximum contribution to patient care.

Effective leaders are consistent in enforcing policies regulating staff conduct. On rare occasions when an exception can be justified, staff members are given an explanation for the exception.

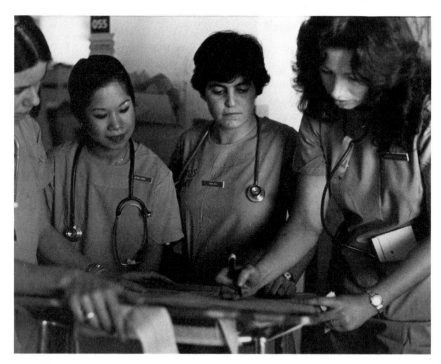

Becoming an effective leader requires study, experience, and the development of a number of personal and interpersonal qualities. (© Richard Wood, Taurus Photos.)

Effective leaders are assertive. They respect the rights of others as well as their own rights. They express how they feel about a situation by using statements that begin with "I." They ask for a certain action and, if not gotten, let it go knowing that they did make their feelings known.

Effective leaders are responsible. They accept responsibility for the actions of their staff members and, when indicated, defend those actions to their superiors. When a staff member is at fault, they try to help that person make positive adjustments rather than dismissing him or her from the team.

An effective leader is courageous. After making a decision, the leader changes the decision only when it is clear that the original decision was a poor one. The courageous leader can admit to having made a poor decision and can offer a sincere apology to an individual who has been offended.

An effective leader has the ability to teach. The leader who has a desire to share knowledge and skills with others is well on the way to becoming a teacher. Patience, tolerance, and praise are qualities that enhance any teaching-learning situation.

An effective leader has developed excellent problem-solving abilities. The effective leader defines the problem, gathers the facts, analyzes the information, proposes several solutions and the consequences of each, makes a decision, and evaluates the effectiveness of that decision.

Effective leaders have excellent clinical skills. They recognize that they "set the standard" of care and serve as role models for staff members. The effective leader offers workable suggestions and techniques to manage difficult nursing care situations.

Effective leaders are critical thinkers. They welcome different points of view and are creative in finding solutions to problems. They collect all the facts about a situation from every available resource, they weigh all of the possible solutions, and they take responsibility for their actions. Critical thinkers learn from their mistakes and use what they have learned in similar or new situations.

Effective leaders are sensitive as well as objective. Although they enforce the rules and regulations of the employer and the unit, they are aware of the special needs and abilities of the people they are leading. They interact with each member of their team as a unique human being with a vast array of personal needs, cultural differences, and interests.

Effective leaders are flexible and match their style of leadership to the situation. During an emergency, an effective leader is decisive and gives direct orders to the team members. In the daily routine, the effective leader follows a fairly well-established and consistent style of leadership. An effective leader who is making long-range plans may encourage suggestions from members of the nursing team and incorporate their recommendations into the plan.

Effective leaders have a sense of humor. Adding humor to an embarrassing, difficult, or tense situation often diffuses the tension and allows everyone to relax. When relaxed, people can think better, make better decisions, and work more effectively.

An effective leader often selects a role model who exemplifies the qualities of an effective leader. By observing the role model's personal and interpersonal relationships with staff members, the inexperienced leader can identify some of the personal qualities that contribute to effective leadership skills.

These are just a few of the personal qualities of an effective leader. These qualities may not come naturally but you can develop them if you make an honest effort to incorporate them into your life and your nursing career. Do this by being aware of what they are, by observing them in yourself, by noting how they change as you practice them, and by making corrections when your actions do not produce the results you want.

It is important to know that leaders, no matter how much education or experience they have, make mistakes. Learning from your mistakes is a quality that will probably contribute most to your development as a leader. Being the leader of a patient care team is a tremendous responsibility but one that can provide equally tremendous rewards. The box on the opposite page summarizes the qualities of an effective leader.

LEADING AND TEAM BUILDING

Having an effective patient care team doesn't just happen. An effective leader creates an environment that encourages team members to work together to do their best so that patients receive the best care possible.

One of the ways the leader can do this is by being a positive role model for the team members. Being a positive role model includes everything from your pro-

---

LEADERSHIP QUALITIES

Effective leaders are:

Emotionally mature	Clinically proficient
Open-minded	Critical thinkers
Fair	Sensitive and objective
Assertive	Flexible
Responsible	Capable of using humor
Courageous	Positive role models
Teachers	Capable of profiting from experience

---

fessional appearance to your desire to provide the best possible care for your patients to your commitment to the nursing profession. Consistently dressing appropriately and being involved in committees, professional organizations, and continuing education programs are all behaviors that you would want from your team members.

To build an effective team, the leader must be able to motivate the team members to achieve their goals. This is easiest when the team members are involved in setting the goals. If one of the goals of the team is that they have no work-related injuries for 1 month, it is likely that all of the team members will work to make that goal a reality. Rewards such as a staff party, a monetary bonus, time off with pay, a recognition banquet, award pins, and so forth often serve to reinforce the motivation to achieve a defined goal.

Building an effective team also requires coaching. It is as important to let the team members know when they have done a good job as it is to let them know when they have not. Praise of good work is highly valued by team members.

Other ways of building an effective team include recognizing the individual strengths and weaknesses of the team members. Capitalizing on an individual's strengths gives opportunities for increased self-esteem. Coaching an individual on how to overcome a weakness will help that individual achieve his or her maximum potential. Even if this results in losing a team member to a promotion, you have the satisfaction of knowing that you were able to help someone else grow in their career.

HANDLING CHANGE

As a leader, you will no doubt be faced with the necessity to cope with change yourself and to explain changes to your team members. In healthcare settings, changes involve policies and procedures, staffing patterns and schedules, work conditions, salary and benefit packages, new equipment, job responsibilities, patient care protocols, government regulations, accrediting agency regulations, and many other things that will affect your work and how you do it.

There are three things you and your team can do when confronted with change. You can resist change, you can accept it, or you can escape it. If a change is unacceptable to you, your best action is to escape it through resignation or transfer. Suppose, for example, that you have been working in an operating room of a hospital that does not perform abortions. The hospital is sold and the new own-ers hire a physician who will begin performing abortions in the operating room in 2 months. You are morally, religiously, and ethically opposed to abortions. In this situation, your best action may be to resign or to request a transfer to another area within the hospital because it is highly unlikely that you will be able to convince the new owners not to make this change.

Resisting change requires a lot of personal energy and can take its toll on your physical and mental health. People often resist change because they fear they will loose their job, that change will require more work for them, or because they do not understand the change. As a leader, it is important for you to make every effort to be involved in planning changes, getting facts related to the change from the source, and in interpreting for your team the effects of the change on them.

How you as a leader handle proposed or real changes will directly influence how your team members handle change. If you accept change and view it as an opportunity to do things differently, as exciting, as progress, as a challenge, and as a way to learn new things, then your team members may also be less resistant to the change. The more involved you and your team members are on your employer's committees, in professional organizations, in continuing education, and in the politics affecting healthcare, the more able you are to influence deci-sions that will change your work environment.

HANDLING CONFLICT

It would be rare to find a nursing team that does not experience conflict. This conflict may be between staff members, between the staff and the leader, or a combination. Team members often look to the leader to resolve team conflict. Unless the leader takes action, conflict will rarely resolve itself. Avoiding the situ-ation or denying that a problem exists will not resolve the issue.

Using the problem-solving approach outlined on page 47, the leader should identify the problem and consider possible solutions. It is often advisable to dis-cuss the problem and proposed action with a supervisor or other nurse manager whom you respect and who can maintain confidentiality of information. Discussing the problem and getting feedback from someone whose judgment you trust often helps you clarify the problem and evaluate your proposed solution before you act.

Once you have chosen a course of action, follow it through to the end. Don't change your mind (unless you are obviously wrong) and don't be influenced by the opinions of others.

Keep disciplinary sessions private and professional. Shouting or threatening will not accomplish a solution. If necessary, involve your supervisor in the session. Have your facts straight, listen to what the individual or team members have to say, clearly state what action will resolve the problem, and specifically identify what you expect in the future.

When conflicts cannot be resolved and you are no longer an effective leader, it may be necessary to request a transfer or to resign from your position. Having effective leadership skills does not guarantee success. To be an effective leader, you must have effective followers as well as an organization that supports your goals as a leader.

FOLLOWERSHIP QUALITIES

A leader cannot be a leader without followers. The success of any patient care team depends to a great extent on the knowledge, experience, and attitudes of the followers.

Followers contribute to the success or failure of a leader. A person with excellent leadership skills will fail miserably if members of the group are not good followers. The box below lists some characteristics of good followers.

An effective follower, one who is competent in performing his or her job responsibilities, who has experience, and who has a positive attitude toward the role of the leader, will help the leader to achieve nursing team goals. A good follower will assist the leader by offering suggestions, giving information, willingly complying with assignments, asking for constructive criticism, and following policies and guidelines of the employer.

On the other hand, a follower who denies his or her incompetence, complains about assignments, withholds important information, rejects constructive criticism, and fails to abide by employer policies and guidelines hinders a leader's effectiveness.

Occasionally, a person in a follower role will take on an informal leadership role with his or her peers. The informal leader has significant power within the group and is in a position to contribute to the leader's effectiveness or destroy the leader. When you are in a follower role, it is important that you avoid behaviors that prevent the leader from leading. If the leader is ineffective in his or her role, the situation should be handled through either the employer grievance procedure or through a supervisor.

SELF-ASSESSMENT

The task of learning to be an effective leader is never done, and there is always room to improve your leadership skills. Take the Leadership and Followership Style Test on pages 206–210 to determine where you are now. If where you are now is not where you want to be, work to make changes.

(text continues on page 210)

FOLLOWERSHIP QUALITIES

Competent	Shares information
Experienced	Willingly accepts assignments
Positive attitude	Asks for constructive criticism
Offers suggestions	Follows policies and guidelines

LEADERSHIP AND FOLLOWERSHIP STYLE TEST

Structural Leadership Profile

The following 20 statements relate to your ideal image of leadership. We ask that as you respond to them, you imagine yourself to be a leader and then answer the questions in a way that would reflect your particular style of leadership. It makes no difference what kind of leadership experience, if any, you have had or are currently involved in. The purpose here is to establish your ideal preference for relating with subordinates.

The format includes a 5-point scale ranging from *strongly agree* to *strongly disagree* for each statement. Please select one point on each scale and mark it as you read the 20 statements relating to leadership. You may omit answers to questions which are confusing or to questions that you feel you cannot answer.

	Strongly Agree	Agree	Mixed Feelings	Disagree	Strongly Disagree
1. When I tell a subordinate to do something I expect him/her to do it with no questions asked. After all, I am responsible for what he/she will do, not the subordinate.	1	2	3	4	5
2. Tight control by a leader usually does more harm than good. People will generally do the best job when they are allowed to exercise self-control.	5	4	3	2	1
3. Although discipline is important in an organization, the effective leader should mediate the use of disciplinary procedures with his/her knowledge of the people and the situation.	1	2	3	4	5
4. A leader must make every effort to subdivide the tasks of the people to the greatest possible extent.	1	2	3	4	5
5. Shared leadership or truly democratic process in a group can only work when there is a recognized leader who assists the process.	1	2	3	4	5
6. As a leader I am ultimately responsible for all of the actions of my group. If our activities result in benefits for the organization I should be rewarded accordingly.	1	2	3	4	5

From "Leadership and Followership," by David R. Frew, copyright February 1977. Reprinted with permission of *Personnel Journal*, Costa Mesa, CA; all rights reserved.

(continued)

LEADERSHIP AND FOLLOWERSHIP STYLE TEST (Continued)

	Strongly Agree	Agree	Mixed Feelings	Disagree	Strongly Disagree
7. Most persons require only minimum direction on the part of their leader to do a good job.	5	4	3	2	1
8. One's subordinates usually require the control of a strict leader.	1	2	3	4	5
9. Leadership might be shared among participants of a group so that at any one time there could be two or more leaders.	5	4	3	2	1
10. Leadership should generally come from the top, but there are some logical exceptions to this rule.	5	4	3	2	1
11. The disciplinary function of the leader is simply to seek democratic opinions regarding problems as they arise.	5	4	3	2	1
12. The engineering problems, the management time, and the worker frustration caused by the division of labor are hardly ever worth the savings. In most cases, workers could do the best job of determining their own job content.	5	4	3	2	1
13. The leader ought to be the group member whom the other members elect to coordinate their activities and to represent the group to the rest of the organization.	5	4	3	2	1
14. A leader needs to exercise some control over his/her people.	1	2	3	4	5
15. There must be one and only one recognized leader in a group.	1	2	3	4	5
16. A good leader must establish and strictly enforce an impersonal system of discipline.	1	2	3	4	5
17. Discipline codes should be flexible and they should allow for individual decisions by the leader, given each particular situation.	5	4	3	2	1

(continued)

LEADERSHIP AND FOLLOWERSHIP STYLE TEST (Continued)

18. Basically, people are responsible for themselves and no one else. Thus, a leader cannot be blamed for or take credit for the work of subordinates.	5	4	3	2	1
19. The job of the leader is to relate to subordinates the task to be done, to ask them for the ways in which it can best be accomplished, and then to help arrive at a consensus plan of attack.	5	4	3	2	1
20. Position of leadership implies the general superiority of its incumbent over his/her workers.	1	2	3	4	5

Structural Followership Profile

This section of the questionnaire includes statements about the type of boss you prefer. Imagine yourself to be in a subordinate position of some kind and use your responses to indicate your preference for the way in which a leader might relate with you. The format will be identical to that within the previous section.

	Strongly Agree	Agree	Mixed Feelings	Disagree	Strongly Disagree
1. I expect my job to be very explicitly outlined for me.	1	2	3	4	5
2. When the boss says to do something, I do it. After all, he/she is the boss.	1	2	3	4	5
3. Rigid rules and regulations usually cause me to become frustrated and inefficient.	5	4	3	2	1
4. I am ultimately responsible for and capable of self-discipline based upon my contacts with the people around me.	5	4	3	2	1
5. My jobs should be made as short in duration as possible, so that I can achieve efficiency through repetition.	1	2	3	4	5
6. Within reasonable limits I will try to accommodate requests from persons who are not my boss since these requests are typically in the best interest of the company anyhow.	5	4	3	2	1
7. When the boss tells me to do something which is the wrong thing to do, it is his/her fault.	1	2	3	4	5

(continued)

LEADERSHIP AND FOLLOWERSHIP STYLE TEST *(Continued)*

8. It is up to my leader to provide a set of rules by which I can measure my performance.	1	2	3	4	5
9. The boss is the boss. And the fact of that promotion suggests that he/she has something on the ball.	1	2	3	4	5
10. I only accept orders from my boss.	1	2	3	4	5
11. I would prefer for my boss to give me general objectives and guidelines and then allow me to do the job my way.	5	4	3	2	1
12. If I do something that is not right it is my own fault, even if my supervisor told me to do it.	5	4	3	2	1
13. I prefer jobs that are not repetitious, the kind of task that is new and different each time.	5	4	3	2	1
14. My supervisor is in no way superior to me by virtue of position. He/she does a different kind of job, one which includes a lot of managing and coordinating.	5	4	3	2	1
15. I expect my leader to give me disciplinary guidelines.	1	2	3	4	5
16. I prefer to tell my supervisor what I will or at least should be doing. It is I who am ultimately responsible for my own work.	5	4	3	2	1

Scoring interpretation

You may score your own leadership and followership styles by simply averaging the numbers below your answers to the individual items. For example, if you scored item number one *strongly agree* you will find the point value of "1" below that answer (Leadership Profile). To obtain your overall leadership style add all the numerical values which are associated with the 20 leadership items and divide by 20. The resulting average is your leadership style. Do the same to score followership.

Score	*Description*	*Leadership Style*	*Followership Style*
Less than 1.9	Very autocratic	Boss decides and announces decisions, rules, orientation	Can't function well without programs and procedures. Needs feedback
2.0–2.4	Moderately autocratic	Announces decisions but asks for questions, makes exceptions to rules	Needs solid structure and feedback but can also carry on independently

(continued)

LEADERSHIP AND FOLLOWERSHIP STYLE TEST (Continued)

Score	Description	Leadership Style	Followership Style
2.5–3.4	Mixed	Boss suggests ideas and consults groups, many exceptions to regulations	Mixture of above and below
3.5–4.0	Moderately participative	Group decides on basis of boss's suggestions, rules are few, group proceeds as they see fit	Independent worker, doesn't need close supervision, just a bit of feedback
4.1 and up	Very democratic	Group is in charge of decisions; boss is coordinator, group makes any rules	Self-starter, likes to challenge new things by him/herself

It should be noted that scores on this instrument will vary depending on mood and circumstances. Your leadership or followership style is best described by the range of scores from several different test times.

Change can occur after you realize that your skills are not what you want them to be. Ask peers or supervisors to help you be more aware of your behaviors as a leader. Ask them to point out behaviors that do not enhance your effectiveness as a leader; then take some calculated risks that include behaviors that are new to you. If you frequently forget to recognize and praise excellent work, remind yourself to look for opportunities to do this. If your team is not working well together, schedule a team meeting to find ways of creating a more pleasant working environment. If you are insensitive to your team members' needs, try to develop a better awareness of their problems and concerns.

Reading journal articles and books on leadership skills can provide insight into your own leadership strengths and weaknesses. Attending workshops and seminars can provide opportunities to learn and practice new leadership skills.

SUMMARY

Whether you prefer being a leader or a follower, it is important that you learn as much about each role as you can. It would be rare to find an individual who possesses all the leadership skills discussed in this chapter. However, to be effective, a leader must know what skills are important and work to acquire as many of these skills as possible. Continue learning about your own strengths and about how you can improve your skills. Don't be afraid to admit when you make mistakes, and don't be afraid to compliment your staff when they earn it.

It would also be rare to find individuals who possess all the followership skills discussed in this chapter. Good followership skills are as important to the team as good leadership skills. Team members must work to develop "following" skills that enhance the leader's effectiveness.

Good leaders who have good followers have the potential to provide excellent patient care in a pleasant working environment. And both leaders and followers can feel satisfaction in knowing that together, they made a patient's stay in the hospital as comfortable as possible.

DISCUSSION QUESTIONS/LEARNING ACTIVITIES

1. Observe two people who you know who are effective leaders. What qualities do they have that make them effective? Are these qualities the same for both leaders? If the qualities are not the same, what are the differences?

2. What are the names of some of the journals that publish articles on leadership and management?

3. Select one or two leadership qualities that you think are important. Practice incorporating these in your relationships with your peers.

4. Interview a nursing leader in your clinical affiliation and ask the following questions:

   How long have you been a leader?
   What education did you have for your position as a leader?
   What advice would you give to someone who wanted to be a team leader?
   What is the most difficult part of your job as a leader?
   What is the most rewarding part of your job as a leader?

5. Get five or six of your classmates together and role play the following situation: You are the team leader and your classmates are the team members. The team members tell you that they want you to schedule a team meeting to discuss their lunch assignments. Currently, you make the lunch assignment by 10 AM and lunch is 30 minutes. Your team members want lunch times assigned by 7:30 AM, and they want 45 minutes for lunch.

READ MORE ABOUT IT

Alfaro-Lefevre R: Critical Thinking in Nursing: A Practical Approach, First Edition. Philadelphia: WB Saunders, 1994.

Bandman EL, Bandman B: Critical Thinking in Nursing, Second Edition, East Norwalk: Appleton and Lange, 1995.

Chenevert M: STAT: Special Techniques in Assertiveness Training for Women in the Health Professions, Fourth Edition. St. Louis: CV Mosby, 1993.

Clark CC: The Nurse As Group Leader, Third Edition. New York: Springer, 1994.

Douglass LM: The Effective Nurse: Leader and Manager, Second Edition. St. Louis: CV Mosby, 1995.

Keenan M: Nursing Leadership and Management Skills, First Edition. St. Louis: CV Mosby, 1995.

Morrison M: Professional Skills for Leadership: Foundations of a Successful Career, First Edition. St. Louis: CV Mosby, 1994.

Miller MA, Babock DE: Critical Thinking Applied to Nursing, First Edition. St. Louis: CV Mosby, 1995.

Northouse PG, Northouse LL: Health Communications: Strategies for Health Professionals, Second Edition. East Norwalk: Appleton and Lange, 1992.

Sullivan MP: Springhouse Notes: Nursing Leadership and Management, Second Edition. Springhouse: Springhouse, 1995.

Yoder-Wise PS: Leading and Managing in Nursing, First Edition. St. Louis: Mosby, 1995.

Management Skills

13

Levels of Management
Managing Patient Care
   Assessing Staff Capabilities
   Diagnosing Patient Needs for
     Nursing Care
   Planning and Delegating Patient Care
   Implementing Assignments
   Evaluating Performance

Managing the Unit
   Ordering Supplies and Equipment
   Maintaining a Safe Environment
Managing Communication
   Communicating With Visitors
   Communicating With Supervisors
   Communicating With Physicians

OBJECTIVES

When you complete this chapter, you should be able to:

Outline the skills associated with managing patient care.

Integrate the knowledge of nurse practice laws, employer policies, job descriptions, and staff capabilities when making patient assignments.

Describe some of the general responsibilities of the charge nurse for maintaining a safe environment.

Suggest techniques for communicating with supervisors, visitors, and physicians.

The entire class seemed to be talking at the same time, but an immediate hush fell over the room when Ms. Donnelly, the teacher, entered. "I could hear you talking all the way down the hall," Ms. Donnelly said. "What is causing all the excitement?" For a few moments no one said anything until Jackie raised her hand. "Yes, Jackie?" "Well," said Jackie, "we were just talking about that assignment you gave us on management. We think that every manager we were assigned to observe has a different style." "Can you be more specific?" asked Ms. Donnelly.

"Our assignment was to observe a nurse manager and to write down how she makes patient assignments, keeps supplies, evaluates performance, manages time, and communicates with others. I was comparing my notes with Robert, and our two managers seemed to be quite different. For example, the

213

manager I observed made patient assignments in the afternoon for the next day, and Robert's manager didn't make assignments until about an hour after the shift started. My manager had plenty of supplies on the utility room shelves, and they were organized and easy to find. Robert said that his manager didn't have many supplies and that the utility room was a mess."

"What you and Robert found was what I had hoped you would find," said Ms. Donnelly. "There are many different styles of management, and you have given us two examples of how different styles could affect the staff. Managing a patient unit is a complex task. Management skills can be learned and, with experience, these skills should improve. Our class today will explore what you found during your observation, how certain manager behaviors can affect the staff, and what you need to know to prepare for a position as a manager."

Management is the coordination of activities associated with providing patient care and delivering nursing services. Being a manager of a patient unit is a responsible position. Managers must have, in addition to leadership skills, skills in planning, organizing, and directing the work of others.

This chapter will introduce you to some of the basic skills involved in managing patient care and a patient unit. Continuing education in management skills, as well as experience and personal evaluation, will help you continue to improve your management skills.

LEVELS OF MANAGEMENT

The first level of management is the head nurse, charge nurse, or nurse manager of a patient care unit. The next level is supervisor, clinical specialists, or assistant director of nursing. The third level of management is chief nurse executive, vice president for nursing, or director of nursing. Each level of manager has specific duties that are generally written in a job or position description.

LP/VNs are most often first-level managers responsible for a specific patient unit, and they most often work in long-term care facilities. It is important for any LP/VN who is considering applying for a management position to know the nurse practice law and the scope of practice permitted in the state in which they work. Most states require that LP/VNs work under the supervision of a registered nurse, a physician, or dentist.

Any LP/VN who is considering a management position should have at least 1 year of experience as a staff nurse. A nurse manager should also complete additional study such as the CEPM-LTC (Chapter 12) to prepare for the role as manager, must thoroughly understand the job requirements, and must honestly assess his or her ability to perform those requirements.

MANAGING PATIENT CARE

The primary responsibility of a nurse manager (team leader, charge nurse, or patient care manager) is to direct patient care on a day-to-day basis. Other functions of the manager include ordering supplies and equipment, maintaining a safe environment, and communicating with other departments and with supervisors, physicians, and visitors.

Directing day-to-day patient care includes assessing staff capabilities, diagnosing patient needs for nursing care, planning and delegating patient care, implementing the assignment, and evaluating performance.

Assessing Staff Capabilities

The first step in directing patient care is to assess staff capabilities. To do this, you will need to know the functions they are legally permitted to perform, their educational preparation, how long they have been working in their position, and what technical and interpersonal skills they have.

The functions your staff are permitted to perform are defined by the nurse practice laws of your state and are also outlined in job descriptions developed by employers. The purpose of the nurse practice laws have been previously discussed and must be adhered to by all licensed nurses. Job descriptions are written documents that outline what is expected from employees in each job title. Job descriptions for a typical nursing team would include separate descriptions for job titles such as LP/VN manager, staff LP/VN, certified nursing assistant, unlicensed assistants, and unit secretary. While not an employee as such, there may also be a job description for volunteers.

Knowing the educational preparation of your staff for their position helps you decide how to best use them on your team. For example, if a new certified nursing assistant joins your staff, it is helpful to know if this person completed a 75-hour or a 480-hour training course. The person who completed the 75-hour course will probably have less experience and skills than the person who completed the 480-hour course. Having this information will help you decide how to best use this person on your team.

You will also need to know how long your team members have been working in their positions. Those who have several years of experience should be capable of working at a level that requires less supervision than those who have been in their position for a short time.

Knowing the technical and interpersonal skills of your staff is also important. There may be those on your team who can not perform all of the tasks listed in their job description. You have a responsibility as a manager to not assign tasks to someone who is incapable of performing them. Some staff members will have excellent interpersonal skills and would be able to work with anyone; others may work better when assigned to work with those with whom they get along.

With experience, you will learn to match your staff and their abilities with the unique needs and personalities of the patients on your unit.

Diagnosing Patient Needs for Nursing Care

The second step in directing patient care is to diagnose the particular nursing care needs of patients on your unit. Does the patient need care that can be provided only by an LP/VN, or can a nursing assistant meet a particular patient's care needs? At this point, you might also consider the personality of the patient. Although all nursing staff members should be able to meet the needs of any patient on your unit, it sometimes improves communication between patient and nurse when personalities are well-matched.

Planning and Delegating Patient Care

The third step in directing patient care is to plan and delegate patient care. This plan is generally communicated through a written assignment sheet or assignment board. The assignment sheet includes the staff members' names, their break and meal times, names and room numbers of patients to whom they are assigned, and any other general duties that staff members are expected to complete during their time on duty.

To delegate patient care means to assign the responsibility you have for the care of all of the patients on your unit to someone else. You have a legal responsibility as a licensed nurse to delegate tasks according to applicable laws, staff capabilities, and patient needs. The National Council of State Boards of Nursing (NCSBN) has identified the five rights of delegation. They are:

Right task
Right circumstances
Right person
Right direction/communication
Right supervision

Appendix K includes the NCSBN document titled "Delegation: Concepts and Decision-Making Process." Before delegating any of your duties as a licensed nurse, whether in a management or staff position, you should read and completely understand the importance of proper and legal delegation of duties.

Implementing Assignments

The fourth step in directing patient care is to post the written assignment sheet. The assignment sheet must be completed and available to staff 15 to 30 minutes before the shift begins so that staff members can determine their priorities and organize their work day. Verbal directions along with written assignments avoids confusion and misunderstanding between staff members and the manager.

On occasion, it may be necessary to change an assignment. When this happens, the manager must verbally tell the staff member of the change, as well as change the written assignment sheet. An effective manager would also explain why the change was necessary and acknowledge how the change affects the staff member.

In summary, these steps will help you plan, organize, and direct patient care on your nursing unit.

Evaluating Performance

The fifth step in directing patient care is to evaluate the performance of your nursing staff. This is done through informal and formal evaluations.

Informal evaluations are those that occur almost daily. As you supervise the work of your staff, you might ask yourself the following evaluation questions about each staff member: Do patients have any comments on their nursing care? Are procedures being done properly? Are assignments being completed on time? Are break and meal times being followed?

For example, suppose you see a nursing assistant piling dirty linen on a chair in the patient's room. The time to confront this breech in procedure is when it occurs. A verbal discussion (informal evaluation) with the nursing assistant should be all that is needed to correct the situation and prevent it from happening again. Remember: conduct such discussions in a private place.

Don't forget to acknowledge excellent judgment or exceptional patient care when it occurs. Managers are often dealing with so many different issues and problems that they forget to tell their staff members when they have done an outstanding job.

Formal evaluations are written and include an assessment of an employee's overall performance over a period of time, usually a year. These formal evaluations may be the basis for an increase in salary so being fair and objective is of utmost importance.

Unless you keep some kind of journal or written notes, chances are that when it comes time for the annual evaluation, you will only remember what that employee did in the last few weeks. Written notes encourage a more objective evaluation and also allow you to furnish dates and specific events upon which you base your comments on the evaluation. An employee may have been early for his or her shift for the past 11 months and late 6 times in the month before the evaluation. Writing on the evaluation that the employee is frequently late would not be a fair statement. It would be more objective to say that the employee was never late for 11 months and was late six times in the past month.

The form on which an evaluation is written is developed by the employer. The first line nurse manager is expected to contribute to the evaluation of his or her staff members. The manager should be familiar with the evaluation form and should make every effort to be objective when writing an evaluation. First line managers should document both positive and negative staff behaviors with examples. When standards of performance are clearly understood by management and staff, evaluating performance is more objective. Managers must keep subjectivity and personal bias out of the evaluation process. It is possible to like a staff member but not his or her job performance, just as it is possible to dislike a staff member but to recognize that his or her job performance is outstanding.

A written evaluation is always reviewed with the staff member. The staff member should be told in advance about the date and location of the review. You should find a quiet, private place for this conference. During this time, you can discuss a staff member's strengths and areas for improvement. Give the staff member an opportunity to respond to the evaluation and to your comments. The evaluation should end on a positive note with goals for the future.

As you evaluate performance of your staff and quality of nursing care each day, you also collect information that will assist you when you begin the same process the next day. Experience as a manager will provide valuable lessons in developing skills that contribute to quality patient care.

If you find it necessary to discuss poor performance with a staff member, do so in a private place. Try to determine the cause of poor performance and if the team member is lacking necessary knowledge or skills, provide information that will help improve performance. Otherwise, suggest that a certain quality of patient care is expected and that you expect everyone to provide that quality.

If a staff member is behaving in a manner that is unsafe and inappropriate, discreetly move the person away from patients and visitors, or call or have someone call for assistance from your supervisor. This difficult situation requires tact and sensitivity on the part of the nurse manager.

MANAGING THE UNIT

In addition to managing patient care, the team leader, charge nurse, or patient care manager has many other functions that contribute indirectly to patient care. These functions are related to the operation of the patient care unit.

Ordering Supplies and Equipment

Supplies and equipment essential for patient care must be available to your nursing staff. Responsibility for having necessary supplies and equipment on the patient unit belongs to the unit manager, or you may delegate (assign) this responsibility to a member of your staff. Regardless of whose responsibility it is to order supplies and equipment, you must periodically check the work to be sure supplies and equipment are being ordered properly.

All supplies, including drugs, must be put away promptly. Storage spaces must be kept neat and orderly so that items needed in an emergency can be quickly located. Equipment must be kept clean and in working order. Requests to repair equipment must be followed until repairs are completed.

Maintaining a Safe Environment

The physical environment consists of the surroundings in which you work. As a manager, you are responsible for seeing to it that unsafe situations are corrected. Although not everything that needs fixing can be fixed immediately, certain measures can be taken to prevent further damage or even injury to people in that environment. You don't have to nag to be persistent.

Carelessness often contributes to injuries to both your patients and staff. Keep clutter to a minimum and clean up spills immediately. Keep bedside cabinet doors and drawers closed when they are not in use. Be sure your staff members remove supplies and equipment from the bedside when a task or procedure is completed. Check that beds and bed rails function properly. Remove broken chairs, wheelchairs, and similar equipment from your unit to prevent accidental use. Require your staff to keep the medication room or medication cart locked when not in use. With experience, common sense, and a concern for the safety of your patients and staff, you will develop a habit of looking for situations that are unsafe. As the manager, you must accept personal responsibility for correcting these situations.

A fire in a healthcare facility is one of the most frightening things that can happen. Require your staff to know the location of fire extinguishers, how to check pressure gauges on fire extinguishers, and how to use them. Be sure they know how to sound an internal fire alarm and when to call the local fire department. Review evacuation procedures and discuss the possibility of having a mock fire drill with your nursing supervisor.

MANAGING COMMUNICATION

As you learned in Chapter 2, good communication skills are essential in nursing. You will want to be sure you understand information you are receiving, and you will want to be clear in information you are giving.

Communicating With Visitors

Visitors are important to your patients and provide a diversion from long hours alone in the healthcare facility. Most visitors are considerate and do not discuss topics that will upset your patients. If the patient does become upset or anxious, you must tactfully ask the visitors to limit their conversations to more neutral subjects.

Use caution when giving information about a patient to a visitor or member of the family. What you know about a patient's diagnosis, laboratory results, or plan of treatment is essentially confidential and not to be shared with anyone. You can tactfully suggest that these kinds of questions are best answered by the patient's physician.

You can discuss nursing concerns such as food likes and dislikes, ambulation, and sleep patterns with the patient's family. If at all possible, this should be done in the patient's presence, and the patient should be included in the conversation.

On occasion, visitors may become disruptive to the unit. As the manager, you must make an attempt to elicit their cooperation in controlling noise. If you are unsuccessful, you should immediately notify your nursing supervisor and ask for assistance.

Communicating With Supervisors

Your relationships with nursing supervisors can be both positive and beneficial to you. It is important to recognize that your nursing supervisor is ultimately responsible for the quality of nursing care that you and your staff provide. You should view your supervisor as a resource person to whom you can go for advice and assistance in managing your patient unit.

To maintain a good working relationship with your nursing supervisor, you must keep the supervisor informed of problems or incidents that occur on your unit. Problems that may seem small and insignificant to you may turn out to be major problems to the institution. You must also report your errors and the errors of your staff to your supervisor and complete a written description of any incident that occurs on your unit.

When you communicate with your nursing supervisor, it is important to present the situation's facts clearly, concisely, and objectively. It is unfair to the supervisor, who will probably have to make a decision related to a situation, to present only what you want the supervisor to know.

Your supervisor is, like you, in a management position. Just as your subordinates will not always like or understand all your decisions, you will not like or understand all the decisions of your supervisor. You must contribute to developing a relationship with your supervisor that is positive and productive, not negative and destructive.

Communicating With Physicians

Communicating with the physician or primary care provider is an essential part of management in nursing. As in communicating with your supervisor, you should keep the physician informed of changes in the condition of his or her patient. You must be able to clearly and concisely describe the facts you are reporting.

If a physician's treatment or medication order is unclear or questionable, it must be verified with the physician. You are not expected to blindly follow orders that you believe could be harmful to your patients. It is important to use tact and good communication skills when requesting verification from the physician.

You, through your staff, are in a position to provide valuable information about patients to their physicians. The nursing team spends a great deal of time with patients and consequently has information that may influence the methods a physician chooses in treating patients. Sharing that information through verbal communication with physicians can make an enormous contribution to the total plan of care for patients. Thus, the team leader, charge nurse, or patient care manager must establish effective methods of communication with physicians.

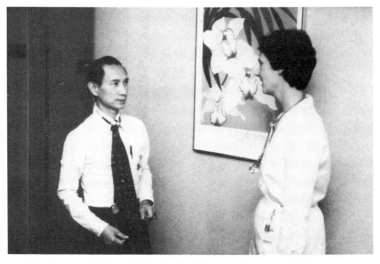

Communicating with the physician is an essential part of management in nursing.

In summary, managing patient care is a tremendous responsibility, but with that responsibility can come equally tremendous rewards. You can enjoy the satisfaction that comes from working with your team, your supervisor, and with physicians to provide the quality of nursing care that you alone could never achieve.

DISCUSSION QUESTIONS/LEARNING ACTIVITIES

1. Obtain the job or position descriptions for members of the nursing team in your clinical affiliation. Analyze each for education, experience, and skills.

2. In addition to the responsibilities of the patient care manager discussed in this chapter, list some of the other duties that might be assigned to this person.

3. Suppose you are the charge nurse of a 20-bed unit in an extended care facility, and one of the nursing assistants has not been coming back from her break on time. Outline what you would do and why.

4. While evaluating the quality of patient care, you notice that a bed rail is broken. What would you do first and why?

5. During your clinical experience, listen carefully to a conversation between a nurse and the nurse's supervisor. Analyze the conversation for its effectiveness in communicating information, ideas, or both. Was the purpose of the conversation understood by both the supervisor and the nurse? Was mutual respect evident? Was the conclusion of the conversation satisfactory to both parties? Were any comments made by either party after the other left?

READ MORE ABOUT IT

Arnold E, Boggs KV: Interpersonal Relationships: Professional Communication Skills for Nurses, Second Edition. Philadelphia: WB Saunders, 1994.

Ellis JR, Hartley CL: Managing and Coordinating Nursing Care. Philadelphia: JB Lippincott, 1991.

Flarey DL: Redesigning Nursing Care Delivery: Transforming Our Future, First Edition. Philadelphia: JB Lippincott, 1995.

Grohar-Murray ME, DiCroce HR: Leadership and Management in Nursing. Norwalk, CT: Appleton & Lange, 1992.

Longest BB: Management Practices for the Health Professional, Fourth Edition, 1990. East Norwalk: Appleton and Lange, 1990.

Loveridge JJ, Cummings CC: Nursing Management: Principles and Practices, First Edition. Sacramento: Aspen, 1996.

Marrelli TM: The Nurse Manager's Survival Guide: Practical Answers to Everyday Problems, First Edition. St. Louis: CV Mosby, 1993.

Porter-O'Grady T: The Nurse Manager's Problem Solver, First Edition. St. Louis: CV Mosby, 1994.

Powell AS: Introduction to Nursing Care Management, First Edition. Philadelphia: JB Lippincott, 1995.

Ringsven MK, Bond D: Gerontology and Leadership Skills for Nurses, First Edition. Albany, NY: Delmar, 1991.

Sullivan EJ, Decker PJ: Effective Management in Nursing, First Edition. Menlo Pa,rk, CA: Addison-Wesley, 1992.

Tamparo CD, Lindh W: Therapeutic Communications for Allied Health Professionals, First Edition. Albany: Delmar, 1993.

Beginning Your Nursing Career

OBJECTIVES

When you complete this chapter, you should be able to:

Compile a list of places, other than hospitals and nursing homes, where an LP/VN could be employed.

Describe some of techniques that ease the transition from student to employee.

Explain the value of a self-assessment before deciding on what type of nursing position to apply for.

(continued)

List several sources of information on available nursing positions.

Prepare a chart that includes areas that should be considered when evaluating positions.

Write a letter of application.

Prepare a personal resumé.

Write a letter of resignation.

Name and give the purposes of the nursing organizations to which LP/VNs usually belong.

Describe the influence of the political process on healthcare.

Compare the advantages and disadvantages of union membership.

Explain the purpose of the grievance process.

Define the term "burnout."

"This is our last class together. Before you leave, I'd like to say a few things that I hope you'll remember. I've enjoyed being your instructor for almost a year now. But I'm not speaking as your instructor today. What I have to say is coming from the heart of someone who cares about nursing and cares about each one of you.

When I became a nurse, the 'field' was more like a small garden. Nursing was basic in those days, in the subjects we studied and in the job opportunities that were available. The world seemed like a much smaller place. There certainly were fewer people. 'Burnout' wasn't a word yet, and if 'substance abuse' and 'hospice care' were, none of us had ever heard of them. But that doesn't mean some of us weren't ready for those and other words when they came. Those who weren't ready—and many of my classmates weren't, I'm sorry to say—have been left behind. And that's the 'message' in what I want to say to you today.

There's no way that all of us on the staff could fully prepare you for the many choices you will face. There are simply too many. You've been busy enough learning what we could teach you. The other things you will have to know—the choices you will be making-are going to be up to you. Once you graduate, you'll be on your own. Oh, we'd love for you to come back anytime, and you know you're always welcome. But out there, out in the world of nursing practice, you won't have someone to remind you to finish an assignment, to practice a procedure until perfect, or to read up on something you're uncertain of. Those things and many more will be expected from you—including things you haven't even heard of yet, just as my class hadn't heard of 'hospice.'

Now, just for a moment, let me pretend I'm one of you. This is what I would say: 'But, Mrs. Fuller, if we haven't heard of something, how are we supposed to know what to do?' Yes, it sounds funny, but isn't that what you were thinking? I thought so. So listen now to the answer.

Nursing is dynamic, growing, and ever expanding. It will never again be what it is today, and what it becomes tomorrow will also change. Nursing moves into the future automatically. Nurses do not. I'll say that again. Nurses do not automatically keep up with nursing. Nurses move into the future by listening, watching, and preparing for it.

All of you are ready for graduation because you have prepared for it, day by day, for almost a year. Those of you who will be in nursing's future have to begin preparing for it, day by day, starting today.

Thank you, class. You've been wonderful."

Although finding a job in the late 1990s is not as easy as it was 5 years ago, today's newly graduated practical/vocational nurse has options undreamed of by those who completed their programs just a few years ago. Finding that first job requires thoughtful preparation on your part and it also requires knowing what career opportunities are available.

CAREER OPPORTUNITIES IN NURSING

Just as you probably evaluated your educational options before you chose your nursing school, you must also evaluate your employment options. Selecting your first nursing position will be an important decision and one that should be made very carefully.

The employment opportunities for licensed practical/vocational nurses (LP/VNs) extend beyond those provided by hospitals and nursing homes. As private businesses and government agencies respond to the growing needs of a complex society, more areas where nursing care is needed are opening. You have an opportunity to look for the type of nursing that best meets your personal interests, needs, and capabilities.

Hospital Nursing

In no work setting has there been more change than in hospitals. Today, people are rarely admitted to hospitals for diagnostic studies or procedures, such as removal of gallstones. Mothers and their babies leave the hospital after 1 or 2 days—not 3 to 5 days as they did just a few years ago. With so many "short" procedures being done on an outpatient basis and with much shorter lengths of stay in the hospital, many hospitals have decreased the number of inpatient beds, as well as the number of staff including nurses. Patients who are admitted to hospitals now are much sicker and many require a level of care that can only be provided by highly trained registered nurses.

While employment opportunities for LP/VNs in inpatient units in acute care hospitals may be declining, there are opportunities for employment for LP/VNs in other areas of hospitals. LP/VNs often work in hospital-based clinics, outpatient same-day surgery units, operating rooms, radiology, hospital-based long-term care units, or in a home health department that is a part of the hospital. If working in a hospital is your career goal, you should look beyond the traditional patient care unit for opportunities for employment.

Hospital work schedules are generally set in three 8½-hour shifts. For example, day (7 AM to 3:30 PM), evening (3 PM to 11:30 PM), and night (11 PM to

7:30 AM) shifts. Shift, weekend, and holiday rotations, time off, and other scheduling procedures are set by the institution. Scheduling may vary from one institution to another to accommodate staffing needs and personal needs of employees.

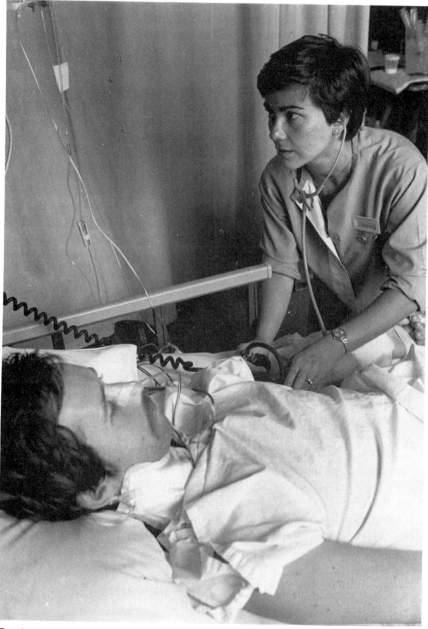

Employment opportunities for licensed practical/vocational nurses continue to expand. (© Richard Wood, Taurus Photos.)

Community and Public Health Nursing

A very different nursing setting is experienced by nurses who work in community or public healthcare. There, nursing is provided to patients under the administration of established healthcare programs. These programs are operated and funded by voluntary agencies or local, state, or federal government agencies.

Nurses employed in public health may work inside community health centers with patients who come to the center, or they may work outside the center, traveling to the patient's home to give care there. Nursing staff of a city department of health clinic, for example, may provide in-clinic immunizations, prenatal care and counseling, and other services to clients who visit the clinic, or they may give the same service at the client's residence.

The LP/VN in public health will work under the direction of a registered nurse or other qualified supervisor. Among the qualifications for this work is the ability to work independently and responsibly when away from the health center.

Office Nursing

An especially challenging opportunity for a licensed P/VN is that of the office nurse. As the employee of a physician, dentist, or other healthcare provider, an office nurse may be responsible for a variety of duties that can include those of receptionist, secretary, lab assistant, bookkeeper, and supply clerk, as well as the nursing skills for which licensure has been granted.

Flexibility, adaptability, and self-direction are assets for the office nurse, who may be required to perform preliminary patient examinations and routine treatments; oversee a waiting room full of patients; assist with treatments; schedule appointments; and collect payment at the end of a patient's visit.

Offices may be large or small, with a staff that matches, so responsibilities may be in the hands of a single nurse, shared with other staff members, or limited to a specific role for each staff member.

Private Duty Nursing

A wholly independent nursing service is given by the private duty nurse, who works directly for a patient. Nursing care may be given in an institution, at the patient's home, or at another place requested by the patient. The patient is the nurse's employer and pays the nurse directly. A self-employed, private duty nurse is responsible for handling taxes, licenses, and other financial matters relating to self-employment.

A private duty nurse in an institution is subject to the institution's policies and direction and is responsible to the physician or other authority in charge of a patient's care. In a home setting, although working under direction of the patient's physician, the nurse must depend on his or her own judgment and experience to provide care.

Home Health Nursing

The principle of home healthcare is to provide nursing services in the patient's home. Because it is far less costly to care for a person in their home than it is to care

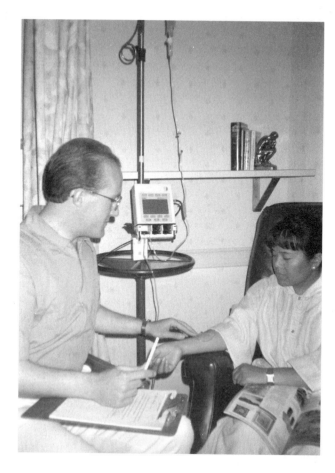

The number of nurses who choose home health nursing is increasing.

for them in a hospital or nursing home, the number of home healthcare agencies and the number of patient they care for each day has increased tremendously over the past few years. Home health agencies deliver a variety of services by a wide range of providers that can include registered nurses, LP/VNs, social workers, home health aides, homemakers, and physical, occupational, and speech therapists.

Nurses who provide nursing care in the patient's home must have excellent assessment skills, as well as good communication and teaching skills. A significant part of the nurse's job in home health is to teach family members to care for the patient at home.

Industrial/Occupational Nursing

Factories and manufacturing plants have had limited in-plant nursing services for years. Generally first-aid oriented (with an emphasis on accident prevention) services were established in response to the influence of labor unions. Today, as business and industry provide more services for their employees, nursing opportunities in the industrial sector are increasing. With a concern for good health now a national issue, other industries, white collar as well as blue collar, have installed health-oriented facilities and staffs that address on-the-job accident treatment and prevention, and broader issues as well. Physical exams, screening tests, diagnostic surveys, and health education are common services offered.

Hospice Nursing

The hospice movement is dedicated to making the inevitable death of terminally ill patients dignified and humane. It provides compassionate care and understanding in settings that are comfortable, familiar, and nonthreatening.

Nurses who work with dying patients require a special understanding of themselves and of their patient's unique place in the world. The nurse in a hospice setting must also be able to interact with the patient's family while not interfering with the patient's and family's personal relationships and business.

Hospice care is based on a philosophy that can be implemented in a variety of settings. Most often hospice services are provided in the home; however, it can also be found in hospitals, long-term care facilities, and other healthcare settings.

School Nursing

School nursing, like nursing services offered by business and industry, has expanded from the delivery of simple first aid, immunizations, and health screenings to a comprehensive program of prevention, treatment, and education. Depending on the size and philosophy of a school district, a school nursing department can be small or extensive. A single nurse may serve a number of schools, or each school may have its own nurse. The registered nurse in a school or schools functions independently and is generally under the authority of a physician appointed by the school district's board of education. LP/VNs assist the registered nurse with routine screening programs and daily activities associated with school nursing.

Nursing Homes

The rise in population of elderly Americans has accounted for a significant increase in the need for nursing and convalescent homes to care for older people who are unable to provide for themselves at home but who do not require hospitalization. The need for nurses to staff these institutions has risen accordingly.

A nursing home may be privately endowed or funded by local or state money. It may be for-profit or not-for-profit, but it must be licensed by the state in which it is located. Services provided may range from simple custodial caretaking to complete medical and rehabilitative care. In general, nursing care is supervised by a registered nurse who is responsible for the overall care of residents under the direction of a physician on call. LP/VNs are often employed as charge nurses and direct day-to-day delivery of nursing care.

Veterans Administration and Armed Forces Nursing

The Veterans Administration's hospital system is the nation's largest, and its hospitals are some of the biggest. They are federally operated hospitals that care for veterans of the U.S. armed forces. Many of them are affiliated with schools of medicine and nursing.

A wide range of job experience, potential for travel, and other benefits are associated with employment in Veterans Administration hospitals.

The U. S. Army offers career opportunities to licensed practical nurses in the Army Medical Corps. Applicants must be U.S. citizens, 17 to 34 years old, and graduates of 1-year practical/vocational nursing programs who hold current licenses. The Army offers active and reserve duty positions with good pay and benefits.

Other Employment Opportunities

LP/VNs often work in shelters for the homeless, boarding homes, group homes for those who are mentally challenged, prisons, outpatient psychiatric clinics, neighborhood health clinics, day care centers for children and older adults, and rehabilitation facilities. While the role of the LP/VNs varies from setting to setting, he or she is in a position to provide a variety of healthcare services from giving medications to performing nursing skills to teaching people how to prevent illness.

LP/VNs are also working for insurance companies and in managed care businesses. In these positions, their responsibilities may include coding treatments and procedures, doing physical examinations for insurance policies, and reviewing medical records.

Many companies that sell medical equipment and supplies find that hiring LP/VNs is cost effective for them. They find it easier to teach someone to sell a product than to teach someone about healthcare.

Getting that first job may not be easy but being aware of the many places where you could work will certainly increase your chances of success.

Regardless of where you choose to work, employers have certain general expectations of their employees. Knowing what employers expect of employees in any work situation will help you understand and accept your new role.

EMPLOYER EXPECTATIONS

Employers expect you to have a theoretical basis for what you do in order for you to understand the care you give, how to give it, what is expected from it, and what the effects of that care are, so that, if necessary, additional action can be taken.

Your nursing skills and how well you perform them will be expected to be comparable with other nurses who have the same level of education and experience. An employer will expect you to complete your assignments within a reasonable period of time.

Employers expect a nurse who does not know how to perform a skill, or who needs help, to ask for assistance. Employers will expect you to function within the law and according to the job description for your position.

Your employer will expect you to contribute to the organization by participating in conferences, serving on committees, and maintaining the skills required of the position.

Your employer will expect you to know how to keep records of your activities. Because medical records are so important to patient care and are legal documents, skills in documenting your activities are definitely expected. Although most employers allow time to learn their specific system, once the system is learned, you will be expected to keep accurate, legible, and technically and grammatically correct records.

Employers expect you to assume responsibility for your work. This includes specific obligations spelled out in the hiring agreement and other implied obligations such as honesty, promptness, and commitment to the job.

Employers expect you to support their philosophy and implement their organization's objectives. They expect you to be loyal to the organization and fair in your relationships with them.

As you begin your career in practical/vocational nursing, your skills and abilities may not yet match all of your employer's expectations. Making the transition from being a student to being a productive employee who is able to meet an employer's expectations can be a difficult process.

If you decide to become an employee in the institution where you were assigned for clinical experience, the transition may be relatively easy. If you decide to accept a position in an institution that is unfamiliar to you, the transition may be more difficult. In either case, there are some transitional challenges that will confront you as a beginning nurse. Being prepared to meet these challenges will help you adjust to your first job as an LPN or an LVN.

TRANSITIONAL CHALLENGES

There are many differences between being a student nurse and being a graduate LP/VN. As a student, the conditions under which you are learning are controlled to provide maximum educational benefit to you and your classmates. Your clinical assignments are selected to contribute to your educational development. Your clinical instructor is legally responsible for your performance in the clinical area and is there to help you resolve problems and answer questions. As a graduate, your assignments will be based on the needs of your patients and employer. You will be responsible and accountable for your own actions. And you will be expected to carry out your assignments within the allotted time.

Making these adjustments from student to employee may be difficult. You will not always have the same amount of time to spend with your patients as you had when you were a student. Your work load and the pace at which you will be expected to carry out your assignments will be increased. Some experienced members of the nursing team may help you during this transition period; others may not.

Expect to have mixed feelings: some very positive and others less so. You will be excited to finally have the chance to put what you have learned to actual use, but you might also be a bit nervous about it. You may feel that there is more work than you can handle. You may have difficulty adjusting to the leadership and management style of your supervisor. But remember, you successfully made similar adjustments when you began your nursing program, and you can do so again.

Some techniques that help ease the transition from student to employee include being honest about your limitations but not shirking your share of the work. If you find that you are getting behind schedule, let your supervisor know. You may want to ask an experienced nursing team member for suggestions on how to better organize your work. Observe how experienced nurses organize their schedules so that assignments are completed on time. You might ask your supervisor to evaluate your performance on a daily or weekly basis and use that information to improve your practice. Take every opportunity you can to learn more about your patient's medical conditions and his or her nursing needs. Admit your mistakes and learn from them. Be prepared to put in the extra time needed to complete your assignments without expecting to be paid for that time. In a surprisingly short time, you will make the adjustment and feel the satisfaction that comes from being accepted as a contributing member of the nursing team.

SELF-ASSESSMENT

Now that you have reviewed some of the career opportunities in nursing, employer expectations, and transitional challenges, you should assess yourself. Self-esteem and sound skills lend encouragement and confidence to one's outlook and tasks, whereas lack of self-esteem and poor skills can undermine one's confidence. The ability to make an objective analysis of yourself will help point out areas of strength and areas that need improvement. The key is to see yourself as best you can without the influence of your own beliefs or wishes about how you think you are or would like to be. An accurate self-assessment is not always easy, but the rewards make the effort worthwhile.

A review of your clinical strengths and weaknesses is an important consideration when thinking about the type of nursing you would prefer to do. If you seem to have a special ability to work with older people, you may consider employment in a long-term care facility. If you enjoyed your clinical experiences with children, perhaps being a school nurse may be the best place for you to begin your career.

You should assess your personal health and physical condition. If you have a health problem or physical condition that limits your activities, you should avoid seeking a position that would adversely affect your own health.

You should assess your work habits, how you prefer to dress, and other personal characteristics. Working in a situation that requires you to behave very differently from the way you usually behave can cause a great deal of stress and personal conflict.

Finally, you should assess your personal and interpersonal characteristics. On page 233 is a list of some characteristics to look for. As you read them, ask yourself how the item applies to you (always, usually, never) and mark the appropriate space next to the item. On completion, review the list with someone who knows you well and ask them what their answer would be. Compare the responses. The results are not scientific, but they will give you an indication of your self-perception and how others may see you. Use them to alter those aspects of yourself that may need changing. Evaluations from instructors during the course of your program can also be used to help judge yourself.

PERSONAL AND INTERPERSONAL CHARACTERISTICS ASSESSMENT

Personal Characteristics	*Always*	*Usually*	*Never*
1. I accept responsibility for my work.	____	____	____
2. I welcome criticism.	____	____	____
3. I tell the truth.	____	____	____
4. I don't waste time.	____	____	____
5. I am patient with myself.	____	____	____
6. I like solving problems.	____	____	____
7. I am organized.	____	____	____
8. I know my own limits.	____	____	____
9. I am comfortable with rules and regulations.	____	____	____
10. I accept change.	____	____	____
11. I do not have to be told what to do.	____	____	____
12. I do more than I'm asked.	____	____	____
13. I control my emotions.	____	____	____
14. I have a good sense of humor.	____	____	____
15. I ask for help when I need it.	____	____	____

Interpersonal Characteristics	*Always*	*Usually*	*Never*
1. I enjoy working with others.	____	____	____
2. I am a good listener.	____	____	____
3. I don't mind sharing credit with others.	____	____	____
4. I am patient with others.	____	____	____
5. I keep promises.	____	____	____
6. I like meeting strangers.	____	____	____
7. I like being in charge.	____	____	____
8. I like talking about work with colleagues.	____	____	____
9. I am tolerant of others' mistakes.	____	____	____
10. I treat everyone as an individual.	____	____	____
11. I go out of my way to help co-workers.	____	____	____
12. I like being a part of a group.	____	____	____
13. I keep judgments of others to myself.	____	____	____

FINDING A POSITION

The job-seeking process should be started in the months preceding your graduation.

Your first task should be to develop a list of names and places where you might expect to find employment opportunities when you complete your program. This list should consist of the names of people you've met and institutions you've learned about while in your program. You might also use the Internet as a source of job availability. As your graduation approaches, check with those on the list from time to time. Ask about the present hiring situation, whether it has changed from the last time you inquired, and what the future looks like. Begin to cultivate relationships with people who are employed at the healthcare facilities where you believe you'd like to work.

According to some statistics, as many as 80% of all jobs are obtained through personal contacts. Networking, the deliberate effort to make connections among people for a variety of interests, including employment opportunities, is a popular method of making personal contacts. Networking may be casual, as when a group of healthcare workers meets from time to time over coffee to talk, or it may be more formal, as when groups meet with the specific intention of exchanging information. Look for networking opportunities in your program, among graduates, and others in the healthcare field in your community.

You'll also learn about employment opportunities by talking with and listening to fellow students, your instructors, and others associated with your program. When you hear something that sounds interesting, make a note to yourself to follow it up with an inquiry.

If your program has a placement service, it can be an invaluable resource. Use it to get information about your local employment market before you're ready to begin applying for a job. Stay in touch with employment developments in your area through the placement service. When the time comes to begin making serious inquiries and applications, you will be up to date.

Most schools have a "Job Opportunities" bulletin board where notices about employment are posted. Make the board a regular stop and watch for new offers to appear.

Begin reading the classified section of your local newspaper. Major papers may have a special section for healthcare. You'll get a good idea of the hiring trends by the number of ads that appear. Even when ads don't apply directly to you, they can be a good source of names of local institutions and private practitioners to add to your contact list.

Most communities have employment agencies, and larger cities have placement agencies that specialize in healthcare personnel. Either kind of agency is a good resource, but those which specialize are likely to have more listings and better contacts with employers because of their specialization. If you register with an agency, your name will be available when applicants are needed to fill newly opened positions. Commercial employment agencies charge for their services, usually a percentage of the first year's salary. In some cases the employer may pay this charge; in others, it is paid by the employee-that is, you. Ask what the fee is and who will pay it before signing an agreement with an employment agency.

THE APPLICATION PROCESS

On graduation, you will have to apply for a job. You can do this informally, by personally visiting prospective places of employment, or more formally (and preferably) by submitting a letter of application with an accompanying resumé. A letter assures you that the prospective employer has a written record of your interest; a resumé provides the prospective employer with an outline of your qualifications.

Large institutions with many employees often have personnel or human resources departments where it is appropriate to "walk in" to fill out an application. Also, some employers who advertise may invite walk-ins.

The Letter of Application

A letter of application should be simple and direct. Its objective is to introduce you, announce your interest in employment (naming the position being applied for), briefly state your qualifications, and express your availability. It should be typewritten on one page in standard business letter form. It should be free of grammatical and spelling errors. Figure 14-1 is an example of an application letter.

The Resumé

The word resumé means summary. Your resumé should include a summary of your previous education and work experience. Like your letter of application, your resumé represents you to your prospective employer. Neatness, clarity, legibility, and organization on paper reflect similar personal qualities. Although you may

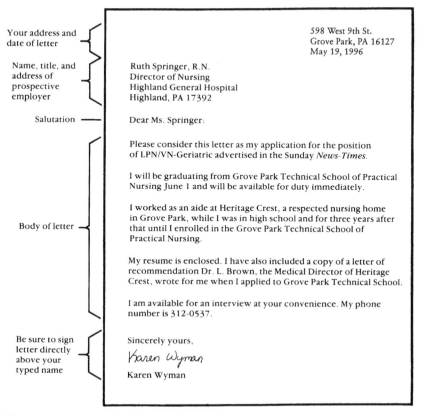

Figure 14-1. Sample application letter.

wish to write your own resumé, the general availability of resumé writing services and computer programs makes the task much simpler.

Whether you prepare your own resumé or have someone prepare it for you, it must be typed and should follow a standardized format. If you're doing your own, get some advice from the reference section of your library or from the placement office at your school. Don't simply prepare a "homemade" resumé; it will stand out, but not in the way a good resumé is intended to. See Figure 14-2 for an example of a solid resumé.

Sandra Melanie Lewis, L.P.N.
1038 University Avenue
Boulder, Colorado 80302
303-264-0537

Immediate Goal:
 Employment as a licensed practical nurse in the geriatric section
 of a major area hospital

Career Goal:
 To provide quality nursing care for older adults in long-term care

Education:
 1989: Arapahoe Hospital, Boulder, Colorado; L.P.N.
 1987: Boulder High School, Boulder, Colorado; H.S. diploma

Licenses:
 Licensed Practical Nurse, State of Colorado, 1989

Experience:
 1984-87: Nurses' aide (part-time), Boulder Nursing Home, Boulder,
 Colorado; long-term care facility for the elderly; assisted LPNs after
 school and weekends

 1987-88: Nurses' aide (full-time), Boulder Nursing Home, Boulder,
 Colorado

Memberships and Honors:
 HOSA Club; Boulder County 4-H Club, Secretary, 1985-87;
 Scholarship, Hopkins Pharmaceutical Company, 1987 (awarded
 to Outstanding Student in Health Occupations Students of
 America)

Availability: Immediate

References:
 Available on request

Figure 14-2. Sample resumé.

The following categories of information should be included on your resumé:

Name, address, and telephone number
Immediate goal
Career goal
Education
Licenses
Experience (work and volunteer)
Memberships and honors
Reference availability

The Interview

The decision to hire a candidate for a job is made within the first 30 seconds of the first meeting between the candidate and the person doing the hiring, according to one report. Whether this finding is completely accurate or not, it underscores the fact that when you go for a job interview, you should assume that your appearance and how you present yourself will make an important impression on the interviewer.

If you've done your "homework" and have taken the time to learn as much as you can about the employer you're seeing, you'll have a good idea of what the interviewer is looking for in an applicant and how you can prepare yourself to meet those expectations. In general, a few simple guidelines will be sufficient:

Dress appropriately. You are applying for a job. This means that what you wear should be businesslike. You should present a serious, capable image that is neither frivolous nor too casual.

Be well-groomed. Combed hair, clean skin, and an overall appearance that shows you take good care of yourself will also signal to an employer what kind of care you are likely to give patients.

Be pleasant and polite but avoid forcing an unnatural charm. Act like yourself, not someone you aren't.

Don't be too concerned about nervousness. Most interviewers expect this, particularly in new entrants to the job market.

The interviewer will no doubt ask you questions that cannot be answered with a simple "yes" or "no." Some of the following are typical questions that might be asked during a job interview:

What are your strong points?
In what areas do you need more experience?
What clinical experiences did you enjoy the most while you were in school?
How do you feel about rotating shifts (working weekends, holidays, overtime, etc.)?
How do you feel about working on a unit to which you are not regularly assigned?
How well do you think you get along with others?
Why do you want to work for us?

What are your long-term career goals?

Where do you see yourself 5 (or 10) years from now?

What would you like to tell me about yourself?

Being prepared ahead of time to answer these and similar questions will demonstrate that you are very interested in your career and in obtaining a position with that employer.

There are a number of questions that are illegal to ask during a pre-employment interview. Questions about your age, marital status, citizenship, birthplace, national or ethnic origin, religion, number of children, living arrangements, sexual preference, and spouse's employment are illegal questions. Rather than tell the interviewer that the question is illegal, be prepared to tactfully respond to such inquiries. If an interviewer asks about your spouse's occupation, you might respond by saying, "My decisions about my career are independent of anyone else and from everything I know, I believe this would be an excellent place to work." Your local Equal Employment Opportunity Commission can provide further guidelines on illegal pre-employment questions.

The Americans with Disabilities Act of 1992 provides those with handicaps or disabilities not directly related to job performance an opportunity for employment. If you have a handicap that does not interfere with job performance and if you expect an employer to take reasonable measures to accommodate your handicap, be prepared to clearly explain what special equipment or supplies you will need to perform your job.

You will show your interest in the employer if you ask questions, but be sure to ask them at appropriate times. Although it is acceptable to inquire about wages and benefits, for example, it is not appropriate to ask about them before the subjects come up. Normally this would be well into the interview. The early part of the interview should focus on the employer, the position offered, its requirements, and your own qualifications for the job.

Prepare a list of good questions ahead of time to avoid the possibility of "going blank," which could be interpreted as disinterest. When given the opportunity to ask questions, you can ask about issues such as staff-to-patient ratios, educational opportunities, orientation programs, and others that apply directly to you.

Avoid asking questions about information that may have been provided in written form unless you need clarification. Most employers provide prospective employees with a fact sheet that answers many of the following questions.

Some questions to investigate include the following:

Vacation, Sick Leave, Holidays, and Leave of Absence
- How much time for each of the above is provided?
- Does the time provided increase with length of employment?
- Is the time with or without pay?
- How many and which holidays are included?
- How is a leave of absence granted?
- Is job status affected by a leave of absence?
- How does a leave affect seniority?
- What are the specific guidelines for Family and Medical Leave?

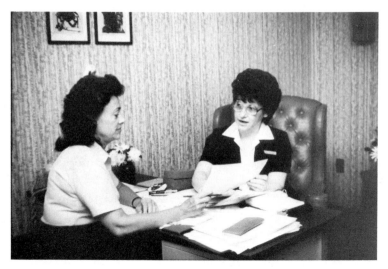

Be prepared to ask questions during the interview.

Insurance, Credit, and Pension
- Are insurance, credit, and pension plans group or individual plans?
- How soon after employment begins do plans become effective?
- What does each plan offer?
- Who is eligible?
- What are the conditions of eligibility?
- Who pays insurance premiums? How much (full or percentage)?
- Are payments automatic (payroll deducted) or voluntary?
- Is interest charged for credit union loans? How much?
- Is interest paid to credit union members? How much?

Work Environment
- Is the facility convenient to public or private transportation?
- Is safe parking provided? Is it free or pay?
- Are uniforms required? If so, what kind and who provides them?
- Is the facility clean and safe?
- Is equipment and care delivery up to date?
- Do present employees exhibit good morale?

Miscellaneous
- What are the work hours, shifts, and rotation schedules?
- Are meals provided, either free or at employee discounts?
- Is there a cafeteria? What is its condition, service, and fare?
- Does the facility have an orientation program or in-service education program? Does it offer advanced educational opportunities at outside institutions?
- Who pays tuition and costs for advanced education programs?

If you are applying for a nontraditional position (ie, not hospital or long-term care facility), there are things you need to know in addition to the above. Is there any flexibility in the starting and ending time? If travel is involved, what is the rate of reimbursement? Will you be expected to be away from home overnight and if so, how often?

The Job Offer

When all of your employment investigation has been done, letters of application written, resumés sent, and interviews completed, one or more of the prospective employers you applied may offer you a job.

Review each offer before accepting or rejecting it to make sure the choice you make is the one you want. If you've already made up your mind that you will accept, do so. If you're uncertain, tell the employer that you will make your decision by a specific date or time. At this point in your career, at the outset of your practice, you must be as sure as possible that your choice of an employer is what you want. It is far better for you to take time at the beginning to assure yourself that the job being offered is what you want than to find out after you're hired that it's not, and then have to face resigning and beginning anew. Avoid "closing the door" to a first job on the basis of unrealistic demands. Although the perfect job may be waiting for you, it's more likely you will have to make some compromises.

EVALUATING POSITIONS

Considering whether or not to accept a position includes weighing all of the information you have about each job offer before making a decision.

Investigate each employment opportunity on its own merits, paying close attention to all its parts. They include the job description, salary, benefits, work hours, and many other matters that will directly influence your working life and often your whole life. For example, poor working conditions can make one unhappy, and unhappiness does not stay at your place of employment when you go home.

Specific items to consider when comparing and evaluating employment opportunities include the following. You may wish to add items of personal concern to the list.

Wages

Your earning power is determined by your credentials on the one hand and by what the job market offers in the form of salary on the other. Ideally, you should earn the maximum salary or wages possible for your level of education and experience, with salary or wages increasing with your level of experience. However, pay rates vary for a number of reasons.

Generally, regional salaries and wages will be similar because employers are competing for the same prospective employees. Where rates vary, other inducements may be offered to make up the difference. Frequently, the inducements (benefits) are as important as the salary or wages alone (sometimes more so).

Be cautious when you see above-average salaries or wages for a position you believe you are qualified for. There is usually a good reason for salaries or wages to be noticeably above a regional average. The position description may call for responsibilities and competencies beyond your qualifications, or the wages may be offered because of high staff turnover resulting from difficult working conditions. In the cost-conscious healthcare field, money that does not have to be spent seldom is.

Carefully study the salary ranges in your area and learn why those that vary do so. Find out what the maximum starting salaries are, what maximum salary can be earned from each employer, how long it takes to reach the maximum salary, and what conditions you have to satisfy to qualify for maximum earnings.

Also, find out what a prospective employer's wage increase policies are. Some may give automatic raises, others may give merit raises, and still others may not give raises at all. Learn how long it takes to qualify for an increase and what is needed to qualify, such as additional education, length of service, or other requirements.

Hours and Shifts

Your intention to work full time or part time, as well as your willingness or ability to work different shifts will have a great bearing on which employment opportunities to consider. The general rule is that employers set the conditions to maintain continuity of services. You may find some flexibility even in those instances, however.

Hospitals and other healthcare agencies that provide round-the-clock nursing services devise schedules in a variety of ways but are usually based on shifts, generally three 8.5-hour shifts per day. Many employers either require or offer rotating shifts. Also, work schedules are often rotated so that all employees have the opportunity to have some weekends and some holidays off.

Your personal circumstances will dictate which schedules you can work. Be certain before accepting a position that you will be available for the hours and shifts being offered or required.

Employer Reputation

Your evaluation of potential employers should include their reputation for upholding high standards. Good and bad reputations are earned for a reason. Learn your prospective employer's reputation and how it was acquired. Don't accept hearsay. Someone may praise or belittle an institution for totally unjustifiable reasons. Find out for yourself. Ask the opinions of those who have worked or received care there. Ask healthcare associations and societies about their members. Also ask the employer; those with good reputations will provide verifiable references, whereas those who have something to hide won't provide such references.

Opportunities for Advancement

Although it may be early in your career to think of advancing beyond the immediate goal of earning your license as a practical/vocational nurse, there may come a time in the future when you'd like to continue your education in nursing. Leave this option open by looking at employment opportunities with employers who offer or encourage employee advancement.

Benefits

Benefits include a wide range of items. Some benefits, such as vacation time, may be considered basic, whereas others, such as daycare facilities for employee's children, may be less standard. Look closely at the benefits package of each employer you are considering. Benefits can be a decisive factor in choosing a position. A high salary without certain benefits may result in a lower overall income for you, whereas a lower salary or wage with good benefits may net you more.

Some benefits to look for are insurance plans (life, health, vision, dental), overtime pay, pension plans, reimbursement for tuition, employee credit union, in-service educational programs, meals, and vacation, leave of absence, and holiday policies.

These are just some of the things you need to consider when evaluating offers of employment. Your personal circumstances will no doubt include the need to have answers to additional questions.

ON THE JOB

Once you are hired, a new round of learning begins. You'll be learning your employer's routine, your specific duties, the names and faces of co-workers and patients, and scores of other details. Your confidence in yourself and your competence will get you through the rough parts, and understanding from those you're working with will help to smooth the transition. You can expect some highs and lows, but you should always know that in a surprisingly short time, the insecurity of being new will be replaced by poise and self-assurance.

However, confidence in yourself alone will not guarantee satisfactory performance. Your own standards should be high, perhaps even higher than those your employer sets, so that your work will never come into question and your ability will never fall short of what's expected.

Accept the responsibilities you are given. Do your work to the best of your ability with interest and commitment. Be punctual and reliable, and if illness or other circumstances prevent you from reporting to work, notify your employer as soon as possible. Show a willingness to learn by asking questions when you are uncertain, and be equally willing to share when someone comes to you for help. Abide by the regulations set by your employer, and if you have serious differences with them, seek to correct the situation through proper channels. Don't snipe, gossip, or bad-mouth about something that upsets you; do something about it, but in the appropriate manner. You are not only working for your employer; you are also working with your employer to provide the service that is the basis for the economic security of both of you.

On the job, you have two roles: yourself as you and yourself as nurse-employee. Your nurse-employee role must come first. When you go to work, leave your personal problems behind. Positive personal characteristics, such as honesty, courtesy, good humor, compassion, and understanding, are valuable assets as an individual and as a nurse, and you should exhibit them at work, just as you would elsewhere.

Politeness in person or on the phone, in greeting people who are new to you, or in your relationships with those you see regularly is also important. Showing good manners on any occasion, whether in an employee cafeteria or in a patient's room, helps to set an example and a tone that inspires similar behavior from others.

Avoiding gossip about your institution, its staff, or your patients is more than desirable; it is essential. Backbiting, grousing, complaining, and speaking ill of anyone or anything not only poisons others' attitudes but darkens your own point of view. Use caution when talking about personal work issues. Others may not share your views, and it is not fair to impose your views if they are negative.

You will always be working directly or indirectly with others. How closely you work together will vary. Some will have authority over you; others will be under your supervision. Some you may rarely see, whereas others may be at your side constantly. Good relationships with others will depend heavily on what you do to keep them good. In general, what you put into a relationship is what you get out of it.

There may be times when you witness care or are asked to deliver care that is below the standards of good nursing or healthcare. Your first obligation is to your patients. If the care you see is truly substandard and can be verified, you should act to prevent it. Report the situation to your supervisor. Don't act on your own to correct the situation because the possibility exists that you're not seeing all the factors involved. Healthcare at any level always includes the potential of serious consequences, the worst being the possibility of death.

Dealing with people will be the major part of your work. However, in the process of providing care, you will also be responsible for such things as dressings, medications, instruments, machines, and a long list of supplies. They belong to your employer and are expressly for use in the delivery of services to patients. Their misuse or misappropriation for a staff member's private use, without permission, is unethical and illegal.

To avoid problems over the use of equipment and supplies, abide by your employer's regulations regarding them. Fill out the forms that may be required. Make accurate counts when taking inventories or requisitioning supplies. Return unused items to their proper place. File breakage or failed equipment reports. In short, do everything you are supposed to do regarding use of facilities and supplies.

Healthcare facilities of every size are continuously battling increasing costs. Any loss, no matter how insignificant it may seem—making an unauthorized long-distance phone call, taking a set of linens or a towel, or using medications for personal use, for example—raises costs. When an employer's costs are excessive, cost-cutting procedures, including staff cuts, may become necessary. Your job will depend on your employer's ability to pay you. How you use your employer's facilities, equipment, and supplies will affect that ability.

With your career aspirations in mind, take advantage of opportunities to advance. If you need additional classes, in-service training, or experience, accept the added effort, knowing that no advancement is possible without it.

RESIGNATION

There may come a time when you decide to leave your position. This decision should never be made without careful study. A brief upset or disagreement with someone is certainly not grounds for leaving, although a long period of inability to get along in an institution or with staff members may suggest a change for the better. If you decide to resign, always do so in the manner set forth by your employer. If no prescribed form is established, write a letter of resignation. Give ample notice (2 weeks is standard) so that your employer can find a replacement for you. No matter what the circumstances of your departure, don't infuse the situation with ill will. You will be looking for another job, if not immediately, then at some time in the future. Your employer's recommendation will be invaluable.

A letter of resignation should be simple and direct, stating the fact that you are resigning, the effective date, giving the reasons (elaborate details are unnecessary), and closing on a positive note. A sample is shown in Figure 14-3.

DISMISSAL

Dismissal from a position is a possibility that is not always based on employer-employee incompatibility. There are economic and other reasons for cutting staff positions, and you have no control over them. If you "fall under the ax" of budget cuts or other administrative changes, such as consolidation of departments, you must accept them. Often an employer who adjusts staff will have alternative jobs within the institution or, if not, will try to help employees find new positions. However, employers are under no obligation to do so.

On the other hand, a dismissal for cause, based on dishonesty, improper performance of duty, insubordination, illegal acts, excessive lateness or absences, or other substantiated causes is something every nurse can do something about before it happens. Adherence to high standards is the best defense against charges of any kind.

If a dismissal is warranted, even though it might be disputed by the employee, the employer has certain options, depending on the nature of the cause for dismissal. Options will vary from employer to employer. A serious charge such as theft can result in an immediate dismissal with forfeiture of all benefits. A less serious matter, such as constantly arriving late for work, although grounds for dismissal if not corrected, is not likely to result in such drastic measures. In most cases, the dismissed employee may have the right to appeal.

YOUR BUDGET

Budgeting your income is largely a personal matter. You may already have a system for managing your money. If not, seek help for your specific needs from someone who understands the process. A budget does not have to be complex, but it should cover all areas of your income and expenses, the two major divisions of any budget.

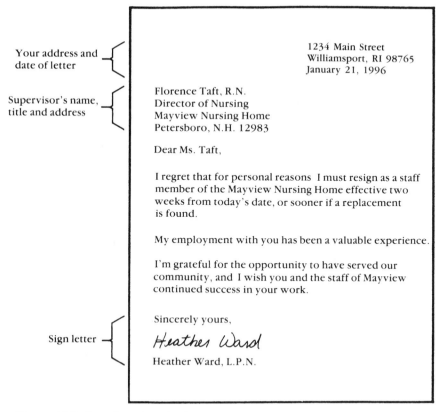

Your address and date of letter

Supervisor's name, title and address

Sign letter

1234 Main Street
Williamsport, RI 98765
January 21, 1996

Florence Taft, R.N.
Director of Nursing
Mayview Nursing Home
Petersboro, N.H. 12983

Dear Ms. Taft,

I regret that for personal reasons I must resign as a staff member of the Mayview Nursing Home effective two weeks from today's date, or sooner if a replacement is found.

My employment with you has been a valuable experience.

I'm grateful for the opportunity to have served our community, and I wish you and the staff of Mayview continued success in your work.

Sincerely yours,

Heather Ward

Heather Ward, L.P.N.

Figure 14-3. Sample resignation letter.

If your position as an LP/VN is your first major employment, be sure to make the distinction between personal and professional (or business) expenses in your budget. Also, since you may be paying local, state, or federal taxes for the first time, get advice from an expert regarding what records you have to keep, how much you must pay, and how the taxes are to be paid. Private duty nurses are responsible for paying their own taxes and for getting licenses required for private duty practice.

Other money matters for you to consider include savings or investment programs, personal insurance (life, health, liability), and the establishment of a good credit rating. Guidance in these matters is recommended, even if you must consult a professional.

CAREER ADVANCEMENT

As your practical nurse program draws to an end, you should feel secure that your career as a nurse is well on its way. Now is a good time to think further in terms of what the future might hold. Goals are incentives to self-fulfillment and to a better, more comfortable life.

Earning your license and a position as an LP/VN may be the goals you have always wanted, and upon reaching those goals, they alone may be totally satisfying to you. However, this accomplishment is proof of what you are capable of achieving. Your success may lead you to strive even higher. If so, numerous opportunities are available.

Higher goals do not necessarily mean the need to earn higher degrees. As you gain experience as an LP/VN, keep an eye on your future by reading professional nursing journals, such as the *Journal of Practical Nursing* and *Nursing*. Stay abreast of developments that affect your work and the healthcare field in general. Attend in-service education programs whenever they are offered, keeping a record of them and updating your credentials.

Various organizations sponsor conventions and workshops. They may be offered locally or in another city. Attend them whenever possible, even if you must do so on your own time. If you show your determination to keep pace with nursing and a willingness to go out of your way to do so, you may get cooperation and time off from your employer. The least you will get will be your employer's respect for your enthusiasm and interest.

Continuing education units (CEUs; one CEU equals 10 hours of qualified instruction in an approved program) are sometimes given by continuing education programs. Earned CEUs are an indication to your employer and others of your career commitment. CEUs are also required for license renewal in some states.

Refresher courses are also a means to maintain and improve skills and knowledge. They may be offered by your own program and by your employer. Treat them as opportunities to advance.

After you've been employed for a time, you may be offered the opportunity to specialize in the care of people with specific healthcare needs. If you think that your theoretical knowledge has not kept up with the practical experience you've gained on the job, and if in-service training, refresher courses, and reading have failed to help you reach the competency level you want, additional study may be the answer. Consider enrolling in an accredited course offered by a college or university. Accredited means that a course or program has been reviewed by an organization or accrediting body and has been found to meet the standards set by that body. Accreditation generally means that standards are above minimum standards as set, for example, by a state licensing authority.

A simple way to maintain your expertise is to take extension courses offered on television, usually on public service channels. Before committing yourself, make certain that you will receive credit for the course.

Finally, you may wish to make a major advance in your nursing career by becoming a registered nurse. Registered nurse (RN) programs vary in length and complexity. A 4-year course of study at a college or university will lead to a bachelor of science in nursing (BSN) degree. An associate degree in nursing (ADN) is usually earned in two years at a college, university, junior or community college. Diploma programs are sponsored by hospitals, last about 26 to 30 months, and generally include up to 60 college credits. Graduates of all three of these types of nursing education programs are qualified to take the NCLEX-RN examination.

You may already be enrolled in an articulated nursing program. An articulated nursing education program provides a sequence of courses that provides flexibility and choice. Some students choose to leave the program after completing the LP/VN portion of the curriculum; others choose to leave after completing the ADN portion of the curriculum; and others choose to leave after completing the BSN portion of the curriculum. These students may also have an option of returning to the next level of nursing education within a specific time period.

The LP/VN who was not enrolled in an articulated program and who wants to enroll in a professional nursing program should look for programs that offer advanced standing. Many professional nursing education programs provide a mechanism for LP/VN students to challenge—by examination, experience, and/or performance—certain professional nursing courses. Those who successfully meet the challenge criteria are exempt from taking the course and granted advanced standing. Most nursing organizations are actively encouraging nursing educators to find innovative ways of providing a nursing career ladder. Some believe the ladder should begin with the certified nursing assistant and continue through doctoral studies. Because the number of innovative programs is rapidly increasing, those who want to continue their education in nursing should review all of their options by carefully studying college catalogs and talking with guidance counselors.

NURSING ORGANIZATIONS

Being active as a nurse and being active in nursing are not the same. Being active as a nurse means working as a nurse. To be active in nursing means participating in nursing organizations. Belonging to nursing organizations is important to your development as an LP/VN and also to the future of practical/vocational nursing as a career. The specific purpose of each organization is unique, but the intention in all such organizations is to benefit the membership.

Practical/Vocational Nursing Organizations

Three national organizations, designed to meet the particular needs of practical/vocational nurses, are the National Federation of Licensed Practical Nurses (NFLPN); the National Association for Practical Nurse Education and Service (NAPNES); and the American Licensed Practical Nurses Association (ALPNA).

The NFLPN was founded in 1949, and membership is limited to LP/VNs and student practical/vocational nurses. This organization's primary purpose is to promote the practice of practical/vocational nursing. NFLPN, through its organizational structure and membership, develops positions on educational requirements for the practice of practical/vocational nursing; makes recommendations related to continuing education; defines ethical conduct; and outlines standards and scope of practical/vocational nursing practice, all of which are based on a clearly defined philosophy of practical vocational nursing. In addition, the NFLPN attempts to influence legislation affecting the LP/VN licensed practical/vocational nurse through national and state lobbying programs.

NAPNES was founded in 1941 to promote the special interests of practical/vocational nurses and to assist schools in developing educational programs. Membership is open to LP/VNs, practical/vocational nursing students, practical/vocational nursing school faculty and directors, and others interested in promoting the practice of practical/vocational nursing. The primary purpose of NAPNES is to promote an understanding of practical/vocational nursing and to develop continuing education opportunities for LP/VNs. NAPNES also develops positions on practical/vocational nurse education, defines ethical conduct, and publishes standards of nursing practice. The NAPNES official publication, the "Journal of Practical Nursing,' and a newsletter, "NAPNES Forum," keep members informed of organizational activities.

ALPNA was founded in 1984 to represent the interests of LP/VNs through lobbying and legislative activities. This organization is also involved in continuing education activities, and holds an annual meeting in August.

Practical/vocational nursing's future depends a great deal on the effectiveness of these three organizations. Since organizations are made up of people who share a common goal, it is important to your future as an LP/VN that you actively participate in one of these organizations. The address of these organizations is listed in Appendix D.

National League for Nursing

The National League for Nursing (NLN) was founded in 1950, and membership is open to anyone interested in promoting healthcare through nursing service. This national organization is primarily concerned with education of nurses and improving quality of healthcare. The official publication of the NLN is "Nursing and Health Care."

The NLN is a large organization, and many of its activities are conducted through special divisions called councils. The Council of Practical Nursing Program (CPNP) is concerned with those issues that affect practical/vocational nursing. This Council accredits practical/vocational nursing education programs and provides continuing education opportunities for faculty and program directors. The CPNP also promotes practical/vocational nursing interests within the NLN. Persons interested in joining the NLN can find its address in Appendix D.

American Nurses Association

The origins of the American Nurses Association (ANA), the professional association for registered nurses and students in professional nursing programs, can be traced to 1890. The ANA is deeply involved in issues such as establishing a credentialing system; developing and administering specialty certification examinations; publishing a Code for Nurses; approving continuing education programs; and lobbying for nurses, nursing, and healthcare, and other issues important to professional nurses. While LP/VNs can not join the ANA, some of the activities of the ANA can have a direct influence on practical/vocational nursing. Reading the ANA official publication, the "American Journal of Nursing," as well as NLN and practical/vocational nursing publications will help you keep informed of the position of all of these national organizations on issues that will affect you and how you practice nursing.

Whichever organizations you choose to join, do so with the intention of being an active member. It can be an investment in your future as well as helping others improve theirs. Remember, organizations depend on members, and the strength of the members will determine the organization's strength.

POLITICAL PROCESS

Healthcare in the next 10 to 20 years will be greatly influenced by local, state, and federal legislative action. As a member of the healthcare team and as a citizen of this country, you are now and will continue to be affected by these political decisions. For example, political efforts to control rising healthcare costs may affect your salary; political efforts to revise the Medicare system may make it necessary for you to care for an aging or ill parent in your home; healthcare services may be reduced as a result of political actions and your job may be eliminated; or political action establishing new healthcare services may increase your personal income taxes.

As a nurse, you are in a unique position to see problems from a patient's point of view, the healthcare system's point of view, and a personal point of view. You must share your opinions and recommendations with your legislators.

You can affect the political process in several ways. The best-known way is to vote. Learn candidates' positions on various issues and vote for those who you think will serve people's interests.

Another way to affect the political process is to write to your legislator. Elected officials need and want to know your views and opinions. Examples of how to address envelopes and letters to state and national legislators are shown below.

FORMS OF ADDRESS

State Senators	The Honorable _____
	Senate Chamber
	City, State, Zip Code
	Dear Senator _____:
State Representatives	The Honorable _____
State Assembly Members	House of Representatives
	City, State, Zip Code
	Dear Representative _____:
U.S. Senators	The Honorable _____
	United States Senate
	Senate Office Building
	Washington, DC 20515
	Dear Senator _____:
U.S. Representatives	The Honorable _____
	House of Representatives
	House of Office Building
	Washington, DC 20515
	Dear Representative _____:

Other ways of affecting the political process include lobbying, negotiating, and demonstrating. Lobbying activities are conducted by organizations on behalf of their members. For example, NFLPN and NAPNES frequently lobby for or against legislation affecting LP/VNs.

Negotiating is the art of persuasion. In the political process, much time and energy is spent negotiating with and between legislators. Promises are made, positions are changed, and decisions are eventually reached.

Demonstrations are techniques that sometimes influence the political process. Demonstrations call attention to a particular problem or issue in a dramatic fashion. Demonstrations, whether peaceful or violent, usually attract public attention.

Demonstrations occur when the political process has been unresponsive to an issue of critical importance to a group of people.

Keeping informed of legislation that may affect you is not as difficult as it may seem. Your organizations, through their publications, keep members informed of current legislative events in both state and national governments. Your local newspaper and national news magazines are also sources of information on political issues.

If you become politically active as a nurse and a concerned citizen, you should exercise care to avoid offending your employer. Your political convictions are personal, and you have no right to impose those convictions on your employer or your patients. For example, if you are actively involved in, and working to pass pro-life legislation and your employer provides legal abortion services, it would be inappropriate for you to conduct political activities against your employer. Such conduct is unethical, and it puts both you and your employer in a difficult position.

The following fundamental tools are at your disposal to help you affect the processes that influence your life and career:

1. Be informed. Stay abreast of what is happening in nursing by reading newspapers and nursing journals, listening to news broadcasts, and watching television programs that address current issues in healthcare.
2. Participate. Join nursing organizations and activist groups and be active in their work.
3. Vote. Express your opinions and vote for those you want to represent you in elections in your organizations, your community, your state, and your country.
4. Communicate. Let your representatives know your views through letters or meetings and support their efforts to pass laws and make changes you favor.
5. Influence Others. Share your opinions with friends, colleagues, neighbors, and others.

To affect the political process, and therefore to affect decisions that have a direct bearing on your life, you must first realize that your opinion is important and that you have the right to express it. Also, even though an individual may seem insignificant in a large group, the group is made of nothing but individuals, and you are one of them.

COLLECTIVE BARGAINING

Certain issues regarding your employment will be out of your direct control but within your indirect control. They are the conditions affecting your job such as wage scales, work hours, working conditions, and other matters that are of daily concern. Nurses' and healthcare workers unions are organizations which, by representing nurses and bargaining with employers, reach agreements that ideally are in everyone's best interest. The process is called *collective bargaining*.

If you join a union, and if that union is acknowledged as the bargaining representative at your place of employment, your wishes will be conveyed to management (your employer) through the activities of the union. But you must first belong to the union and then be active in it for the process to be effective.

Unions work for the benefit of their members. Any issue can be advanced by a union, but in general, unions are involved in wage and hour matters, health and safety issues, discrimination issues of all kinds, and formulation of contracts between employers and union members that incorporate these items.

Joining a union is a personal choice. Whether or not you accept an offer to join is up to you. Before deciding either to join or not to join, look closely into what your decision would mean to you, your employment, and your career.

GRIEVANCES

No occupation or job is without its grievances (problems). It's not a good idea to look for them, especially at the beginning of your career when your attention should be on learning and performance, but you should be aware that they may appear from time to time. They may cover a range of serious matters, such as health and safety or discrimination on the basis of sex, race, religion or other factors. There may be less serious issues of only passing concern. Some can be solved on the spot; others may require a lengthy process to settle.

Most employers will have some form of grievance procedure (problem resolution process) for employees to rectify problems. In some institutions, the process may be a part of a contract worked out by the union representing workers there. At other establishments it may be as simple as calling the problem to the attention of a supervisor.

Learn the process used at your institution or place of employment because without it, small, even petty, problems could grow out of proportion, and already large problems could become serious. Complaining about a problem accomplishes nothing if it's not done through the proper channels, whereas a legitimate complaint that reaches an authority who can do something about it gets action.

BURNOUT

The term *burnout* describes a condition characterized by a sense of hopelessness about one's job brought about by chronic stress. It decreases performance on the job and carries over into one's personal life. It can be the result of highly stressful working conditions or stressful relationships among staff.

Physical and psychological symptoms accompany burnout. Physical symptoms may include exhaustion, fatigue, headaches, susceptibility to colds, and the inability to sleep. Psychological symptoms may include quick loss of temper, decreased ability to make decisions, guilt, anger, and depression.

At least part of the stress that produces burnout comes from the inability of those who suffer it to match what they expect of themselves to what time and conditions let them deliver. Candidates for burnout include the nurse who wants to provide ideal nursing care but is prevented from doing so because there isn't enough time for each patient, or the nurse who wants to promote health but is faced every day with dying patients.

Often a nurse who has reached this point quits nursing to resolve the problem. This is a dramatic and unnecessary solution.

The issue of burnout is a growing concern in healthcare. As a new member of the healthcare team, you can do something now to manage possible future stress by being prepared. Discuss problems openly with co-workers and supervisors. Learn to share your feelings and listen to others in return. If the area of healthcare you are about to enter is one of known high stress, find out from the beginning what those who are already in it do to manage theirs. Don't shoulder a burden that is not yours to carry alone.

DISCUSSION QUESTIONS/LEARNING ACTIVITIES

1. In addition to nursing opportunities listed in this chapter, list other places where LP/VNs may work in your community. (Your local newspaper may help you with this question.)

2. What is the salary range for LP/VNs in various healthcare facilities in your community? (Your local newspaper and health facility personnel offices can help you answer this question.)

3. Prepare your resumé for a prospective employer.

4. Ask a classmate to conduct a mock interview with you. Videotape the session then critique how well you presented yourself.

5. Think about how you will dress for an interview. Your librarian can direct you to reference books that discuss dressing for an interview.

6. Ask one or two experienced nurses about their transition from student to employee. What did they find most difficult? What would they recommend to make this transition less difficult?

7. List several things that you can do now to prepare for the transition from student to employee.

8. Select a problem related to healthcare that is currently being discussed in your state legislature. What are the issues? What are the positions of various special interest groups on the proposed legislation? Some topics that may be appropriate are catastrophic health insurance, regulating the cost of health insurance, laws affecting nursing practice (nurse practice acts), seat belt laws, and funding for nursing education.

9. After you investigate a political issue and reach a personal conclusion, write a letter to your congressperson, giving your reasons for urging support or nonsupport of the proposed legislation.

10. Review the stress management techniques in Appendix A. How could you use some of these techniques to help you avoid burnout?

11. Prepare a list of the pros and cons of union membership. Compare your list with those of your classmates.

12. Describe your nursing career goals. What position and responsibility do you want in 1 year, in 5 years, and in 10 years? What will you have to do to achieve these goals? Are these goals realistic? Do you have the ability to achieve them? What changes (personal, educational, social) might you have to make to achieve your goals?

READ MORE ABOUT IT

Benner P: From Novice to Expert: Excellence and Power in Clinical Nursing Practice. Menlo Park, CA: Addison-Wesley, 1984.

Drafke MW: Working in Health Care: What You Need to Know, First Edition. Philadelphia: FA Davis, 1994.

Eyler DA: Resumés that Mean Business. New York: Random House, 1990.

Grippando GM: Nursing Perspective and Issues, Fifth Edition. Albany, NY: Delmar, 1992.

Hamilton JM, Kiefer ME: Survival Skills for the New Nurse. Philadelphia: JB Lippincott, 1986.

Lindberg JB, et al: Introduction to Nursing: Concepts, Issues, and Opportunities, Second Edition. Philadelphia: JB Lippincott, 1994.

Marno K: Resumés for the Health Care Professional, First Edition. New York: Wiley, 1993.

Yate MJ: Resumés that Knock 'em Dead. Boston: Bob Adams, 1992.

Current Issues and Future Concerns

15

OBJECTIVES

When you complete this chapter, you should be able to:

List techniques that will help you adapt to future changes in the workplace.

Identify sources of information related to occupational risks.

Discuss several methods through which you can maintain your competence in nursing practice.

Critically analyze an announcement for a continuing education program.

Identify the advantages and disadvantages of mandatory continuing education for nurse license renewal.

Analyze how changes in the healthcare system and new categories of healthcare workers affect patient care.

Value the cultural diversity of nursing team members.

List and describe some of the major issues and future concerns of nurses and nursing.

Take and defend your position on current issues in nursing.

It is impossible in one chapter to present or thoroughly discuss all the current issues and future concerns that face you as you begin your career in practical/vocational nursing. What you know today will get you started, but you will have to continually strive to adapt to social, cultural, and scientific changes. You must actively participate in resolving issues and concerns that will affect your career as a licensed practical/vocational nurse (LP/VN) now and in the future.

CHANGE

The one thing that will remain constant during your career in nursing is change. Those who see change as an opportunity to do things more efficiently and better will make better personal adjustments in the workplace. Those who do not like change and either actively or passively resist it will experience a tremendous amount of stress and many will prematurely end their career in nursing.

It will help you in your career as a nurse to learn to expect changes in how you work and to do all that you can to be involved in helping to decide what those changes may be. You can do this through political activities, voting in political elections, membership on policy and procedure committees, continuing your education both formally and informally, membership in your professional organizations, and by being positive and optimistic that proposed changes will improve how things are done.

People who have difficulty accepting change often make statements like, "We've never done it that way before," "We don't have enough staff to do that," "Sounds good, but...," and "I've always done it this way and it worked just fine." Just imagine where we would be today if everyone thought this way.

New technology, invention of new equipment, new categories of healthcare workers, and new diseases are just a few changes that nurses will experience in the next 10 years. Those who ask questions like, "How can we do this better?" "What are the alternatives to how things are now?" "How many different methods can we think of to achieve our goal?" are open-minded and able to accept change in stride.

Now is the time, when confronted with change, to respond with positive thoughts and behaviors. Consider change as an opportunity to grow as a person and to learn as a nurse.

OCCUPATIONAL RISKS

Working in healthcare imposes a number of risks to nurses. Accidental needle sticks are of extreme concern. Back injuries, overexposure to radiation, acquired immunodeficiency syndrome (AIDS), hepatitis B, tuberculosis, rare viruses and as yet unknown diseases are concerns that will be with us for many years.

The Occupational Safety and Health Administration (OSHA) develops guidelines that employers must follow to ensure the safety of healthcare workers but not even OSHA can prevent nurses from contracting diseases or being exposed to environmental toxins that have not yet been identified. New products used in new ways have the potential to cause harm to those who handle them.

Occupational risks will increase in the future. The prudent nurse will do everything he or she can to know as much as possible about his or her working environment. Careful attention to handling medications, using new self-protection techniques as soon as they become available, and understanding the implications of a medical diagnosis will go a long way toward helping you maintain your own health.

CHEMICALLY IMPAIRED NURSES

The number of nurses who are illegally using drugs and abusing alcohol will continue to increase over the next years. Some of the reasons so many nurses resort to using drugs, alcohol, or both include job-related stress, inability to cope with changes in the workplace, overwhelming personal responsibilities, a feeling of frustration and helplessness in their personal and professional lives, and easy access to drugs.

The model Disciplinary Diversion Act developed by the American Nurses Association (ANA) and recommended to State Boards of Nursing includes a voluntary treatment and rehabilitation program for addicted nurses. It is expected that more and more State Boards of Nursing will include these recommendations in their Nurse Practice Acts in the future, just as more and more employers will begin random drug testing of those who provide healthcare services.

It is your responsibility to yourself, your family, and your patients to avoid the use of nonprescription medications. If you or someone you know does become addicted to drugs or alcohol, the only option is to seek immediate assistance. Referring yourself or someone else to your State Board of Nursing for the voluntary treatment and rehabilitation program may not only save a career—it may save a life.

DISCRIMINATION

Discrimination in the workplace is perhaps more common than many people think. As workers become more assertive and confident that their rights will be protected in courts of law, more and more cases of discrimination will be filed.

It is illegal to use age, race, color, sex, national origin, religion, marital status, pregnancy, sexual orientation, membership in organizations, or handicaps to deny employment and promotion. It is also illegal for someone to use a position of power to intimidate and sexually harass someone in a subordinate position.

Although it may not yet be illegal, a common discriminatory practice is for female nurses to always ask male nurses for assistance in lifting and moving patients. It is also discriminatory to always assign the nurse who doesn't complain to those patients who are the most difficult or require the most care. It is discriminatory to always fulfill all of the most difficult staff member's requests.

As the workplace becomes increasingly complex, more rules and laws governing relationships between employers and employees and between managers and staff members will be developed. Whether a manager or staff member, future rules and laws will have an impact on your professional relationships in the workplace.

MAINTAINING COMPETENCE

Several sources predict that much of what you learn this year will be obsolete in less than 6 years. Your nursing program has prepared you with the minimum competencies needed to enter the practice of practical/vocational nursing but maintaining and expanding your competencies will require attention throughout your entire career.

Maintaining competence through informal educational experiences is one of the most frequently used methods for keeping up with changes in nursing. Reading journals, attending staff development programs offered by your employer, learning new procedures or techniques from those skilled in their performance, reading patient charts, listening to physicians as they discuss treatment options, and learning to use new and different equipment will help you remain competent in your nursing skills.

Another method for maintaining competence is through formal continuing education. Formal continuing education includes lectures, workshops, seminars, college courses, and independent study programs. Sponsors of continuing education programs include hospitals, nursing homes, colleges and universities, and nursing and healthcare associations. Sponsors can apply to nursing organizations, such as the American Nurses Association, the National Federation of Licensed Practical Nurses, the National Association for Practical Nurse Education and Service, the National League for Nursing, and the State Board of Nursing for program approval. Approved programs may offer continuing education units (CEUs). A CEU is the equivalent of 10 contact hours of participation in an approved continuing education program. A contact hour is equal to 50 minutes.

The National Association for Practical Nurse Education and Service (NAPNES) offers several formal continuing education opportunities. NAPNES also pro-

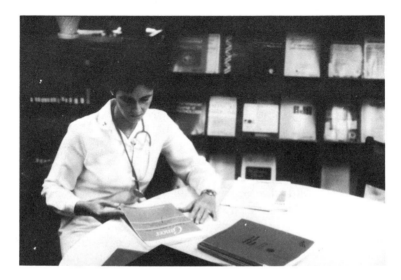

Journals provide current information that can help you keep up with changes in the field of nursing.

vides a Continuing Education Record Keeping System (CERKS) for both members and nonmembers. This system records your continuing education contact hours and supplies transcripts when you want or need to document your participation in continuing education programs. For additional information on continuing education programs or CERKS, you can write to NAPNES. (Refer to Appendix D for the NAPNES address.)

When selecting a continuing education program, you should consider those which apply directly to your learning needs. You will want to determine the program's purpose, objectives, content, teaching-learning methods, and faculty qualifications. You will also want to know whether the program is approved to offer CEUs and what organization gave that approval.

CONTINUING EDUCATION
FOR LICENSE RENEWAL

A current issue that will no doubt become more important in the future is the controversy over whether continuing education should be voluntary or mandated by law. Those who believe that continuing education should be voluntary assert that continuing education is a responsibility of all nurses and that laws should not dictate how this responsibility is met. Those who favor defining, in the law, the minimum hours of continuing education required for license renewal believe this is the only way to ensure that nurses will keep their knowledge current.

The nurse practice acts of at least 15 states require a specific number of contact hours in continuing education for license renewal as a practical/vocational nurse. Several additional states require continuing education, as well as a minimum number of hours of practice as a nurse for license renewal. If you practice nursing in a state that does not yet have a mandatory continuing education requirement for license renewal, this is one of the current issues that will affect your nursing practice and one in which you should become involved. Learn the reasons for both mandatory and voluntary continuing education and the implications of each. When this issue is presented in your state or place of employment, you will be prepared to help influence decisions that will benefit you, your colleagues, and your future.

COMPUTERS IN HEALTHCARE

Continued advances in computer technology will drastically change how nurses do much of their work. Computers will provide the technology for voice-activated charting, customized nursing care plans, assessing acuity levels, and for reminding staff of treatment and medication schedules. Computer technology will aid in ordering supplies, equipment, diagnostic tests, and medications. Computer programs will provide quick access to drug incompatibilities and food interactions, treatment modalities, and suggested interventions related to specific nursing diagnoses.

The widespread use of computer technology in healthcare poses many future concerns. Questions about how to maintain the confidentiality of the patient's medical record and how to protect the integrity of the system are already of concern. What effect the even temporary failure of a system upon which the staff is totally dependent have on the ability of the nursing staff to carry out scheduled medication and treatment plans remains to be answered.

Being proficient in using current computer technology in healthcare settings today does not guarantee success in the future. New programs, new systems, and new applications will require continued education and training in the future.

EMPLOYMENT

The employment outlook for nurses in the late 1990s is different from any time in the past. Before the 1990s, the majority of nurses worked in hospitals. In the future, the majority of nurses will be working outside hospitals. It is estimated that 60 percent of the beds in acute care hospitals that were in use in 1994 will be closed by the year 2000.

Now is the time, when you are defining your clinical interests and exploring your employment options, to think about what you want to be doing 5 years and 10 years from now. If working in a hospital is your goal and if you obtain employment in a hospital, you should be aware that downsizing and closing patient beds may force you to look elsewhere for employment in the future.

Opportunities for employment in long-term and community health facilities will be plentiful. If you have limited knowledge and experience in these areas, you will need to prepare yourself with the special skills needed in these settings. You can do this by volunteering your services a few hours a week, through continuing education activities, by finding a mentor (a tutor or coach) in the setting in which you want to work, and by accepting a position on a trial basis at perhaps a lower rate of pay.

Getting a job in the future, especially when the healthcare system is uncertain of its own future, will not be as easy as it once was. Your nursing education probably included experiences in a variety of clinical settings. It is well known that most new graduates get their first job through contacts made during a clinical rotation. It is in your best interest to demonstrate to the staff and supervisors in these clinical rotations that you have the characteristics and qualities of an effective team member. When the time comes for you to seek employment, you will be remembered.

Many healthcare facilities are reducing the number of employees as a way of controlling costs. When job openings do occur, employers have many applicants from which to choose. Having an excellent academic background, strong clinical skills, and an ability to present yourself well during an interview; being flexible in the hours and shifts you can work; and demonstrating a strong desire to learn will go a long way toward securing employment now and in the future.

EDUCATION

The curricula of nursing education programs will also change in the future. These curricula changes, which have already begun, will prepare nurses to work not only in acute care but also in long-term care and community healthcare settings. The 1993 National League for Nursing publication titled "An Agenda for Nursing

Education Reform" outlines how changes in nursing curricula must be made to prepare nurses to work in a variety of nursing practice settings.

The use of computer technology in nursing education will provide opportunities for learners, through CD-ROM technology, to be actively involved in acquiring knowledge and skills. Traditional lectures in which the teacher talks and the learner listens will become a rare rather than usual method of teaching. Nursing students, as well as graduate nurses, will have access to learning modules which they can complete at their own pace 24 hours a day, 7 days a week.

LONG-TERM CARE

The number of long-term care facilities, as well as the number of residents living in these facilities, is expected to continue increasing rapidly over the next 40 years. Several factors will contribute to these increases. First, there are now approximately 31 million Americans over the age of 65; 3 million of these are over the age of 85. As the number of older people increases over the next 40 years, especially of those over the age of 85, the number of people who will need to live in long-term care facilities will increase.

Second, many younger people with Parkinson's disease, Alzheimer's disease, other chronic and crippling diseases, and AIDS, who can no longer be cared for at home by their families, will need the services available in long-term care facilities.

AIDS alone will account for a need to increase the number of long-term care facilities or beds. There were 56,782 new cases of AIDS reported in 1995 and to date, 501,310 total cases have been reported to the Centers for Disease Control.

A third factor that will affect long-term care is the addition of sub-acute units. Traditionally, resident units were classified as either skilled care, intermediate care, or custodial care. Those living in custodial care units usually need some assistance with a few activities of daily living; those living in intermediate care units need assistance with several activities of daily living plus medications and minor treatments; those living in skilled care units are those who need treatments, procedures, and frequent assessments that must be performed by licensed nurses.

These relatively new sub-acute units in long-term care facilities will care for people who, in the past, were often admitted to acute care hospitals. Those who are ventilator-dependent, those who need monitoring during medication adjustments, and unstable diabetic patients are just a few examples of those who might be admitted to a sub-acute unit.

These changes in the types of healthcare services provided in long-term care facilities will provide many employment opportunities for LP/VNs in the future.

CULTURAL DIVERSITY AND THE NURSING TEAM

The U.S. Bureau of the Census (1990) predicts that by the year 2080, about 51.1 percent of the total population of the United States will be from culturally diverse backgrounds. It is logical to expect that similar ratios will be found in the members of the nursing team.

Working with people who have different values, attitudes, religions, social systems, beliefs about health and illness, food preferences, languages, and role relationships offers many opportunities to explore our own values and beliefs and to learn to accept and appreciate the values and beliefs of others.

Resolving conflicting cultural manifestations will be a continuing challenge for all of the nursing team members. For example, the cultural manifestations of time are different for different cultural groups. For some groups, time is flexible and arriving at work around 7 AM (6:30–7:30) is acceptable while for other groups, time is not flexible and arriving after 7 AM is unacceptable. These cultural differences, unless discussed and understood, can create tension among the nursing team members.

A challenge for the future will be for nurses to not only include an awareness of how culture affects a patient's response to healthcare but also how cultural diversity affects their own relationships with their co-workers.

NURSING TEAM MEMBERS

Legal issues related to crosstraining and the use of multipurpose workers and unlicensed assistive personnel will continue to concern licensed nurses well into the future.

We have already discussed how healthcare facilities are attempting to reduce costs by decreasing the number of employees. Another way they are attempting to reduce costs is by crosstraining current employees, using multipurpose workers to perform a variety of tasks, and assigning unlicensed personnel to assist licensed staff. (See Chapter 7 for a discussion of multipurpose workers and unlicensed assistive personnel.)

The legal issues associated with assigning tasks that by law belong to licensed nurses to multipurpose workers and unlicensed personnel will expose the patient to a multitude of caregivers, each with their own tasks to perform. Employers who expect to save money by replacing licensed nurses with other less skilled workers may in the long run loose money because of patient dissatisfaction with the quality of their care, the number of people who provide that care, and claims of malpractice as a result of negligent care.

Crosstraining of nurses and other healthcare workers is an issue that is stimulating a lot of discussion. The LP/VN who is working in a hospital and can provide respiratory therapy treatments, do electrocardiograms (EKGs), draw blood, and start intravenous (IV) therapy fluids may be considered crosstrained. The LP/VN in this scenario is performing jobs normally performed by the respiratory care practitioner, the EKG technician, and the IV team. Crosstraining is also used to describe the nurse who is trained to work in several different clinical specialties, such as the postpartum unit, the normal and intensive care nursery, and the delivery room.

There are advantages and disadvantages to being crosstrained. One advantage is that the person who is crosstrained is a valuable employee. If the time comes to decrease the size of the staff, the crosstrained person may be retained while those who have limited skills would be let go. A second advantage is for the employer. Because the crosstrained person can work in several different areas of the facility or do the jobs of several other people, an employer can save the money that would be paid to others.

A major disadvantage to crosstraining is based on the quality of the training the person receives for his or her additional duties. Almost anyone can quickly learn the manipulative skills needed to perform treatments and procedures. Acquiring the knowledge essential to understanding the implications, side effects, and how to cope with potential complications does not occur quickly. The respiratory care practitioner, for example, spends up to 4 years learning to safely provide respiratory therapy services.

Another disadvantage to crosstraining is related to quality and safety. The nurse who is crosstrained to work in the four different divisions of the maternity department may have difficulty maintaining expertise in all four areas. The LP/VN who can, in addition to providing patient care, provide respiratory therapy treatments, do EKGs, draw blood, and start IV therapy fluids may find that this added work load is more than he or she can safely handle.

It is likely that you will be personally confronted with the issue of crosstraining as you continue in your career in nursing. Remember to base your actions on state nursing practice laws as well as your competence to perform additional duties.

ALTERNATE THERAPIES

Aromatherapy, basic neuromuscular integration, foot reflexology, hypnotherapy, massage, therapeutic touch, meditation, and Reiki are a few of the alternate therapies being offered today.

Public interest in alternative therapies is increasing and the National Institute of Health, recognizing the potential of these alternatives, has established an Office of Alternative Medicine. Nurses who provide alternate therapies emphasize that these techniques and procedures are intended as adjuncts to, not substitutes for, traditional medical treatment. Proponents of alternate therapies believe that the mind and body work together and their focus on the mind, along with the medical focus on the body, gives the patient an opportunity for improved health.

As a person, you may or may not at some time in the future consider alternate therapies in conjunction with traditional medical treatment for yourself and your family. As a nurse, you will probably have more and more patients who find that combining these two therapies is best for them. Continuing your education in this area will help you incorporate your patient's preferences in your nursing care.

CRITICAL THINKING

Those who work in healthcare in the future will be required to improve their critical thinking skills. So much knowledge in nursing and medicine is available and healthcare situations are so complex that being able to identify problems, propose solutions, and make good decisions will be an essential characteristic of tomorrow's nurse.

New nursing textbooks, journal articles, and computer simulations on the subject of critical thinking in nursing, as well as practice in applying what you learn, will help you to continue to improve your critical thinking skills.

BIOETHICS

Advances in science and technology are continuing to create new ethical issues every day. Many of the issues in the future will be related to death and dying. Advanced directives, physician-assisted suicide, "do not resuscitate" orders, withholding food and fluids, and forgoing life-sustaining treatment are all issues that continue to be of concern.

Maternal-fetal issues are continuing to increase in complexity. Sperm banks create questions about paternal rights. Questions about the rights of surrogate mothers, the ethics of genetic counseling and genetic engineering, termination of pregnancy, rights of the father, and rights of the fetus will continue to be asked in the future.

Transplants of organs is not new but certainly new sources of donor organs and new ways of obtaining donor organs will present an ethical concern for many. Killing animals for their organs and buying and selling organs are real issues that will face us more frequently in the future.

Learn as much as you can about these and other issues. Look at each issue from your personal point of view and from society's point of view. When you can accept the right of people and society to have opinions different from yours, you will be able to provide nursing care to all your patients, regardless of their personal decisions.

THE HEALTHCARE SYSTEM

President Clinton's 1993 proposal to provide affordable and permanent healthcare for every citizen was a response to public concern about access to and cost of healthcare. As the government is continuing to work to find solutions to this national problem, insurance companies and providers are beginning to work together to attempt to address the issue.

Managed care, which includes case management, utilization review, and quality assurance programs, have demonstrated an ability to drastically reduce costs and at the same time provide quality care. More and more people are choosing a managed care insurance plan.

Traditional fee-for-service insurance plans continue to be offered, however, the cost of this type of insurance has become so expensive that few can afford it.

While managed care and traditional fee-for-service plans provides for those who can afford the insurance premiums, providing care for those who can not afford health insurance remains a huge burden to the healthcare system.

There is no doubt that during your career as a nurse you will see many changes in the healthcare system. It is likely that more care will be provided outside hospitals, limits on how much money will be spent for healthcare for one's entire life may be defined, healthcare may be rationed, and restrictions on the use of expensive technology to maintain life may be imposed.

What the future healthcare system will look like is unknown at this time but it is certain, however, that it will never again be what it is today.

SUMMARY

This chapter has only touched on a few current issues and future concerns. What the future holds is unknown. There will no doubt be new issues and new concerns. Technology will continue to have an impact on how we live our lives and where. Some ethical dilemmas will be resolved and new ones will develop. The healthcare system will be different from what it is today. How you practice your profession and where you practice it will continue to change over time.

Your only chance of enjoying a long and rewarding career in nursing is to take advantage of every educational opportunity that you can and to be deeply involved in anything and everything that affects you as a nurse and your patient as a person.

DISCUSSION QUESTIONS/LEARNING ACTIVITIES

1. Assess how well you think you adapt to change. What makes you uncomfortable when a change is about to occur? What can you do to make better adjustments to change?

2. Make a list of things you can do if you think your working environment is hazardous to your health.

3. Review several brochures announcing continuing education programs. How much do these programs cost, where are they held, are continuing education credits offered, and what audience are they designed to attract? Would attending any of these programs improve your nursing practice?

4. Prepare a list of states that require continuing education for renewal of the LP/VN license. How many hours are required? Are the requirements specific or general? (Your librarian can assist you in finding this information in your library.)

5. Write to your state board of nursing and ask for a summary of their activities related to mandatory continuing education for license renewal.

6. Plan a debate on proposed changes in the healthcare system with your classmates.

7. In addition to the issues discussed in this chapter, what other issues and future concerns can you identify and describe?

8. Take a position on any current issue in nursing and defend it. When appropriate, include facts and figures to support your position.

9. What is your greatest concern for your future as a nurse? What can you do to influence the outcome?

READ MORE ABOUT IT

Aiken LH, Fagin CM: Charting Nursing's Future: Agenda for the 1990s. Philadelphia: JB Lippincott, 1992.

Bullough B, Bullough V: Nursing Issues for the Nineties and Beyond, First Edition. New York: Springer, 1994.

Curtin L: Nursing Into the 21st Century, First Edition. Springhouse: Springhouse, PA: 1995.

Deloughery GL: Issues and Trends in Nursing, Second Edition. St. Louis: CV Mosby, 1995.

Ellis JR, Hartley CL: Nursing in Today's World: Challenges, Issues, and Trends, Fifth Edition. Philadelphia: JB Lippincott, 1995.

Grippando GM: Nursing Perspectives and Issues, Fifth Edition. Albany, NY: Delmar, 1992.

Harrington N, et al: LPN to RN Transitions, First Edition. Philadelphia: JB Lippincott, 1995.

Kelly K: Health Care Rationing: Dilemma and Paradox, First Edition. St. Louis: Mosby, 1994.

Kelly LY, Joel LA: The Nursing Experience: Trends, Challenges, Transitions, Third Edition. Blacklick, OH: McGraw-Hill, 1996.

McCloskey G: Current Issues in Nursing, Fourth Edition. St. Louis: CV Mosby, 1994.

Zerwekh J, Claborn JC: Nursing Today: Transition and Trends, First Edition. Philadelphia: WB Saunders, 1994.

Appendix A
Stress Management Techniques

The following techniques can be taught to provide an individual with an opportunity to control his or her response to stressors and, in turn, increase his or her ability to manage stress constructively. Suggested readings are listed at the end to provide more specific information.

PROGRESSIVE RELAXATION TECHNIQUE

Progressive relaxation is a self-taught exercise that involves learning to constrict and relax muscle groups in a systematic way, beginning with the face and finishing with the feet. This exercise may be combined with breathing exercises that focus on inner body processes. It usually takes 15 to 30 minutes and may be accompanied by a taped instruction that directs the person concerning the sequence of muscles to be relaxed.

1. Wear loose clothing; remove glasses and shoes.
2. Sit or recline in a comfortable position with neck and knees supported; avoid lying completely flat.
3. Begin with slow, rhythmic breathing.
   a. Close your eyes or stare at a spot and take in a slow deep breath.
   b. Exhale the breath slowly.
4. Continue rhythmic breathing at a slow steady pace and feel the tension leaving your body with each breath.
5. Begin progressive relaxation of muscle groups.
   a. Breathe in and tense (tighten) your muscles and then relax the muscles as you breathe out.
   b. Suggested order for tension-relaxation cycle (with tension technique in parentheses):
      - Face, jaw, mouth (squint eyes, wrinkle brow)
      - Neck (pull chin to neck)
      - Right hand (make a fist)
      - Right arm (bend elbow in tightly)

From Carpenito L: Nursing Diagnosis: Application to Clinical Practice, Sixth Edition. Philadelphia: JB Lippincott, 1995, pp 1146–1147.

- Left hand (make a fist)
- Left arm (bend elbow in tightly)
- Back, shoulders, chest (shrug shoulders up tightly)
- Abdomen (pull stomach in and bear down on chair)
- Right upper leg (push leg down)
- Right lower leg and foot (point toes toward body)
- Left upper leg (push leg down)
- Left lower leg and foot (point toes toward body)

6. Practice technique slowly.
7. End relaxation session when you are ready by counting to three, inhaling deeply, and saying, "I am relaxed."

SELF-COACHING

Self-coaching is a procedure to decrease anxiety by understanding one's own signs of anxiety (such as increased heart rate or sweaty palms) and then coaching oneself to relax.

For example, "I am upset about this situation but I can control how anxious I get. I will take things one step at a time, and I won't focus on my fear. I'll think about what I must do to finish this task. The situation will not be forever. I can manage until it is over. I'll focus on taking deep breaths."

THOUGHT STOPPING

Thought stopping is a self-directed behavioral procedure learned to gain control of self-defeating thoughts. Through repeated systematic practice, a person does the following:

1. Says "Stop" when a self-defeating thought crosses the mind (*eg,* "I'm not smart enough" or "I'm not a good nurse")
2. Allows a brief period—15 to 30 seconds—of conscious relaxation (because of an increased focus on negative thoughts, it may seem at first that self-defeating thoughts increase; however, eventually the self-defeating thoughts will decrease)

ASSERTIVE BEHAVIOR

Assertive behavior is the open, honest, empathetic sharing of your opinions, desires, and feelings. Assertiveness is not a magical acquisition but a learned behavioral skill. Assertive persons do not allow others to take advantage of them and thus are not victims. Assertive behavior is not domineering but remains controlled and nonaggressive. An assertive person:

Does not hurt others
Does not wait for things to get better

Does not invite victimization
Listens attentively to the desires and feelings of others
Takes the initiative to make relationships better
Remains in control or uses silences as an alternative
Examines all the risks involved before asserting
Examines personal responsibilities in each situation before asserting

Refer to suggested readings for specific techniques or participate in an assertiveness training course led by a competent instructor. Assertive behavior is best learned slowly in several sessions rather than in one lengthy session or workshop.

GUIDED IMAGERY

This technique is the purposeful use of one's imagination in a specific way to achieve relaxation and control. The person concentrates on the image and pictures himself or herself involved in the scene. The following is an example of the technique.

1. Discuss with person an image he or she has experienced that is pleasurable and relaxing, such as
   a. Lying on a warm beach
   b. Feeling a cool wave of water
   c. Floating on a raft
   d. Watching the sun set
2. Choose a scene that will involve at least two senses.
3. Begin with rhythmic breathing and progressive relaxation.
4. Have a person travel mentally to the scene.
5. Have the person slowly experience the scene; how does it look? sound? smell? feel? taste?
6. Practice the imagery.
   a. Suggest tape-recording the imagined experience to assist with the technique.
   b. Practice the technique alone to reduce feelings of embarrassment.
7. End the imagery technique by counting to three and saying, "I am relaxed" (if the person does not utilize a specific ending, he may become drowsy and fall asleep, which defeats the purpose of the technique).

BIBLIOGRAPHY

Alberti RE, Emmons L: Your Perfect Right: A Guide to Assertive Behavior, Second Edition. San Luis Obispo, CA: Impact, 1974.
Bloom L, Coburn K, Pearlman J: The New Assertive Woman. New York: Dell, 1976.
Chenevert M: Special Techniques in Assertiveness Training for Women in the Health Professions. St. Louis: Mosby, 1978.

Chenevert M: Pro-nurse Handbook. St. Louis: Mosby, 1985.

Gridano D, Everly G: Controlling Stress and Tension. Englewood Cliffs, NJ: Prentice-Hall, 1979.

Herman S: Becoming Assertive: A Guide for Nurses. New York: Van Nostrand, 1978.

Hill L, Smith N: Self-care Nursing. Englewood Cliffs, NJ: Prentice-Hall, 1985 (especially Part II, Self-care primarily associated with the mind).

McCafferty M: Nursing Management of the Patient with Pain, Second Edition. Philadelphia: JB Lippincott, 1979 (especially Chapter 9, Relaxation; Chapter 10, Imagery).

Appendix B
Controlled Substances—
Uses and Effects

Drugs CSA Schedules	Trade or Other Names	Medical Uses	Dependence	
			Physical	*Psychological*
Stimulants				
Cocaine[1] II	Coke, Flake, Snow, Crack	Local anesthetic	Possible	High
Amphetamines II	Biphetamine, Delcobase, Desoxyn, Dexedrine, Obetrol	Attention deficit disorders, narcolepsy, weight control	Possible	High
Phenmetrazine II	Preludin	Weight control	Possible	High
Methylphenidate II	Ritalin	Attention deficit disorders, narcolepsy	Possible	Moderate
Other Stimulants III, IV	Adipex, Cylert, Didrex, Ionamin, Mellat, Plagine, Sanorex, Tenuate, Taperul, Prelu-2	Weight control	Possible	High
Hallucinogens				
LSD I	Acid, Microdot	None	None	Unknown
Mescaline and Peyote I	Mexc, Buttons, Cactus	None	None	Unknown
Amphetamine Variants I	2,5-DMA, PMA, STP, MDA, MDMA, TMA, DOM, DOB	None	Unknown	Unknown
Phencyclidine II	PCP, Angel Dust, Hog	None	Unknown	High
Phencyclidine Analogues I	PCE, PCPy, TCP	None	Uknown	High
Other Hallucinogens I	Buloterine, Ibogaine, DMT, DET, Psilocybin, Psilocyn	None	None	Unknown
Cannabis				
Marijuana I	Pot, Acapulco Gold, Grass, Reefer, Sinsemila, Thai Sticks	None	Unknown	Moderate
Tetrahydrocannabinol I, II	THC, Marinol	Cancer chemotherapy, antinauseant	Unknown	Moderate
Hashish I	Hash	None	Unknown	Moderate
Hashish Oil I	Hash Oil	None	Unknown	Moderate

[1]Designated a narcotic under the GSA.

[2]Not designated a narcotic under the GSA.

From U.S. Department of Justice: *Drugs of Abuse (1989 Edition)*.

Tolerance	Duration (Hours)	Usual Methods of Administration	Possible Effects	Effects of Overdose	Withdrawal Syndrome
Yes	1–2	Sniffed, smoked, injected	Increased alertness, excitation, euphoria, increased pulse rate and blood pressure, insomnia, loss of appetite	Agitation, increase in body temperature, hallucinations, convulsions, possible death	Apathy, long periods of sleep, irritability, depression, disorientation
Yes	2–4	Oral, injected			
Yes	2–4	Oral, injected			
Yes	2–4	Oral, injected			
Yes	2–4	Oral, injected			
Yes	8–12	Oral	Illusions and hallucinations, poor perception of time and distance	Longer, more intense "trip" episodes, psychosis, possible death	Withdrawal syndrome not reported
Yes	8–12	Oral			
Yes	Variable	Oral, injected			
Yes	Days	Smoked, oral, injected			
Yes	Days	Smoked, oral, injected			
Possible	Variable	Smoked, oral, injected, sniffed			
Yes	2–4	Smoked, oral	Euphoria, reduced inhibitions, increased appetite, disoriented behavior	Fatigue, paranoia, possible psychosis	Insomnia, hyperactivity, and decreased appetite occasionally reported
Yes	2–4	Smoked, oral			
Yes	2–4	Smoked, oral			
Yes	2–4	Smoked, oral			

Drugs CSA Schedules	Trade or Other Names	Medical Uses	Dependence	
			Physical	*Psychological*
Narcotics				
Opium II, III, V	Dover's Powder, Paregoric, Parepectolin	Analgesic, antidiarrheal	High	High
Morphine II, III	Morphine, MS-Contin, Roxanol, Retinol-SR	Analgesic, antitussive	High	High
Codeine	Tylenol w/Codeine, Empirin w/Codeine, Robitussin A-C, Fiorinal w/Codeine	Analgesic, antitussive	Moderate	Moderate
Heroin I	Diacetylmorphine, Horse, Smack	None	High	High
Hydromorphone II	Dilaudid	Analgesic	High	High
Meperidine (Pethidine) II	Demerol, Mepergan	Analgesic	High	High
Methadone II	Dolophine, Methadone, Methadose	Analgesic	High	High-Low
Other Narcotics I, II, III, IV, V	Numorphan, Percodan, Percocet, Tylox, Tussionex, Fentanyl, Darvon, Lomotil, Talwin[2]	Analgesic, antidiarrheal, antitussive	High-Low	High-Low
Depressants				
Chloral Hydrate IV	Noctec	Hypnotic	Moderate	Moderate
Barbiturates II, III, IV	Amytal, Butisol, Florinal, Lotusate, Nembutal, Seconal, Tuinal, Phenobarbital	Anesthetic, anticonvulsant, sedative, hypnotic, veterinary euthenasic agent	High-Moderate	High-Moderate
Benzodiazepines IV	Ativan, Dalmane, Diazepam, Librium, Xanax, Serax, Valium, Tranxene, Verstran, Versed, Halcion, Paxipam, Restoril	Antianxiety, anticonvulsant, sedative, hypnotic	Low	Low
Methaquaione I	Quaalude	Sedative, hypnotic	High	High
Glutethimide III	Doriden	Sedative, hypnotic	High	Moderate
Other Depressants III, IV	Equanil, Miltown, Noludar, Placidyl, Valmid	Antianxiety, sedative, hypnotic	Moderate	Moderate

[1]Designated a narcotic under the GSA.

[2]Not designated a narcotic under the GSA.

Tolerance	Duration (Hours)	Usual Methods of Administration	Possible Effects	Effects of Overdose	Withdrawal Syndrome
Yes	3–6	Oral, smoked	Euphoria, drowsiness, respiratory depression, constricted pupils, nausea	Slow and shallow breathing, clammy skin, convulsions, coma, possible death	Watery eyes, runny nose, yawning, loss of appetite, irritability, tremors, panic, cramps, nausea, chills, and sweating
Yes	3–6	Oral, smoked, injected			
Yes	3–6	Oral, injected			
Yes	3–6	Injected, sniffed, smoked			
Yes	3–6	Oral, injected			
Yes	3–4	Oral, injected			
Yes	12–24	Oral, injected			
Yes	Variable	Oral, Injected			
Yes	5–8	Oral	Slurred speech, disorientation, drunken behavior without odor of alcohol	Shallow respiration, clammy skin, dilated pupils, weak and rapid pulse, coma, possible death	Anxiety, insomnia, tremors, delirium, convulsions, possible death
Yes	1–16	Oral			
Yes	4–8	Oral			
Yes	4–8	Oral			
Yes	4–8	Oral			
Yes	4–8	Oral			

ALCOHOL

Effects

Alcohol consumption causes a number of marked changes in behavior. Even low doses significantly impair the judgement and coordination required to drive a car safely, increasing the likelihood that the driver will be involved in an accident. Low to moderate doses of alcohol also increase the incidence of a variety of aggressive acts, including spouse and child abuse. Moderate to high doses of alcohol cause marked impairments in higher mental functions, severely altering a person's ability to learn and remember information. Very high doses cause respiratory depression and death. If combined with other depressants of the central nervous system, much lower doses of alcohol will produce the effects just described.

Repeated use of alcohol can lead to dependence. Sudden cessation of alcohol intake is likely to produce withdrawal symptoms, including severe anxiety, tremors, hallucinations, and convulsions. Alcohol withdrawal can be life-threatening. Long-term consumption of large quantities of alcohol, particularly when combined with poor nutrition, can also lead to permanent damage to vital organs such as the brain and the liver.

Mothers who drink alcohol during pregnancy may give birth to infants with fetal alcohol syndrome. These infants have irreversible physical abnormalities and mental retardation. In addition, research indicates that children of alcoholic parents are at greater risk than other youngsters of becoming alcoholics.

From U.S. Department of Education. *What Works: Schools Without Drugs (1989 Edition).*

Appendix C
Common Sexually
Transmitted Diseases

Disease	Usual Time from Contact to First Symptoms	Usual Symptoms	Complications
Gonorrhea Cause: bacterium	2–10 days; sometimes 30 days	Local, genital discharge, pain, often no symptoms in men; usually no symptoms in women	Pelvic inflammatory disease, sterility, arthritis, blindness, eye infection in newborns
Syphilis Cause: spirochete	3–5 weeks; average 21 days	First stage: painless pimple that disappears without treatment on genitals, fingers, lips, breast. Second stage: rash, fever, flu-like illness. Latent stage: none	Brain damage, insanity, paralysis, heart disease, death, damage to skin, bones, eyes, liver, teeth of fetus and newborns
Genital Herpes Cause: virus	About 1 week	Swollen, tender, painful blisters on genitals	Strong evidence linking infection to cervical cancer; severe central nervous system damage or death in infants infected during birth
Nonspecific Vaginitis Cause: (7) bacterium	1–2 weeks	Gray offensive vaginal discharge, usually no itching	Medical complications unknown
Nonspecific Urethritis Cause: Chlamydia	1–3 weeks	Penile discharge, frequent urination; usually no itching	Pelvic inflammatory disease in women, possible eye infections or pneumonia in newborns

Disease	Incubation	Symptoms	Complications
Trichomonas Cause: protozoon	1–4 weeks	Discharge, intense itching, burning and redness of genitals and thighs; painful intercourse; usually no symptoms in men	Gland infections in females, prostatitis in men
Monilia Cause: fungus	Varies	Thick, cheesy, offensive vaginal discharge; itching, skin irritation; usually no symptoms in men	Secondary infections by bacteria; mouth and throat infections of newborn
Venereal Warts Cause: virus	Up to 2 months	Local irritation, itching	Highly contagious; can spread enough to block vaginal opening
Pediculosis Pubis Cause: louse	4–5 weeks	Intense itching, pinhead blood spots on underwear; small eggs or nits on pubic hair	No medical complications
Scabies Cause: itch mite	4–6 weeks	Severe nighttime itching, raised gray lines in skin where mite burrows	May infest elbows, hands, breasts, and buttocks as well as genitals
AIDS (acquired immune deficiency syndrome) Cause: HIV virus	Not established. Seroconversion may occur in 5 days to 3 months; time from seroconversion to AIDS averages 10 years	Lymph gland swelling (swollen glands), flu-like illness of long duration, purplish discolorations on arms and legs, unexplained weight loss, persistent cough, loss of appetite	Kaposi's sarcoma (a form of cancer), pneumonia, tuberculosis, various other life-threatening infections, death

Appendix D
Directory of Nursing
and Health-Related
Organizations

This Appendix is divided into four parts. Part I lists state boards of nursing alphabetically by state and territory. Part II lists Canadian associations and boards of nursing. Part III is a list of national practical/vocational nursing organizations. Part IV is a listing of additional organizations of particular interest to practical nurses.

(Note: These addresses were current as of 1996.)

STATE AND TERRITORIAL BOARDS OF NURSING

Alabama Board of Nursing
PO Box 303900
Montgomery, Alabama 36130-3900
Phone: (334) 242-4060
FAX: (334) 242-4360

Alaska Board of Nursing
PO Box 110806
Juneau, Alaska 99811
Phone: (907) 465-2544
FAX: (907) 465-2974

American Samoa Health Service
Regulatory Board
LBJ Tropical Medical Center
Pago Pago, American Samoa 96799
Phone: (684) 633-1221 x206
FAX: 011-684-633-1869

Arizona State Board of Nursing
1651 E. Morten Ave., Suite 150
Phoenix, Arizona 85020
Phone: (602) 255-5092
FAX: (602) 255-5130

Arkansas State Board of Nursing
University Tower Building, Suite 800
1123 South University
Little Rock, Arkansas 72204
Phone: (501) 686-2700
FAX: (501) 686-2714

California Board of Registered Nursing
PO Box 944210
Sacramento, California 94244-2100
Phone: (916) 322-3350
FAX: (916) 327-4402

California Board of Vocational
    Nurse and Psychiatric
    Technician Examiners
2535 Capitol Oaks Drive
Suite 205
Sacramento, California 95833
Phone: (916) 263-7800
FAX: (916) 263-7859

Colorado Board of Nursing
1560 Broadway, Suite 670
Denver, Colorado 80202
Phone: (303) 894-2430
FAX: (303) 894-2821

Connecticut Board of Examiners
    for Nursing
Department of Public Health
    Nurse Licensure
150 Washington Street
Hartford, Connecticut 06106
Phone: (860) 566-1041
FAX: (860) 566-1032

Delaware Board of Nursing
Cannon Building, Suite 203
PO Box 1401
Dover, Delaware 19903
Phone: (302) 739-4522
FAX: (302) 739-2711

District of Columbia Board
    of Nursing
614 H Street, NW
Washington, DC 20001
Phone: (202) 727-7468
FAX: (202) 727-7662

Florida Board of Nursing
4080 Woodcock Drive, Suite 202
Jacksonville, Florida 32207
Phone: (904) 858-6940
FAX: (904) 858-6964

Georgia Board of Nursing
166 Pryor Street, SW
Atlanta, Georgia 30303
Phone: (404) 656-3943
FAX: (404) 656-7489

Georgia State Board of Licensed
    Practical Nurses
166 Pryor Street, SW
Atlanta, Georgia 30303
Phone: (404) 656-3903
FAX: (404) 651-9532

Guam Board of Nurse Examiners
PO Box 2816
Agana, Guam 96910
Phone: 011-671-475-0251
FAX: 011-671-477-4733

Hawaii Board of Nursing
PO Box 3469
Honolulu, Hawaii 96801
Phone: (808) 586-2695
FAX: (808) 586-2689

Idaho Board of Nursing
PO Box 83720
Boise, Idaho 83720-0061
Phone: (208) 334-3110
FAX: (208) 334-3262

Illinois Department of
    Professional Regulation
320 West Washington Street
3rd Floor
Springfield, Illinois 62786
Phone: (217) 782-8556
FAX: (217) 782-7645

Indiana State Board of Nursing
Health Professions Bureau
402 West Washington Street, Room #041
Indianapolis, Indiana 46204
Phone: (317) 232-2960
FAX: (317) 232-4236

Iowa Board of Nursing
State Capitol Complex
1223 East Court Avenue
Des Moines, Iowa 50319
Phone: (515) 281-3255
FAX: (515) 281-4825

Kansas State Board of Nursing
Landon State Office Building
900 SW Jackson, Suite 551-S
Topeka, Kansas 66612-1230
Phone: (913) 296-4929
FAX: (913) 296-3929

Kentucky Board of Nursing
312 Wittington Parkway, Suite 300
Louisville, Kentucky 40222-5172
Phone: (502) 329-7000
FAX: (502) 329-7111

Louisiana State Board of
    RN Nursing
912 Pere Marquette Building
150 Baronne Street
New Orleans, Louisiana 70112
Phone: (504) 568-5464
FAX: (504) 568-5467

Louisiana State Board of
    Practical Nurse Examiners
3421 N. Causeway Boulevard
Suite 203
Metairic, Louisiana 70002
Phone: (504) 838-5791
FAX: (504) 838-5279

Maine State Board of Nursing
State House Station #158
Augusta, Maine 04333-0158
Phone: (207) 624-5275
FAX: (207) 624-5290

Maryland Board of Nursing
4140 Patterson Avenue
Baltimore, Maryland 21215-2299
Phone: (410) 764-5124
FAX: (410) 358-3530

Massachusetts Board of Registration
    in Nursing
Leverett Saltonstall Building
100 Cambridge Street, Room 1519
Boston, Massachusetts 02202
Phone: (617) 727-9961
FAX: (617) 727-2197

Michigan Department of Commerce
Bureau of Occupational and
    Professional Regulation
Ottawa Towers North
611 West Ottawa
Lansing, Michigan 48933
Phone: (517) 373-1600
FAX: (517) 373-2179

Minnesota Board of Nursing
2700 University Avenue, West #108
St. Paul, Minnesota 55114
Phone: (601) 359-6170
FAX: (601) 359-6185

Missouri State Board of Nursing
PO Box 656
Jefferson City, Missouri 65102
Phone: (314) 751-0681
FAX: (314) 751-0075

Montana State Board of Nursing
111 North Jackson
PO Box 200513
Helena, Montana 59620-0513
Phone: (406) 444-2071
FAX: (406) 444-7759

Nebraska Department of Health
Bureau of Examining Boards
PO Box 95007
Lincoln, Nebraska 68509
Phone: (402) 471-2115
FAX: (402) 471-3577

Nevada State Board of Nursing
PO Box 46886
Las Vegas, Nevada 89114
Phone: (702) 739-1575
FAX: (702) 739-0298

New Hampshire Board of Nursing
Health & Welfare Building
6 Hazen Drive
Concord, New Hampshire 03301-6527
Phone: (603) 271-2323
FAX: (603) 271-6605

New Jersey Board of Nursing
PO Box 45010
Newark, New Jersey 07101
Phone: (201) 504-6493
FAX: (201) 648-3481

New Mexico Board of Nursing
4206 Louisiana Boulevard, NE
Suite A
Albuquerque, New Mexico 87109
Phone: (505) 841-8340
FAX: (505) 841-8347

New York State Board of Nursing
State Education Department
Cultural Education Center
Room 3023
Albany, New York 12230
Phone: (518) 474-3843/3845
FAX: (518) 473-0578

North Carolina Board of Nursing
PO Box 2129
Raleigh, North Carolina 27602
Phone: (919) 782-3211
FAX: (919) 781-9461

North Dakota Board of Nursing
919 South 7th Street, Suite 504
Bismarck, North Dakota 58504-5881
Phone: (701) 328-9777
FAX: (701) 328-4614

Northern Mariana Islands
Commonwealth Board of Nurse Examiners
Public Health Center
PO Box 1458
Saipan, MP 96950
Phone: 011-670-234-8950
FAX: 011-670-234-8930

Ohio Board of Nursing
77 South High Street, 17th Floor
Columbus, Ohio 43226-0316
Phone: (614) 466-3947
FAX: (614) 466-0388

Oklahoma Board of Nursing
2915 North Classen Blvd., Suite 524
Oklahoma City, Oklahoma 73106
Phone: (405) 525-2076
FAX: (405) 521-6089

Oregon State Board of Nursing
Suite 465
800 NE Oregon Street, Box 25
Portland, Oregon 97232
Phone: (503) 731-4745
FAX: (503) 731-4755

Pennsylvania State Board of Nursing
PO Box 2649
Harrisburg, Pennsylvania 17105-2649
Phone: (717) 783-7142
FAX: (717) 787-7769

Commonwealth of Puerto Rico
Board of Nurse Examiners
Call Box 10200
Santurce, Puerto Rico 00908
Phone: (809) 725-8161
FAX: (809) 725-7903

Rhode Island Board of Nurse
Registration & Nursing Education
Cannon Health Building
Three Capitol Hill, Room 104
Providence, Rhode Island 02908-5097
Phone: (401) 277-2827
FAX: (401) 277-1272

South Carolina State Board of Nursing
220 Executive Center Drive
Suite 220
Columbia, South Carolina 29210
Phone: (803) 731-1648
FAX: (803) 731-1647

South Dakota Board of Nursing
3307 South Lincoln Avenue
Sioux Falls, South Dakota 57105-5224
Phone: (605) 367-5940
FAX: (605) 367-5945

Tennessee State Board of Nursing
283 Plus Park Blvd.
Nashville, Tennessee 37217-1010
Phone: (615) 367-6232
FAX: (615) 367-6397

Texas Board of RN Nurse Examiners
PO Box 140466
Austin, Texas 78714
Phone: (512) 305-7400
FAX: (512) 305-7401

Texas Board of Vocation Nurse Examiners
William P. Hobby Building, Tower 3
333 Guadalupe Street, 3-400
Austin, Texas 78701
Phone: (512) 305-8100
FAX: (512) 305-8101

Utah State Board of Nursing
Division of Occupational & Professional
    Licensing
PO Box 45805
Salt Lake City, Utah 84145-0805
Phone: (801) 530-6628
FAX: (801) 530-6511

Vermont State Board of Nursing
109 State Street
Montpelier, Vermont 05609-1106
Phone: (802) 828-2396
FAX: (802) 828-2853

Virgin Islands Board of Nurse Licensure
PO Box 4247, Veterans Drive Station
St. Thomas, US Virgin Islands 00803
Phone: (809) 776-7397
FAX: (809) 777-4003

Virginia Board of Nursing
6606 West Broad Street, 4th Floor
Richmond, Virginia 23230-1717
Phone: (804) 662-9909
FAX: (804) 662-9943

Washington State Nursing Care
Quality Assurance Commission
Department of Health
PO Box 47864
Olympia, Washington 98504-7864
Phone: (360) 753-2686
FAX: (360) 586-5935

West Virginia Board of Examiners
    for Registered Professional Nurses
100 Dee Drive
Charleston, West Virginia 25311-1620
Phone: (304) 558-3596
FAX: (304) 558-3666

West Virginia State Board of Examiners for
    Practical Nurses
101 Dee Drive
Charleston, West Virginia 25311-1620
Phone: (304) 558-3572
FAX: (304) 558-3666

Wisconsin Department of Regulation &
    Licensing
1400 East Washington Avenue
PO Box 8935
Madison, Wisconsin 53708-8935
Phone: (608) 266-0257
FAX: (608) 267-0644

Wyoming State Board of Nursing
2020 Carey Avenue, Suite 110
Cheyenne, Wyoming 82002
Phone: (307) 777-7601
FAX: (307) 777-3519

CANADIAN ASSOCIATIONS AND BOARDS OF NURSING

National Organizations

Canadian Nurses Association
50 The Driveway
Ottawa, ON, Canada K2P 1E2
Phone: (613) 237-2133
FAX: (613) 237-3520

Professional Associations/Boards of Nursing

Alberta Association of Registered Nurses
11620 168th Street
Edmonton, Alberta T5M 4A6
Phone: (403) 426-0160

Alberta Association of Registered Nursing
    Assistants
10615 170th Street
Edmonton, Alberta T5S 1P3
Phone: (403) 483-8126

Registered Nurses' Association of
    British Columbia
2855 Arbutus Street
Vancover, British Columbia V6J 3Y8
Phone: (605) 736-7331

British Columbia Council of Licensed Practical
    Nurses
3405 Willingdon Ave.
Burnaby, British Columbia V5G 3H4
Phone: (604) 660-5750

Manitoba Association of Licensed
    Practical Nurses
615 Kernaghan Ave.
Winnipeg, Manitoba R2C 2Z4
Phone: (204) 222-6743

Manitoba Association of Registered Nurses
647 Broadway Avenue
Winnipeg, Manitoba R3C 0X2
Phone: (204) 774-3477

New Brunswick Association of
    Registered Nurses
231 Saunders Street
Fredericton, New Brunswick E3B 1N6
Phone: (506) 454-5591

Association of New Brunswick Registered
    Nursing Assistants
384 Smythe Street
Fredericton, New Brunswick E3B 3E4
Phone: (506) 454-0747

Association of Registered Nurses of
    Newfoundland
55 Military Rd.
P.O. Box 6116
Saint John's, Newfoundland A1C 5X8
Phone: (709) 753-6040

Northwest Territory Registered Nurses'
    Association
Box 2757
Yellowknife, Northwest Territory X0E 1H0
Phone: (403) 873-2745

Registered Nurses' Association of Nova Scotia
6035 Coburg Road
Halifax, Nova Scotia B3H 1Y8
Phone: (902) 423-6156

Nova Scotia Board of Registration for
    Nursing Assistants
404-2021 Brunswick St.
Halifax, Nova Scotia B3K 2X5
Phone: (902) 423-8517

College of Nurses of Ontario
101 Davenport Road
Toronto, Ontario M5R 3P1
Phone: (416) 928-0900

Association of Nurses of Prince Edward Island
P.O. Box 1838
Charlottetown, Prince Edward Island C1A 7N5
Phone: (902) 892-6322

Prince Edward Island Licensed Nursing
    Assistants Association
P.O. Box 1253
Charlottetown, Prince Edward Island C1A 7M8
Phone: (902) 566-1512

Order of Nurses of Quebec
4200 Dorchester Boulevard West
Montreal, Quebec H3Z 1V4
Phone: (514) 935-2501

Professional Alliance of Quebec Nurses Aides
531 est, rue Sherbrooke
Montreal, Quebec H2L 1K2
Phone: (514) 282-9511

Saskatchewan Registered Nurses Association
2066 Retallack Street
Regina, Saskatchewan S4T 2K2
Phone: (306) 527-4643

Saskatchewan Nursing Assistants Association
2310 Smith Street
Regina, Saskatchewan S4P 2P6
Phone: (306) 525-1436

Yukon Government of Justice
J-6
P.O. Box 2703
Whitehorse, Yukon Y1A 2C6
Phone: (403) 667-5124

NATIONAL PRACTICAL/VOCATIONAL NURSING ORGANIZATIONS

American Licensed Practical
    Nurses Association
1090 Vermont Ave. NW
Suite 1200
Washington, DC 20005
Phone: (202) 682-9000

National Association for Practical
    Nurse Education and Service
1400 Spring Street
Suite 310
Silver Spring, Maryland 20910
Phone: (301) 588-2491

National Federation of Licensed
    Practical Nurses
1418 Aveesboro Rd.
Garner, North Carolina 27529-4547
Phone: (919) 779-0046

Other Organizations

American Hospital Association
Division of Nursing
840 North Lake Shore Drive
Chicago, Illinois 60611
Phone: (312) 280-6000

American Nurses Association
600 Maryland Avenue, SW
Suite 100W
Washington, DC 20024-2571
Phone: (202) 651-7000

American Red Cross
431 18th Street, NW
Washington, DC 20006
Phone: (202) 737-8300

American Vocational Association
1410 King Street
Alexandria, Virginia 22314
Phone: (703) 683-3111

Army Nurse Corp
Office of the Surgeon General
Department of the Army
5111 Leesburg Pike
Falls Church, Virginia 22031-3258
Phone: (202) 756-0045

Catholic Health Association of the
  United States
4455 Woodson Road
Saint Louis, Missouri 63134-0889
Phone: (314) 427-2500

Federation for Accessible Nursing
Education and Licensure
P.O. Box 1418
Lewisburg, West Virginia 24901
Phone: (304) 645-4357

Federation of Nurses and Health Professionals
555 New Jersey Avenue, NW
Washington, DC 20001
Phone: (202) 879-4491

Health Occupations Students of America
National Headquarters
6309 North O'Connor Road
Suite 215, LB-117
Irving, Texas 75039-3510
Phone: (214) 506-9780

National Black Nurses Association
1511 K Street, SW
Suite 415
Washington, DC 20005
Phone: (202) 393-6870

National Council of State Boards of Nursing
676 North Saint Clair Street
Suite 550
Chicago, Illinois 60611-2921
Phone: (312) 787-6555

National League for Nursing
350 Hudson Street
New York, New York 10014
Phone: (800) 669-1656

National Nurses Society on Addictions
4101 Lake Boone Trail
Suite 201
Raleigh, North Carolina 27607
Phone: (919) 783-5871

North American Nursing Diagnosis
  Association
1211 Locust St.
Philadelphia, Pennsylvania 19107
Phone: (215) 545-8105

Pan American Health Organization
WHO Regional Office for the Americas
525 23rd Street, NW
Washington, DC 20037
Phone: (202) 861-3200

People to People Health Foundation
  (Project Hope)
Health Sciences Education Center
Center Hall
Millwood, Virginia 22646
Phone: (703) 837-2100

World Health Organization
20, Ave. Appia
CH-1211
Geneva 27, Switzerland
Phone: (022) 791-21-11

Appendix E
NFLPN Nursing Practice Standards for the Licensed Practical/Vocational Nurse

PREFACE

The Standards were developed and adopted by the NFLPN to provide a basic model whereby the quality of health service and nursing service and nursing care given by LP/VNs may be measured and evaluated.

These nursing practice standards are applicable in any practice setting. The degree to which individual standards are applied will vary according to the individual needs of the patient, the type of healthcare agency or services and the community resources.

The scope of licensed practical nursing has extended into specialized nursing services. Therefore, specialized fields of nursing are included in this document.

THE CODE FOR LICENSED PRACTICAL/VOCATIONAL NURSES

The Code, adopted by NFLPN in 1961 and revised in 1979, provides a motivation for establishing, maintaining and elevating professional standards. Each LP/VN, upon entering the profession, inherits the responsibility to adhere to the standards of ethical practice and conduct as set forth in this code.

1. Know the scope of maximum utilization of the LP/VN as specified by the nursing practice act and function within this scope.
2. Safeguard the confidential information acquired from any source about the patient.

Reprinted with permission of the National Federation of Licensed Practical Nurses, Inc. Copyright 1991.

3. Provide healthcare to all patients regardless of race, creed, cultural background, disease, or lifestyle.
4. Refuse to give endorsement to the sale and promotion of commercial products or services.
5. Uphold the highest standards in personal appearance, language, dress, and demeanor.
6. Stay informed about issues affecting the practice of nursing and delivery of healthcare and, where appropriate, participate in government and policy decisions.
7. Accept the responsibility for safe nursing by keeping oneself mentally and physically fit and educationally prepared to practice.
8. Accept responsibility for membership in NFLPN and participate in its efforts to maintain the established standards of nursing practice and employment policies which lead to quality patient care.

INTRODUCTORY STATEMENT

Definition

Practical/Vocational nursing means the performance for compensation of authorized acts of nursing which utilize specialized knowledge and skills and which meet the health needs of people in a variety of settings under the direction of qualified health professionals.

Scope

Practical/Vocational nursing comprises the common core of nursing and, therefore, is a valid entry into the nursing profession.

Opportunities exist for practicing in a milieu where different professions unite their particular skills in a team effort for one common objective—to preserve or improve an individual patient's functioning.

Opportunities also exist for upward mobility within the profession through academic education and for lateral expansion of knowledge and expertise through both academic and continuing education.

STANDARDS

Education

The Licensed Practical/Vocational Nurse
1. Shall complete a formal education program in practical nursing approved by the appropriate nursing authority in a state.
2. Shall successfully pass the National Council Licensure Examination for Practical Nurses.
3. Shall participate in initial orientation within the employing institution.

Legal/Ethical Status

The Licensed Practical/Vocational Nurse
1. Shall hold a current license to practice nursing as an LP/VN in accordance with the law of the state wherein employed.
2. Shall know the scope of nursing practice authorized by the Nursing Practice Act in the state wherein employed.
3. Shall have a personal commitment to fulfill the legal responsibilities inherent in good nursing practice.
4. Shall take responsible actions in situations wherein there is unprofessional conduct by a peer or other healthcare provider.
5. Shall recognize and have a commitment to meet the ethical and moral obligations of the practice of nursing.
6. Shall not accept or perform professional responsibilities which the individual knows (s)he is not competent to perform.

Practice

The Licensed Practical/Vocational Nurse
1. Shall accept assigned responsibilities as an accountable member of the healthcare team.
2. Shall function within the limits of educational preparation and experience as related to the assigned duties.
3. Shall function with other members of the healthcare team in promoting and maintaining health, preventing disease and disability, caring for and rehabilitating individuals who are experiencing an altered health state, and contributing to the ultimate quality of life until death.
4. Shall know and utilize the nursing process in planning, implementing, and evaluating health services and nursing care for the individual patient or group.
   a. Planning: The planning of nursing includes:
      1. assessment of health status of the individual patient, the family and community groups
      2. an analysis of the information gained from assessment
      3. the identification of health goals.
   b. Implementation: The plan for nursing care is put into practice to achieve the stated goals and includes:
      1. observing, recording and reporting significant changes which require intervention or different goals
      2. applying nursing knowledge and skills to promote and maintain health, to prevent disease and disability and to optimize functional capabilities of an individual patient
      3. assisting the patient and family with activities of daily living and encouraging self-care as appropriate
      4. carrying out therapeutic regimens and protocols prescribed by an RN, physician, or other persons authorized by state law.

      c. Evaluations: The plan for nursing care and its implementations are evaluated to measure the progress toward the stated goals and will include appropriate persons and/or groups to determine:
        1. the relevancy of current goals in relation to the progress of the individual patient
        2. the involvement of the recipients of care in the evaluation process
        3. the quality of the nursing action in the implementation of the plan
        4. a re-ordering of priorities or new goal setting in the care plan.
5. Shall participate in peer review and other evaluation processes.
6. Shall participate in the development of policies concerning the health and nursing needs of society and in the roles and functions of the LP/VN.

Continuing Education

The Licensed Practical/Vocational Nurse
1. Shall be responsible for maintaining the highest possible level of professional competence at all times.
2. Shall periodically reassess career goals and select continuing education activities which will help to achieve these goals.
3. Shall take advantage of continuing education opportunities which will lead to personal growth and professional development.
4. Shall seek and participate in continuing education activities which are approved for credit by appropriate organizations, such as the NFLPN.

Specialized Nursing Practice

The Licensed Practical/Vocational Nurse
1. Shall have had at least 1 year's experience in nursing at the staff level.
2. Shall present personal qualifications that are indicative of potential abilities for practice in the chosen specialized nursing area.
3. Shall present evidence of completion of a program or course that is approved by an appropriate agency to provide the knowledge and skills necessary for effective nursing services in the specialized field.
4. Shall meet all of the standards of practice as set forth in this document.

GLOSSARY

Authorized (acts of nursing)—Those nursing activities made legal through State Nurse Practice Acts or other laws.

Lateral Expansion of Knowledge—An extension of the basic core of information learned in the school of practical nursing.

Peer Review—A formal evaluation of performance on the job by other LP/VNs.

Specialized Nursing Practice—A restricted field of nursing in which a person is particularly skilled and has specific knowledge.

Therapeutic Regimens—Regulated plans designed to bring about effective treatment of disease.

Upward Mobility—A change of career goal, eg, Licensed Practical/Vocational Nurse to Registered Nurse.

LP/VN—A combined abbreviation for Licensed Practical and Licensed Vocational Nurse. The LVN title is used in California and Texas for the nurses who are called LPNs in other states.

Milieu—One's environment and surroundings.

Protocols—Courses of treatment which include specific steps to be performed in a stated order.

Appendix F
NAPNES Standards of Practice for Licensed Practical/Vocational Nurses

THE LP/VN PROVIDES INDIVIDUAL AND FAMILY-CENTERED NURSING CARE. THE LP/VN SHALL:

A. Utilize principles of nursing process in meeting specific patient needs of patients of all ages in the areas of:
   1. Safety
   2. Hygiene
   3. Nutrition
   4. Medication
   5. Elimination
   6. Psycho-social and cultural
   7. Respiratory needs
B. Utilize appropriate knowledge, skills and abilities in providing safe, competent care.
C. Utilize principles of crisis intervention in maintaining safety and making appropriate referrals when necessary.
D. Utilize effective communication skills.
   1. Communicate effectively with patients, family members of the health team, and significant others.
   2. Maintain appropriate written documentation.
E. Provide appropriate health teaching to patients and significant others in the areas of:
   1. Maintenance of wellness
   2. Rehabilitation
   3. Utilization of community resources

Reprinted with permission of the National Association for Practical Nurse Education and Service. Copyright 1992.

    F. Serves as a patient advocate:
      1. Protect patient rights
      2. Consult with appropriate others when necessary

THE LP/VN FULFILLS THE PROFESSIONAL RESPONSIBILITIES OF THE PRACTICAL/VOCATIONAL NURSE. THE LP/VN SHALL:

    A. Know and apply the ethical principles underlying the profession.
    B. Know and follow the appropriate professional and legal requirements.
    C. Follow the policies and procedures of the employing institution.
    D. Cooperate and collaborate with all members of the healthcare team to meet the needs of family-centered nursing care.
    E. Demonstrate accountability for his/her nursing actions.
    F. Maintain currency in terms of knowledge and skills in the area of employment.

    Adopted 1992

THE LP/VN FOLLOWS THE NAPNES CODE OF ETHICS. THE LP/VN SHALL:

    1. Consider as a basic obligation the conservation of life and the prevention of disease.
    2. Promote and protect the physical, mental, emotional, and spiritual health of the patient and his family.
    3. Fulfill all duties faithfully and efficiently.
    4. Function within established legal guidelines.
    5. Accept personal responsibility (for his/her acts) and seek to merit the respect and confidence of all members of the health team.
    6. Hold in confidence all matters coming to his/her knowledge, in the practice of his profession, and in no way at no time violate this confidence.
    7. Give conscientious service and charge just remuneration.
    8. Learn and respect the religious and cultural beliefs of his/her patient and of all people.
    9. Meet his/her obligation to the patient by keeping abreast of current trends in healthcare through reading and continuing education.
    10. As a citizen of the United States of America, uphold the laws of the land and seek to promote legislation which shall meet the health needs of its people.

Appendix G
NLN Entry-Level Competencies of Graduates of Educational Programs in Practical Nursing

The graduate practical/vocational nurse demonstrates the following entry-level competencies:

ASSESSMENT

- Assesses basic physical, emotional, spiritual, and socio-cultural needs of the healthcare client.
- Collects data within established protocols and guidelines from various sources: client interviews; observations/measurements; healthcare team members, family, and significant others; and health records.
- Utilizes knowledge of normal values to identify deviations in health status.
- Documents data collection.
- Communicates findings to appropriate healthcare personnel.

PLANNING

- Contributes to the development of nursing care plans utilizing established nursing diagnoses for clients with common, well-defined health problems.
- Prioritizes nursing care needs of clients.
- Assists in the review and revision of nursing care plans to meet the changing needs of clients.

Reprinted with permission of the National League for Nursing, Council of Practical Nursing Programs, 350 Hudson Street, New York, NY 10014; Phone: (800) 669-1656. Copyright 1994.

IMPLEMENTATION

- Provides nursing care according to: accepted standards of practice; priority of client needs; and individual and family rights to dignity and privacy.
- Utilizes effective communication in: recording and reporting; and establishing and maintaining therapeutic relationships with clients, families, and significant others.
- Collaborates with healthcare team members to coordinate the delivery of nursing care.
- Instructs clients regarding health maintenance based on client needs and nurse's knowledge level.

EVALUATION

- Seeks guidance as needed in evaluating nursing care.
- Modifies nursing approaches based on evaluation of nursing care.
- Collaborates with other health team members in the revision of nursing care plans.

MEMBER OF THE DISCIPLINE

- Complies with the scope of practice as outlined in the nurse practice act of the state in which licensed.
- Describes the role of the licensed practical/vocational nurse in the healthcare delivery system.
- Utilizes educational opportunities for continued personal and professional growth.
- Identifies personal potential and considers career mobility options.
- Identifies personal strengths and weaknesses for the purpose of improving performance.
- Adheres to a nursing code of ethics.
- Functions as an advocate for the healthcare consumer.

MANAGING/SUPERVISION

- Assumes responsibility for managing his/her own actions when providing nursing care for individuals and groups of clients.
- Is accountable for nursing care delegated to unlicensed healthcare providers.

POLITICAL ACTIVISM

- Is aware that the practical nurse, through political, economic, and societal activities, can affect nursing and health.

DEFINITIONS

Basic A word synonymous with fundamental, initial, elementary, essential, and necessary.

Client A person who is a recipient of nursing care.

Competency Cognitive, affective, and/or psychomotor capability demonstrated in various roles in the practice setting.

Nursing Care Plan Written plan incorporating data obtained from utilization of the nursing process.

Nursing Diagnosis A statement that describes an existing or potential health problem that nurses can treat separately from physician orders.

Nursing Process The nursing process is the core of the practice of nursing. The four phases of the nursing process—assessment, planning, implementation, and evaluation—are the framework around which competencies have been developed.

Practical Nursing Program An educational program under the control of a hospital, vocational-technical institute, community college, or, in some instances, independently incorporated that awards a certificate or diploma in practical nursing and prepares the graduate to be eligible for licensure as a practical/vocational nurse.

Structured Care Setting An environment in which the policies, procedures, and protocols for provision of healthcare are established. The amount of structure may vary among individual agencies, such as hospitals, nursing homes, and home health settings.

Appendix H
Overview of the NCLEX-PN Test Plan

Among the functions of the National Council of State Boards of Nursing (NCSBN) is the development of nurse licensing examinations. One of these examinations is called the National Council Licensure Examination for Practical Nurses (NCLEX-PN).

Participating state boards of nursing use the results of the NCLEX-PN plus other factors when making decisions related to issuing practical/vocational nursing licenses.

The content of the NCLEX-PN is based on an in-depth job analysis of entry-level practical/vocational nurses. This job analysis is conducted every 3 years. Information collected from this analysis is used to review and revise the NCLEX-PN. The most recent job analysis was conducted in 1994.

Each question in the NCLEX-PN consists of two interrelated elements. One element is the phases of the nursing process and the other element is client needs.

The percentages of questions related to the phases of the nursing process are as follows:

Data collection	27% to 33%
Planning	17% to 23%
Implementation	27% to 33%
Evaluation	17% to 23%

The percentages of questions related to client needs are as follows:

Safe and effective care environment	16% to 22%
Physiological integrity	49% to 55%
Psychosocial integrity	8% to 14%
Health promotion and maintenance	15% to 21%

For detailed information on the general content of each of these areas, please refer to the October, 1996 Test Plan for the National Council Licensure Examination for Practical Nurses. This document is available for a fee from the National Council of State Boards of Nursing.

Appendix I
Andrews/Boyle
Transcultural Nursing
Assessment Guide

CULTURAL AFFILIATIONS

With what cultural group(s) does the client report affiliation (eg, American, Hispanic, Navajo, or combination)? To what degree does the client identify with the cultural group (eg, "we" concept of solidarity or as a fringe member)?

Where was the client born?

Where has the client lived (country, city) and when (during what years)? *Note:* If a recent relocation to the United States, knowledge of prevalent diseases in country of origin may be helpful. Current residence? Occupation?

VALUES ORIENTATION

What are the client's attitudes, values, and beliefs about developmental life events such as birth and death, health, illness, and healthcare providers?

Does culture affect the manner in which the client relates to body image change resulting from illness or surgery (eg, importance of appearance, beauty, strength, and roles in cultural group)? Is there a cultural stigma associated with the client's illness (ie, how is the illness or client condition viewed by the larger culture)?

How does the client view work, leisure, education?

How does the client perceive change?

How does the client perceive changes in lifestyle relating to current illness or surgery?

How does the client value privacy, courtesy, touch, and relationships with individuals of different ages, social class (or caste), and gender?

How does the client view biomedical/scientific healthcare (eg, suspiciously, fearfully, accepting)? How does the client relate to persons outside of his or her cultural group (eg, withdrawal, verbally or nonverbally expressive, negatively or positively)?

Andrews MM, Boyle JS: Transcultural Concepts in Nursing Care, Second Edition. Philadelphia: JB Lippincott, 1995.

CULTURAL SANCTIONS AND RESTRICTIONS

How does the client's cultural group regard expression of emotion and feelings, spirituality, and religious beliefs? How are dying, death, and grieving expressed in a culturally appropriate manner?

How is modesty expressed by men and women? Are there culturally defined expectations about male-female relationships, including the nurse-client relationship?

Does the client have any restrictions related to sexuality, exposure of body parts, certain types of surgery (eg, amputation, vasectomy, hysterectomy)?

Are there any restrictions against discussion of dead relatives or fears related to the unknown?

COMMUNICATION

What language does the client speak at home? What other languages does the client speak or read? In what language would the client prefer to communicate with you?

What is the fluency level of the client in English—both written and spoken use of the language? Remember that the stress of illness may cause clients to use a more familiar language and to temporarily forget some English.

Does the client need an interpreter? If so, is there a relative or friend whom the client would like to interpret? Is there anyone whom the client would prefer did not serve as an interpreter (eg, member of the opposite sex, a person younger/older than the client, member of a rival tribe or nation)?

What are the rules (linguistics) and modes (style) of communication? How does the client prefer to be addressed?

Is it necessary to vary the technique of communication during the interview and examination to accommodate the client's cultural background (eg, tempo of conversation, eye contact, sensitivity to topical taboos, norms of confidentiality, and style of explanation)?

How does the client's nonverbal communication compare with that of individuals from other cultural backgrounds? How does it affect the client's relationship with you and with other members of the healthcare team?

How does the client feel about healthcare providers who are not of the same cultural background (eg, black, middle-class nurse and Hispanic of a different social class)?

Does the client prefer to receive care from a nurse of the same cultural background, gender, and/or age?

What are the overall cultural characteristics of the client's language and communication processes?

HEALTH-RELATED BELIEFS AND PRACTICES

To what cause(s) does the client attribute illness and disease (eg, divine wrath, imbalance in hot/cold or yin/yang, punishment for moral transgressions, hex, soul loss, pathogenic organism)?

What are the client's cultural beliefs about ideal body size and shape? What is the client's self-image vis-à-vis the ideal?

What name does the client give to his or her health-related condition?

What does the client believe promotes health (eating certain foods, wearing amulets to bring good luck, sleep, rest, good nutrition, reducing stress, exercise, prayer, rituals to ancestors, saints, or intermediate deities)?

What is the client's religious affiliation (eg, Judaism, Islam, Pentacostalism, West African voodooism, Seventh-Day Adventism, Catholicism, Mormonism)? How actively involved in the practice of this religion is the client?

Does the client rely on cultural healers (eg, curandero, shaman, spiritualist, priest, minister, monk?) Who determines when the client is sick and when he or she is healthy? Who influences the choice/type of healer and treatment that should be sought?

In what types of cultural healing practices does the client engage (use of herbal remedies, potions, massage, wearing of talismans, copper bracelets or charms to discourage evil spirits, healing rituals, incantations, prayers)?

How are biomedical/scientific healthcare providers perceived? How does the client and his or her family perceive nurses? What are the expectations of nurses and nursing care?

What comprises appropriate "sick role" behavior? Who determines what symptoms constitute disease/illness? Who decides when the client is no longer sick? Who cares for the client at home?

How does the client's cultural group view mental disorders? Are there differences in acceptable behaviors for physical versus psychological illnesses?

NUTRITION

What nutritional factors are influenced by the client's cultural background? What is the meaning of food and eating to the client?

With whom does the client usually eat? What types of foods are eaten? What is the timing and sequencing of meals?

What does the client define as food? What does the client believe comprises a "healthy" versus an "unhealthy" diet?

Who shops for food? Where are groceries purchased (eg, special markets or ethnic grocery stores)? Who prepares the client's meals?

How are foods prepared at home (type of food preparation, cooking oil(s) used, length of time foods are cooked, especially vegetables, amount and type of seasoning added to various foods during preparation)?

Has the client chosen a particular nutritional practice such as vegetarianism or abstinence from alcoholic or fermented beverages?

Do religious beliefs and practices influence the client's diet (eg, amount, type, preparation, or delineation of acceptable food combinations, eg, kosher diets)? Does the client abstain from certain foods at regular intervals, on specific dates determined by the religious calendar, or at other times?

If the client's religion mandates or encourages fasting, what does the term *fast* mean (eg, refraining from certain types or quantities of foods, eating only during certain times of the day)? For what period of time is the client expected to fast?

During fasting, does the client refrain from liquids/beverages? Does the religion allow exemption from fasting during illness? If so, does the client believe that an exemption applies to him or her?

SOCIOECONOMIC CONSIDERATIONS

Who comprises the client's social network (family, friends, peers, and cultural healers)? How do they influence the client's health or illness status?

How do members of the client's social support network define caring (eg, being continuously present, doing things for the client, providing material support, looking after the client's family)? What is the role of various family members during health and illness?

How does the client's family participate in the promotion of health (eg, lifestyle changes in diet, activity level, etc.) and nursing care (eg, bathing, feeding, touching, being present) of the client?

Does the cultural family structure influence the client's response to health or illness (eg, beliefs, strengths, weaknesses, and social class)? Is there a key family member whose role is significant in health-related decisions (eg, grandmother in many African-American families or eldest adult son in Asian families)?

Who is the principal wage earner in the client's family? What is the total annual income? (*Note:* This is a potentially sensitive question.) Is there more than one wage earner? Are there other sources of financial support (extended family, investments)?

What insurance coverage (health, dental, vision, pregnancy) does the client have?

What impact does economic status have on lifestyle, place of residence, living conditions, ability to obtain healthcare? How does the client's home environment (eg, presence of indoor plumbing, handicap access) influence nursing care?

ORGANIZATIONS PROVIDING CULTURAL SUPPORT

What influence do ethnic/cultural organizations have on the client's receiving healthcare (eg, Organization of Migrant Workers, National Association for the Advancement of Colored People [NAACP], Black Political Caucus, churches such as African-American, Muslim, Jewish, and others, schools including those which are church-related, Urban League, community-based healthcare programs and clinics).

EDUCATIONAL BACKGROUND

What is the client's highest educational level obtained?

Does the client's educational background affect his or her knowledge level concerning the healthcare delivery system, how to obtain the needed care, teaching-learning, and any written material that he or she is given in the healthcare set-ting (eg, insurance forms, educational literature, information about diagnostic procedures and laboratory tests, admissions forms)?

Can the client read and write English, or is another language preferred? If English is the client's second language, are materials available in the client's pri-mary language?

What learning style is most comfortable/familiar? Does the client prefer to learn through written materials, oral explanation, or demonstration?

RELIGIOUS AFFILIATION

How does the client's religious affiliation affect health and illness (eg, life events such as death, chronic illness, body image alteration, cause and effect of illness)?

What is the role of religious beliefs and practices during health and illness? Are there special rites or blessings for those with serious or terminal illnesses?

Are there healing rituals or practices that the client believes can promote well-being or hasten recovery from illness? If so, who performs these?

What is the role of significant religious representatives during health and illness? Are there recognized religious healers (eg, Islamic imams, Christian Scientist practitioners or nurses, Catholic priests, Mormon elders, Buddhist monks)?

CULTURAL ASPECTS OF DISEASE INCIDENCE

Are there any specific genetic or acquired conditions that are more prevalent for a specific cultural group (eg, hypertension, sickle cell anemia, Tay Sachs, G6PD, lactose intolerance)?

Are there socioenvironmental diseases more prevalent among a specific cul-tural group (eg, lead poisoning, alcoholism, HIV/AIDS, drug abuse, ear infec-tions, family violence)?

Are there any diseases against which the client has an increased resistance (eg, skin cancer in darkly pigmented individuals, malaria for those with sickle cell anemia)?

BIOCULTURAL VARIATIONS

Does the client have distinctive physical features characteristic of a particular eth-nic or cultural group (eg, skin color, hair texture)? Does the client have any varia-tions in anatomy characteristic of a particular ethnic or cultural group (eg, body structure, height, weight, facial shape and structure [nose, eye shape, facial con-tour], upper and lower extremities)?

How do anatomic and racial variations affect the physical examination?

DEVELOPMENTAL CONSIDERATIONS

Are there any distinct growth and development characteristics that vary with the client's cultural background (eg, bone density, psychomotor patterns of development, fat-folds)?

What factors are significant in assessing children of various ages from the newborn period through adolescence (eg, expected growth on standard grid, culturally acceptable age for toilet training, introducing various types of foods, gender differences, discipline, socialization to adult roles)?

What is the cultural perception of aging (eg, is youthfulness or the wisdom of old age more highly valued)?

How are elderly persons handled culturally (eg, cared for in the home of adult children, placed in institutions for care)? What are culturally acceptable roles for the elderly?

Does the elderly person expect family members to provide care, including nurturance and other humanistic aspects of care?

Is the elderly person isolated from culturally relevant supportive persons or enmeshed in a caring network of relatives and friends?

Has a culturally appropriate network replaced family members in performing some caring functions for the elderly person?

Appendix J
A Patient's Bill
of Rights

INTRODUCTION

Effective healthcare requires collaboration between patients and physicians and other healthcare professionals. Open and honest communication, respect for personal and professional values, and sensitivity to differences are integral to optimal patient care. As the setting for the provision of health services, hospitals must provide a foundation for understanding and respecting the rights and responsibilities of patients, their families, physicians, and other caregivers. Hospitals must ensure a healthcare ethic that respects the role of patients in decision making about treatment choices and other aspects of their care. Hospitals must be sensitive to cultural, racial, linguistic, religious, age, gender, and other differences as well as the needs of persons with disabilities.

The American Hospital Association presents *A Patient's Bill of Rights* with the expectation that it will contribute to more effective patient care and be supported by the hospital on behalf of the institution, its medical staff, employees, and patients. The American Hospital Association encourages healthcare institutions to tailor this bill of rights to their patient community by translating and/or simplifying the language of this bill of rights as may be necessary to ensure that patients and their families understand their rights and responsibilities.

BILL OF RIGHTS*

1. The patient has the right to considerate and respectful care.
2. The patient has the right to and is encouraged to obtain from physicians and other direct caregivers relevant, current, and

*These rights can be exercised on the patient's behalf by a designated surrogate or proxy decision maker if the patient lacks decision-making capacity, is legally incompetent, or is a minor.

A patient's Bill of Rights was first adopted by the American Hospital Association in 1973. This revision was approved by the AHA Board of Trustees on October 21, 1992.

understandable information concerning diagnosis, treatment, and prognosis.

Except in emergencies when the patient lacks decision-making capacity and the need for treatment is urgent, the patient is entitled to the opportunity to discuss and request information related to the specific procedures and/or treatments, the risks involved, the possible length of recuperation, and the medically reasonable alternatives and their accompanying risks and benefits.

Patients have the right to know the identity of physicians, nurses, and others involved in their care, as well as when those involved are students, residents, or other trainees. The patient also has the right to know the immediate and long-term financial implications of treatment choices, insofar as they are known.

3. The patient has the right to make decisions about the plan of care prior to and during the course of treatment and to refuse a recommended treatment or plan of care to the extent permitted by law and hospital policy and to be informed of the medical consequences of this action. In case of such refusal, the patient is entitled to other appropriate care and services that the hospital provides or transfer to another hospital. The hospital should notify patients of any policy that might affect patient choice within the institution.

4. The patient has the right to have an advance directive (such as a living will, health care proxy, or durable power of attorney for healthcare) concerning treatment or designating a surrogate decision maker with the expectation that the hospital will honor the intent of that directive to the extent permitted by law and hospital policy.

Healthcare institutions must advise patients of their rights under state law and hospital policy to make informed medical choices, ask if the patient has an advance directive, and include that information in patient records. The patient has the right to timely information about hospital policy that may limit its ability to implement fully a legally valid advance directive.

5. The patient has the right to every consideration of privacy. Case discussion, consultation, examination, and treatment should be conducted so as to protect each patient's privacy.

6. The patient has the right to expect that all communications and records pertaining to his/her care will be treated as confidential by the hospital, except in cases such as suspected abuse and public health hazards when reporting is permitted or required by law. The patient has the right to expect that the hospital will emphasize the confidentiality of this information when it releases it to any other parties entitled to review information in these records.

7. The patient has the right to review the records pertaining to his/her medical care and to have the information explained or interpreted as necessary, except when restricted by law.

8. The patient has the right to expect that, within its capacity and policies, a hospital will make reasonable response to the request of a patient for appropriate and medically indicated care and services. The hospital must provide evaluation, service, and/or referral as indicated by the urgency of the case. When medically appropriate and legally permissible, or when a patient has so requested, a patient may be transferred to another facility. The institution to which the patient is to be transferred must first have accepted the patient for transfer. The patient must also have the benefit of complete information and explanation concerning the need for, risks, benefits, and alternatives to such a transfer.

9. The patient has the right to ask and be informed of the existence of business relationships among the hospital, educational institutions, other healthcare providers, or payers that may influence the patient's treatment and care.

10. The patient has the right to consent to or decline to participate in proposed research studies or human experimentation affecting care and treatment or requiring direct patient involvement, and to have those studies fully explained prior to consent. A patient who declines to participate in research or experimentation is entitled to the most effective care that the hospital can otherwise provide.

11. The patient has the right to expect reasonable continuity of care when appropriate and to be informed by physicians and other caregivers of available and realistic patient care options when hospital care is no longer appropriate.

12. The patient has the right to be informed of hospital policies and practices that relate to patient care, treatment, and responsibilities. The patient has the right to be informed of available resources for resolving disputes, grievances, and conflicts, such as ethics committees, patient representatives, or other mechanisms available in the institution. The patient has the right to be informed of the hospital's charges for services and available payment methods.

The collaborative nature of healthcare requires that patients, or their families/surrogates, participate in their care. The effectiveness of care and patient satisfaction with the course of treatment depend, in part, on the patient fulfilling certain responsibilities. Patients are responsible for providing information about past illnesses, hospitalizations, medication, and other matters related to health status. To participate effectively in decision making, patients must be encouraged to take responsibility for requesting additional information and instructions. Patients are also responsible for ensuring that the healthcare institution has a copy of their written advance directive if they have one. Patients are responsible for informing their physicians and other caregivers if they anticipate problems in following prescribed treatment.

Patients should also be aware of the hospital's obligation to be reasonably efficient and equitable in providing care to other patients and the community. The hospital's rules and regulations are designed to help the hospital meet this obligation. Patients and their families are responsible for making reasonable accommodations to the needs of the hospital, other patients, medical staff, and hospital employees. Patients are responsible for providing necessary information for insurance claims and for working with the hospital to make payment arrangements, when necessary.

A person's health depends on much more than healthcare services. Patients are responsible for recognizing the impact of their life-style on their personal health.

CONCLUSION

Hospitals have many functions to perform, including the enhancement of health status, health promotion, and the prevention and treatment of injury and disease; the immediate and ongoing care and rehabilitation of patients; the education of health professionals, patients, and the community; and research. All these activities must be conducted with an overriding concern for the values and dignity of patients.

Appendix K
Delegation: Concepts and Decision-Making Process

INTRODUCTION

To meet the public's increasing need for accessible, affordable, quality healthcare, providers of health care must maximize the utilization of every healthcare worker and ensure appropriate delegation of responsibilities and tasks. Nurses, who are uniquely qualified for promoting the health of the whole person by virtue of their education and experience, must be actively involved in making healthcare policies and decisions; they must coordinate and supervise the delivery of nursing care, including the delegation of nursing tasks to others.

Issues related to delegation have become more complex in today's evolving healthcare environment, creating a need for practical guidelines to direct the process for making delegatory decisions. Accordingly, this paper expands and builds upon the National Council's 1987 and 1990 conceptual and historical papers on delegation by presenting a dynamic decision-making process and practical guidelines for delegation.

PURPOSE

The purpose of this paper is to provide a resource for Boards of Nursing, health policy makers, and healthcare providers on delegation and the roles of licensed and unlicensed healthcare workers. The paper emphasizes and clarifies the responsibility of Boards of Nursing for the regulation of nursing, including nursing tasks performed by unlicensed healthcare workers, and the responsibility of licensed nurses to delegate nursing tasks in accord with their legal scopes of practice. It provides a decision-making tool which can be used in clinical and administrative settings to guide the process of delegation. This paper also describes the accountability of each person involved in the delegation process and potential liability if competent, safe care is not provided.

Reprinted with permission of the National Council of State Boards of Nursing, Inc.

PREMISES

The following premises constitute the basis for the delegation decision-making process.

1. All decisions related to delegation of nursing tasks must be based on the fundamental principle of protection of the health, safety and welfare of the public.

2. Boards of Nursing are responsible for the regulation of nursing. Provision of any care which constitutes nursing or any activity represented as nursing is a regulatory responsibility of Boards of Nursing.

3. Boards of Nursing should articulate clear principles for delegation, augmented by clearly defined guidelines for delegation decisions.

4. A licensed nurse must have ultimate responsibility and accountability for the management and provision of nursing care.

5. A licensed nurse must be actively involved in and be accountable for all managerial decisions, policy making and practices related to the delegation of nursing care.

6. There is a need and a place for competent, appropriately supervised, unlicensed assistive personnel in the delivery of affordable, quality healthcare. However, it must be remembered that unlicensed assistive personnel are equipped to assist—not replace—the nurse.

7. Nursing is a knowledge-based process discipline and cannot be reduced solely to a list of tasks. The licensed nurse's specialized education, professional judgment and discretion are essential for quality nursing care.

8. While nursing tasks may be delegated, the licensed nurse's generalist knowledge of patient care indicates that the practice-pervasive functions of assessment, evaluation and nursing judgment must not be delegated.

9. A task delegated to an unlicensed assistive person cannot be redelegated by the unlicensed assistive person.

10. Consumers have a right to healthcare that meets legal standards of care. Thus, when a nursing task is delegated, the task must be performed in accord with established standards of practice, policies and procedures.

11. The licensed nurse determines and is accountable for the appropriateness of delegated nursing tasks. Inappropriate delegation by the nurse and/or unauthorized performance of nursing tasks by unlicensed assistive personnel may lead to legal action against the licensed nurse and/or unlicensed assistive personnel.

DEFINITIONS

Accountability   Being responsible and answerable for actions or inactions of self or others in the context of delegation.

Delegation   Transferring to a competent individual the authority to perform a selected nursing task in a selected situation. The nurse retains accountability for the delegation.

Delegator   The person making the delegation.

Delegatee   The person receiving the delegation. (a.k.a. Delegate)

Supervision   The provision of guidance or direction, evaluation and follow-up by the licensed nurse for accomplishment of a nursing task delegated to unlicensed assistive personnel.

Unlicensed Assistive Personnel (UAP)   Any unlicensed personnel, regardless of title, to whom nursing tasks are delegated.

REGULATORY PERSPECTIVE: A FRAMEWORK FOR MANAGERIAL POLICIES

Boards of Nursing have the legal responsibility to regulate nursing and provide guidance regarding delegation. Registered Nurses (RNs) may delegate certain nursing tasks to Licensed Practical Nurses/Vocational Nurses (LPN/VNs) and unlicensed assistive personnel (UAP). In some jurisdictions, LPN/VNs may also delegate certain tasks within their scope of practice to unlicensed assistive personnel. The licensed nurse has a responsibility to assure that the delegated task is performed in accord with established standards of practice, policies and procedures. The nurse who delegates retains accountability for the task delegated.

The regulatory system serves as a framework for managerial policies related to the employment and utilization of licensed nurses and unlicensed assistive personnel. The nurse who assesses the patient's needs and plans nursing care should determine the tasks to be delegated and is accountable for that delegation. It is inappropriate for employers or others to require nurses to delegate when, in the nurse's professional judgment, delegation is unsafe and not in the patient's best interest. In those instances, the nurse should act as the patient's advocate and take appropriate action to ensure provision of safe nursing care. If the nurse determines that delegation may not appropriately take place, but nevertheless delegates as directed, the nurse may be disciplined by the Board of Nursing.

ACCEPTABLE USE OF THE AUTHORITY TO DELEGATE

The delegating nurse is responsible for an individualized assessment of the patient and situational circumstances, and for ascertaining the competence of the delegatee before delegating any task. The practice-pervasive functions of assessment, evaluation and nursing judgment must not be delegated. Supervision, monitoring, evaluation and follow-up by the nurse are crucial components of delegation. The delegatee is accountable for accepting the delegation and for his/her own actions in carrying out the task.

The decision to delegate should be consistent with the nursing process (appropriate assessment, planning, implementation and evaluation). This necessarily precludes a list of nursing tasks that can be routinely and uniformly delegated for all patients in all situations. Rather, the nursing process and decision to delegate must be based on careful analysis of the patient's needs and circumstances. Also critical to delegation decisions are the qualifications of the proposed delegatee, the nature of the nurse's delegation authority set forth in the law of the jurisdiction, and the nurse's personal competence in the area of nursing relevant to the task to be delegated.

DELEGATION DECISION-MAKING PROCESS

In delegating, the nurse must ensure appropriate assessment, planning, implementation and evaluation. The delegation decision-making process, which is continuous, is described by the following model:

  I. Delegation criteria
   A. Nursing Practice Act
      1. Permits delegation
      2. Authorizes task(s) to be delegated or authorizes the nurse to decide delegation
   B. Delegator qualifications
      1. Within scope of authority to delegate
      2. Appropriate education, skills and experience
      3. Documented/demonstrated evidence of current competency
   C. Delegatee qualifications
      1. Appropriate education, training, skills and experience
      2. Documented/demonstrated evidence of current competency

Provided that this foundation is in place, the licensed nurse may enter the continuous process of delegation decision-making.

  II. Assess the situation
   A. Identify the needs of the patient, consulting the plan of care
   B. Consider the circumstances/setting
   C. Assure the availability of adequate resources, including supervision

If patient needs, circumstances, and available resources (including supervisor and delegatee) indicate patient safety will be maintained with delegated care, proceed to III.

III. Plan for the specific task(s) to be delegated
- A. Specify the nature of each task and the knowledge and skills required to perform it
- B. Require documentation or demonstration of current competence by the delegatee for each task
- C. Determine the implications for the patient, other patients, and significant others

If the nature of the task, competence of the delegatee, and patient implications indicate patient safety will be maintained with delegated care, proceed to IV.

IV. Assure appropriate accountability
- A. As delegator, accept accountability for performance of the task(s)
- B. Verify that delegatee accepts the delegation and the accountability for carrying out the task correctly

If delegator and delegatee accept the accountability for their respective roles in the delegated patient care, proceed to V.

V. Supervise performance of the task
- A. Provide directions and clear expectations of how the task(s) is to be performed
- B. Monitor performance of the task(s) to assure compliance to established standards of practice, policies and procedures
- C. Intervene if necessary
- D. Ensure appropriate documentation of the task(s)

VI. Evaluate the entire delegation process
- A. Evaluate the patient
- B. Evaluate the performance of the task(s)
- C. Obtain and provide feedback

VII. Reassess and adjust the overall plan of care as needed

The Five Rights of Delegation provide an additional resource to facilitate decisions about delegation.

THE FIVE RIGHTS OF DELEGATION

- ▪ **Right Task**—one that is delegable for a specific patient.
- ▪ **Right Circumstances**—appropriate patient setting, available resources, and other relevant factors considered.
- ▪ **Right Person**—right person is delegating the right task to the right person to be performed on the right person.
- ▪ **Right Direction/Communication**—clear, concise description of the task, including its objective, limits and expectations.
- ▪ **Right Supervision**—appropriate monitoring, evaluation, intervention, as needed, and feedback.

CONCLUSION

The guidelines presented in this paper provide a decision-making process that facilitates the provision of quality care by appropriate persons in all healthcare settings. The National Council of State Boards of Nursing believes that this paper will assist all healthcare providers and healthcare facilities in discharging their shared responsibility to provide optimum healthcare that protects the public's health, safety and welfare.

Approved November 21, 1995.

Index

Page numbers followed by *f* indicate illustrations; *t* following a page number indicates tabular material.

American Journal of Nursing, 248
American Licensed Practical Nurses
        Association (ALPNA), 76, 247
American Medical Association (AMA), 64*t*
American Nurses' Association (ANA)
    continuing education and, 258
    Disciplinary Diversion Act developed by, 257
    Mary Mahoney Award of, 61
    membership and purpose of, 248
    nursing education policies of, 63*t*
    standards for nursing care set by, 182
American Nursing Assistant's Association, 285
American Osteopathic Association, standards
        for nursing care set by, 77, 182
American Red Cross, 60, 61, 285
Americans with Disabilities Act of 1992, 238
American Vocational Association, 286
Amniocentesis, as ethical issue, 173
Amphetamines, uses and effects of, 272*t*–273*t*
ANA. *See* American Nurses' Association (ANA)
Ancient civilizations, nursing in, 51–53
Andrews/Boyle Transcultural Nursing
        Assessment Guide, text of, 301–306
Angel of the Battlefield, 60
Anger, as dying stage, 160
Anxiety. *See also* Stress management
    about tests, overcoming of, 17–18
Appendix, textbook, 15
Application for job, 234–240
    interview, 237–240
    letter, 235
    resumé, 235–237, 235*f*–236*f*
Approval, of nursing programs, 72
Armed Forces, opportunities for LP/VNs in,
        230
Army Nurse Corp, 286
Army School of Nursing, 61
Articulated nursing program, defined, 246–247
Artificial insemination, as ethical issue,
        172–173
Aseptic surgical techniques, Joseph Lister and,
        60
Assault, defined, 186
Assertive behavior
    in effective leaders, 201
    requirements of, 199–200
    in stress management, 268–269
Assessment
    as step in nursing process, 92, 95*f*
    transcultural, Andrews/Boyle guide for, text
        of, 301–306
Assignment(s)
    academic
        reading, 13–14
        written, 14–15
    patient-care, implementation of, 216

Assisi, St. Francis of, 55
Associate degree in nursing (ADN)
    programs leading to, 69–70
    requirements for, 246
Association of Collegiate Schools of Nursing, 63*t*
Association of Practical Nursing Schools,
        62–64, 63*t*
Associations, nursing and health-related, listing
        of, 284–286
Attendant. *See* Nurse aide(s)
Attendant Nursing, Household Nursing
        Association School of, 62, 63*t*
Audiovisual (A/V) instruction, 13
Augustinian Sisters, 54
Authoritarian leader, 197–199, 198*f*
Authorized, defined, 291
A/V (audiovisual) instruction, 13

B
Babylon, nursing in, 51
Bachelor of science in nursing (BSN), require-
        ments for, 246
Ballard, Lucinda, 62, 63*t*
Ballard School, 62, 63*t*
    YWCA program at, 68
Baptism
    Catholic, 139
    Protestant, 140–141
Baptist Church, basic practices of, 140
Barbiturates
    use and abuse of, 34–35
    uses and effects of, 274*t*–275*t*
Bargaining
    collective, 251
    as dying stage, 160
Barton, Clara, 60
Basic, defined, 297
Battery, 186
Bed rails, 152
Behavior
    aggressive, 199
    assertive, 199–201
        in stress management, 268–269
    passive, 199
Beliefs, cultural
    assessment of, 302–303
    nursing care and, 38
Bellevue Hospital, New York Training School
        of, 60
Belonging, human need for, 26–27, 27*f*
Benefits, job search and, 242
Benzodiazepines, uses and effects of, 274*t*–275*t*
"Bill of Rights, Patient's" (AHA)
    right to informed consent specified by,
        185–186